W9-ATY-521

Sleep Disorders in Women

CURRENT CLINICAL NEUROLOGY

Daniel Tarsy, MD, SERIES EDITOR

Sleep Disorders
in Women
A Guide to Practical Management

Edited by

Hrayr P. Attarian, MD

Vermont Regional Sleep Center
Department of Neurology
University of Vermont College
of Medicine/Fletcher Allen Health Care
Burlington, VT

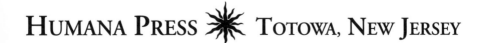

HUMANA PRESS ✳ TOTOWA, NEW JERSEY

Cover design by Patricia F. Cleary

Production Editor: Robin B. Weisberg

For additional copies, pricing for bulk purchases, and/or information about other Humana titles, contact Humana at the above address or at any of the following numbers: Tel.: 973-256-1699; Fax: 973-256-8341; E-mail: orders@humanapr.com; or visit our Website: www.humanapress.com

Printed in the United States of America. 10 9 8 7 6 5 4 3 2 1
e-ISBN 1-59745-115-0

Library of Congress Cataloging-in-Publication Data

Sleep disorders in women : a guide to practical management / edited by Hrayr P. Attarian.
    p. ; cm. -- (Current clinical neurology)
  Includes bibliographical references and index.
  ISBN 1-58829-592-3 (alk. paper)
  1. Sleep disorders. 2. Women--Health and hygiene.
  [DNLM: 1. Sleep Disorders. 2. Hormone Replacement Therapy. 3. Menopause--physiology.
4. Postpartum Period--physiology. 5. Pregnancy--physiology. 6. Sex Factors. 7. Women.
WL 108 S63039 2006] I. Attarian, Hrayr P. II. Series.
  RC547.S528 2006
  616.8'4980082--dc22

                                                                    2005028675

Dedication

To my parents, Angele and Pierre Attarian, with extreme gratitude

Series Editor's Introduction

Increasing attention is currently being directed to a variety of health disorders that are either unique to or more common among women than men. This volume adds sleep disorders to the list of those in which important gender differences have been neglected. *Sleep Disorders in Women: A Guide to Practical Management* explores the reasons for gender bias in this area of research and provides a comprehensive and in-depth review of what is currently known and what still remains to be studied concerning this important topic.

As several contributors to this volume indicate, numerous misconceptions exist due, not surprisingly, to a shortage of reliable data in the field. As an example, obstructive sleep apnea (OSA) is typically thought to be far more common in men than in women. However, as contributors to this volume carefully document, the prevalence of OSA in women varies considerably depending on the specific female population that is studied. It is low in premenopausal women, higher in postmenopausal women, particularly high in women with polycystic ovary syndrome, and of uncertain prevalence in pregnancy. This exemplifies the fact that as women move through varying hormonal environments including puberty, the menstrual cycle, use of oral contraceptives, pregnancy, the postpartum period, and menopause, their risk for a variety of sleep disorders varies considerably. As pointed out in Dr. Attarian's earlier volume in the Current Clinical Neurology Series, *Clinical Handbook of Insomnia*, the physiological causes of insomnia and excessive daytime sleepiness have been underestimated. In the current volume we are now presented with evidence that endocrinological causes play a particularly significant role in women.

This volume certainly does not limit itself to sleep disorders unique to women. Very useful chapters deal with the usual fare of restless legs syndrome, insomnia, excessive daytime sleepiness, and OSA. Less commonly appreciated circadian rhythm disorders in adolescents such as delayed sleep phase syndrome and insomnia are also addressed. A real bonus is provided by a particularly fascinating chapter concerning the phenomenology of the parasomnias! *Sleep Disorders in Women: A Guide to Practical Management* fills an important gap in the literature concerning sleep disorders, which will be invaluable for health care workers who advise and treat such patients.

Daniel Tarsy, MD
Parkinson's Disease and Movement Disorders Center
Beth Israel Deaconess Medical Center
Harvard Medical School
Boston, MA

Preface

Gender bias in medical research and care is a well-established fact. It has, fortunately, become less prevalent now than in the past, but still is a significant problem, especially in conditions traditionally thought of as male illnesses. Sleep medicine, a relatively young field, has not been immune to gender bias. It has been a well-established fact that symptoms of obstructive sleep apnea (OSA) do not necessarily differ between genders, yet until recently it took twice as long for a woman with OSA to get correctly diagnosed than a man with the same condition. In certain circles, unfortunately, it has been a common practice to attribute any type of sleep symptom in women to a psychiatric illness, which leads to delay in diagnosis and treatment. Thanks to pioneers in sleep research, such as Dr. Terry Young and others, these trends are slowly changing. OSA was first described in middle-aged overweight men and because it was only looked for in that population group for a long time, no one looked for it in women or other population groups. Certain features associated with OSA unique to middle-aged men were automatically assumed to be applicable to other population groups. Research in the past 10–15 years, however, has produced a wealth of data regarding the prevalence and uniqueness of sleep disorders in women. The interplay of reproductive hormones, the endocrinological changes that women go through during various life stages, and both normal and disordered sleep is being explored more in depth. Despite all these advances in our understanding of sleep disorders in women, we are still just scratching the surface of this fascinating and multifaceted field.

Sleep Disorders in Women: A Guide to Practical Management is divided into five parts. The first part is an overview discussing epidemiology, workup, and normal sleep changes, with chapters devoted to adolescence, premenopausal state, pregnancy, and menopause. The last four sections are divided into illness-specific chapters.

In order to write a book that covers the multifaceted aspect of sleep medicine, one needs a multidisciplinary team of specialists. The authors of these chapters are well-respected and well-published researchers and clinicians in this field and come from a variety of backgrounds, making the book multidisciplinary.

Sleep Disorders in Women: A Guide to Practical Management is intended to help introduce primary care physicians and health care providers to the multifaceted discipline of sleep disorders in women. It summarizes the latest, cutting-edge research and presents it in a succinct and clinically relevant manner. Its goals are to help physicians recognize the symptoms patterns of sleep disorders in their female patients, guide them in diagnosing and treating these patients in a timely fashion, and help in the elimination of gender bias in sleep medicine research and care.

ix

I hope that *Sleep Disorders in Women: A Guide to Practical Management* will fill an important niche in the medical literature by being the first multidisciplinary comprehensive review written for physicians on sleep disorders in women.

Hrayr P. Attarian, MD

Contents

Contributors

PETER ANDERER, PhD • Department of Psychiatry, University of Vienna, Vienna, Austria

HRAYR P. ATTARIAN, MD • Vermont Regional Sleep Center, Department of Neurology, University of Vermont College of Medicine/Fletcher Allen Health Care, Burlington, VT

MIRA AUBUCHON, MD • Department of Obstetrics and Gynecology, University of Cincinnati College of Medicine, Cincinnati, OH

KANIKA BAGAI, MD • Department of Neurology, Vanderbilt University School of Medicine, Nashville, TN

LAUREN BROCH, PhD • Sleep Disorders Institute, Good Samaritan Hospital, Suffern, NY

AARON B. CAUGHEY, MD, MPP, MPH • Department of Obstetrics & Gynecology, University of California, San Francisco, CA

NANCY S. COLLINS, MD • Department of Neurology, The Chicago Medical School, Rosalind Franklin University of Medicine and Science, North Chicago, IL

JOHN GARCIA, MD • Departments of Pediatrics and Neurology, Minnesota Regional Sleep Center, Hennepin County Medical Center/University of Minnesota, Minneapolis, MN

ROCHELLE GOLDBERG, MD, FCCP • Department of Internal Medicine, Main Line Health System, Wynnewood, PA

ELISABETH GRÄTZHOFER, Mag • Department of Psychiatry, University of Vienna, Vienna, Austria

GEORG GRUBER, Mag • Department of Psychiatry, University of Vienna, Vienna, Austria

DAVID M. HIESTAND, MD, PhD • Division of Pulmonary, Critical Care and Sleep Medicine, University of Kentucky Medical Center and Samaritan Sleep Disorders Center, Lexington, KY

JOHANNES HUBER, MD, PhD • Department of Gynecological Endocrinology, University of Vienna, Vienna, Austria

KATHRYN A. LEE, RN, PhD, FAAN • Department of Family Health Care Nursing, School of Nursing, University of California, San Francisco, CA

MARK W. MAHOWALD, MD • Department of Neurology, Hennepin County Medical Center, and University of Minnesota Medical School, Minneapolis, MN

BETH A. MALOW, MD, MS • Department of Neurology, Vanderbilt University School of Medicine, Nashville, TN

MARKUS METKA, MD • Department of Gynecological Endocrinology, University of Vienna, Vienna, Austria

MARGARET MOLINE, PhD • Eisai Medical Research, Ridgefield Park, NJ

DIANA MONAGHAN, PA-C • Fairfax Associates in Medicine/Department of Surgery, Fletcher Allen Health Care, Burlington, VT

KEITH J. NAGLE, MD • Department of Neurology, Vermont Regional Sleep Center, University of Vermont College of Medicine, Burlington, VT

BARBARA PHILLIPS, MD, MSPH, FCCP • Division of Pulmonary, Critical Care and Sleep Medicine, University of Kentucky Medical Center and Samaritan Sleep Disorders Center, Lexington, KY

GRACE PIEN, MD • Division of Sleep Medicine, Department of Medicine, Center for Sleep and Respiratory Neurobiology, University of Pennsylvania School of Medicine, Philadelphia, PA

ALISON QUINN, BA • Department of Psychology, College of the Holy Cross, Worcester, MA

BERND SALETU, MD • Department of Psychiatry, University of Vienna, Vienna, Austria

GERDA SALETU-ZYHLARZ, MD • Section of Sleep Research and Pharmacopsychiatry, Department of Psychiatry, University of Vienna, Vienna, Austria

CARLOS H. SCHENCK, MD • Department of Psychiatry, Hennepin County Medical Center, and University of Minnesota Medical School, Minneapolis, MN

HELENA SCHOTLAND, MD • Division of Sleep Medicine, Department of Medicine, University of Pennsylvania School of Medicine, Philadelphia, PA

CATHERINE C. SCHUMAN, PhD • Departments of Neurology and Psychiatry, University of Vermont College of Medicine and Fletcher Allen Health Care, Burlington, VT

ANNA VANNUCCI • Department of Psychology, College of the Holy Cross, Worcester, MA

SIGRID CARLEN VEASEY, MD • Division of Sleep Medicine, Department of Medicine, Center for Sleep and Respiratory Neurobiology, University of Pennsylvania School of Medicine, Philadelphia, PA

AMY WOLFSON, PhD • Department of Psychology, College of the Holy Cross, Worcester, MA

ROCHELLE ZAK, MD • Sleep–Wake Disorders Center, New York Weill Cornell Medical Center, White Plains, NY

I Overview

1

Introduction

Hrayr P. Attarian

In general, sleep complaints are common in the health care field and they are twice as prevalent in women *(1)*. Women with sleep disorders have been persistently underdiagnosed. This is primarily owing to a strong gender bias when it comes to both diagnosing and researching sleep disorders *(2)*, and partially because of a difference in the way symptoms are perceived by women as opposed to men *(3)*. Furthermore, most norms considered to be representative are from studies based primarily on men *(4–6)* despite the recognition that there are important sleep-related physiological differences in women. Women are generally underrepresented in sleep and sleep disorders research; in fact 75% of sleep research has been conducted in men *(7)*. This has gradually started to change since the late 1990s, however, gender differences in sleep and sleep-disorder characteristics, are still underappreciated. This volume includes a chapter on the epidemiology of sleep disorders in women. It discusses and summarizes the latest research results from around the world.

It is a clearly established fact that sex hormones influence sleep and circadian rhythms, and sleep in turn affects the episodic secretion of gonadotropin hormones *(8,9)*.

Gender-related differences in sleep and its regulation therefore influence the risk for and mechanisms of sleep disorders *(1,10)*.

Physiological changes that occur during puberty, the menstrual cycle, pregnancy, and menopause can sometimes have profound effects on sleep quality, daytime functioning, and quality of life in women from adolescence throughout adulthood *(1,10)*. We have also included a chapter describing the effects of those physiological changes on normal sleep and one on their impact on different sleep disorders. Although some women may not experience premenstrual symptoms and secondary insomnia, insomnia and associated symptoms often occur with onset of menses *(1,11–15)*.

These repetitive bouts of insomnia, occurring once a month for the greater portion of a woman's life, can have potential health consequences *(1)*. This volume includes a chapter that discusses insomnia in the adolescent girl, one that focuses on insomnia in the premenopausal woman and its relation to premenstrual symptoms, as well as a chapter on insomnia treatment modalities.

From: *Current Clinical Neurology: Sleep Disorders in Women: A Guide to Practical Management*
Edited by: H. P. Attarian © Humana Press Inc., Totowa, NJ

Menstrual cycle symptoms and premenstrual dysphoria correlate with excessive daytime sleepiness as well, so a chapter specifically discussing this issue is included here *(16–18)*.

During pregnancy, sleep is affected by both hormonal changes and physical discomfort. Despite the paucity of research studies in this population, it is well known that nearly all pregnant women will experience disturbed sleep by the third trimester *(19–22)*.

In addition, history of sleep disruptions in late-stage pregnancy are associated with a higher incidence of postpartum blues *(13,19)*. Thus, this volume includes a chapter that specifically discusses insomnia and sleep disturbances in pregnancy. Certain sleep disorders, such as restless legs syndrome (RLS; *20,22–25*), periodic limb movement disorder *(20,22–25)*, and obstructive sleep apnea syndrome (OSAS; *20,22,26*), are more prevalent and in fact may start during pregnancy. Although the extent to which these disorders resolve or place women at higher risk for sleep disorders later in life is not known, it is clear that they have significant adverse consequences during pregnancy. Pregnancy-induced changes in the upper airway make women more prone to snoring, OSAS, and decreased oxygen saturations *(20,22,26–28)*. Pregnant women who snore may be at risk for pre-eclampsia and pregnancy-induced hypertension *(20,22,26–28)*. Both of these conditions have been associated with adverse fetal outcomes *(29–31)*. This volume includes chapters on OSAS in nonpregnant and prepregnant women, and chapters on RLS in both pregnant and nonpregnant women of childbearing age. Many women during the menopausal transition (perimenopause, menopause, postmenopause) complain of sleep disturbances *(32–34)*, some of which are attributed to hot flashes and night sweats rather than to menopause itself *(35,36)*. Insomnia is reported in about 46% of menopausal women *(37)*.

Research has shown that short-term hormone replacement therapy (HRT) may have beneficial effects for improving subjective and objective sleep quality in women with menopausal symptoms *(33,38,39)*. Included in this volume is a chapter on insomnia in perimenopausal women and another on RLS in menopause.

Menopause may also be a significant risk factor for OSAS *(10,40–47)*. It has been suggested that one of the reasons for increased prevalence of OSAS in postmenopausal women is sex-hormone deficiency *(47–50)*. Some studies have shown that women on HRT might be at lower risk *(51–55)*. Given the obvious concerns about risk of other diseases associated with HRT for the treatment of menopausal symptoms, fewer women in the future may receive HRT. Hence, more women may experience menopause-related sleep problems *(1)*. Finally, surveys show that more than 80% of working women complain of fatigue, and half of them get inadequate sleep *(14)*. Shift-working women have altered sleep and circadian rhythms and are at increased risk for menstrual irregularities, infertility, miscarriage, and low birthweight infants *(29)*. In most societies, in addition to working outside the home, women remain the main caregivers for children and elderly family members. These responsibilities may add a significant stress burden and increase their risk for sleep deprivation and sleep disturbances with negative impacts on health and quality of life *(56)*. In addition, significant life events, such as sudden death of a loved one, have been associated with development of posttraumatic symptoms, including sleep disturbances *(1)*. Women who use alcohol as a coping method for demands of work, family, and social obligations are at increased risk for alcohol-induced sleep disturbances *(57)*.

In the last several years, there has been an increase in the number of mid-level primary care providers (nurse practitioners and physician assistants). An overview chapter geared toward these mid-level professionals is included in this volume in order to help them best diagnose and treat sleep complaints in women. Polycystic ovarian syndrome has been associated with higher risk of OSAS *(58,59)* in premenopausal women. As such, a chapter on that relationship in addition to one on OSAS in otherwise healthy premenopausal women is provided here. Finally, chapters on parasomnias and delayed sleep phase syndrome in adolescents are also included.

REFERENCES

1. *National sleep disorders research plan* 2nd ed. 2003, Bethesda: National Center on Sleep Disorders Research, U. S. Department of Health and Human Services, National Institutes of Health, National Heart, Lung and Blood Institute. 152.
2. Young, T., R. Hutton, L. Finn, S. Badr, and M. Palta, The gender bias in sleep apnea diagnosis. Are women missed because they have different symptoms? *Arch Intern Med*, 1996;**156**(21):2445–2451.
3. Shepertycky, M., K. Banno, and M. Kryger. Differences between men and women in the clinical presentation of patients diagnosed with obstructive sleep apnea syndrome. *Sleep*, 2005;**28**(3):309–314.
4. Mohsenin, V., Effects of gender on upper airway collapsibility and severity of obstructive sleep apnea. *Sleep Med*, 2003;**4**(6):523–529.
5. O'Connor, C., K.S. Thornley, and P.J. Hanly, Gender differences in the polysomnographic features of obstructive sleep apnea. *Am J Respir Crit Care Med*, 2000;**161**(5):1465–1472.
6. Rowley, J.A., X. Zhou, I. Vergine, M.A. Shkoukani, and M.S. Badr, Influence of gender on upper airway mechanics: upper airway resistance and Pcrit. *J Appl Physiol*, 2001;**91**(5):2248–2254.
7. Driver, H., J. Cachon, L. Dableh, et al., Gender representation in sleep research. *J Sleep Res*, 1999;**8**(2):157–159.
8. Hall, J.E., J.P. Sullivan, and G.S. Richardson, Brief wake episodes modulate sleep-inhibited luteinizing hormone secretion in the early follicular phase. *J Clin Endocrinol Metab*, 2005;**90**(4):2050–2055.
9. Rossmanith, W.G., S. Boscher, W. Kern, and H.L. Fehm, Impact of sleep on the circadian excursions in the pituitary gonadotropin responsiveness of early follicular phase women. *J Clin Endocrinol Metab*, 1993;**76**(2):330–336.
10. Moline, M.L., L. Broch, and R. Zak, Sleep in women across the life cycle from adulthood through menopause. *Sleep Med Rev*, 2003;**7**(2):155–177.
11. Freeman, E.W., M.D. Sammel, P.J. Rinaudo, and L. Sheng, Premenstrual syndrome as a predictor of menopausal symptoms. *Obstet Gynecol*, 2004;**103**(5 Pt 1):960–966.
12. Kageyama, T., N. Nishikido, T. Kobayashi, J. Oga, and M. Kawashima, Cross-sectional survey on risk factors for insomnia in Japanese female hospital nurses working rapidly rotating shift systems. *J Hum Ergol* (Tokyo), 2001;**30**(1–2):149–154.
13. Krystal, A.D., Depression and insomnia in women. *Clin Cornerstone*, 2004;**6 Suppl 1B**:S19–S28.
14. Lee, K.A., Self-reported sleep disturbances in employed women. *Sleep*, 1992;**15**(6):493–498.
15. Manber, R. and R.R. Bootzin, Sleep and the menstrual cycle. *Health Psychol*, 1997;**16**(3):209–214.
16. Bamford, C.R., Menstrual-associated sleep disorder: an unusual hypersomniac variant associated with both menstruation and amenorrhea with a possible link to prolactin and metoclopramide. *Sleep*, 1993;**16**(5):484–486.

17. Hart, W.G. and J.W. Russell, A prospective comparison study of premenstrual symptoms. *Med J Aust*, 1986;**144**(9):466–468.

18. Sachs, C., H.E. Persson, and K. Hagenfeldt, Menstruation-related periodic hypersomnia: a case study with successful treatment. *Neurology*, 1982;**32**(12):1376–1379.

19. Wolfson, A.R., S.J. Crowley, U. Anwer, and J.L. Bassett, Changes in sleep patterns and depressive symptoms in first-time mothers: last trimester to 1-year postpartum. *Behav Sleep Med*, 2003;**1**(1):54–67.

20. Sharma, S. and R. Franco, Sleep and its disorders in pregnancy. *Wmj*, 2004;**103**(5):48–52.

21. Lee, K.A., Alterations in sleep during pregnancy and postpartum: a review of 30 years of research. *Sleep Med Rev*, 1998;**2**(4):231–242.

22. Pien, G.W. and R.J. Schwab, Sleep disorders during pregnancy. *Sleep*, 2004;**27**(7):1405–1417.

23. Manconi, M., V. Govoni, A. De Vito, et al., Restless legs syndrome and pregnancy. *Neurology*, 2004;**63**(6):1065–1069.

24. Suzuki, K., T. Ohida, T. Sone, et al., The prevalence of restless legs syndrome among pregnant women in Japan and the relationship between restless legs syndrome and sleep problems. *Sleep*, 2003;**26**(6):673–677.

25. Manconi, M., V. Govoni, A. De Vito, et al., Pregnancy as a risk factor for restless legs syndrome. *Sleep Med*, 2004;**5**(3):305–308.

26. Young, T., P.E. Peppard, and D.J. Gottlieb, Epidemiology of obstructive sleep apnea: a population health perspective. *Am J Respir Crit Care Med*, 2002;**165**(9):1217–1239.

27. Izci, B., S.E. Martin, K.C. Dundas, W.A. Liston, A.A. Calder, and N.J. Douglas, Sleep complaints: snoring and daytime sleepiness in pregnant and pre-eclamptic women. *Sleep Med*, 2005;**6**(2):163–169.

28. Hannhart, B., C.K. Pickett, and L.G. Moore, Effects of estrogen and progesterone on carotid body neural output responsiveness to hypoxia. *J Appl Physiol*, 1990;**68**(5):1909–1916.

29. Mozurkewich, E.L., B. Luke, M. Avni, and F.M. Wolf, Working conditions and adverse pregnancy outcome: a meta-analysis. *Obstet Gynecol*, 2000;**95**(4):623–635.

30. Loube, D.I., et al., Self-reported snoring in pregnancy. Association with fetal outcome. *Chest*, 1996;**109**(4):885–889.

31. Franklin, K.A., P.A. Holmgren, F. Jonsson, N. Poromaa, H. Stenlund, and E. Svanborg, Snoring, pregnancy-induced hypertension, and growth retardation of the fetus. *Chest*, 2000;**117**(1):137–141.

32. Guilleminault, C., L. Palombini, D. Poyares, and S. Chowdhuri, Chronic insomnia, postmenopausal women, and sleep disordered breathing: part 1. Frequency of sleep disordered breathing in a cohort. *J Psychosom Res*, 2002;**53**(1):611–615.

33. Saletu-Zyhlarz, G., P. Anderer, G. Gruber, et al., Insomnia related to postmenopausal syndrome and hormone replacement therapy: sleep laboratory studies on baseline differences between patients and controls and double-blind, placebo-controlled investigations on the effects of a novel estrogen-progestogen combination (Climodien, Lafamme) versus estrogen alone. *J Sleep Res*, 2003;**12**(3):239–254.

34. Krystal, A.D., J. Edinger, W, Wohlgemuth, and G.R. Marsh, Sleep in peri-menopausal and post-menopausal women. *Sleep Med Rev*, 1998;**2**(4):243–253.

35. Shanafelt, T.D., D.L. Barton, A.A. Adjei, and C.L. Loprinzi, Pathophysiology and treatment of hot flashes. *Mayo Clin Proc*, 2002;**77**(11):1207–1218.

36. Polo-Kantola, P., E. Rauhala, T. Saaresranta, T. Aittokallio, R. Erkkola, and O. Polo, Climacteric vasomotor symptoms do not predict nocturnal breathing abnormalities in postmenopausal women. *Maturitas*, 2001;**39**(1):29–37.

37. Owens, J.F. and K.A. Matthews, Sleep disturbance in healthy middle-aged women. *Maturitas*, 1998;**30**(1):41–50.

38. White, D.P., The hormone replacement dilemma for the pulmonologist. *Am J Respir Crit Care Med*, 2003;**167**(9):1165–1166.

39. Jones, C.R. and L. Czajkowski, Evaluation and management of insomnia in menopause. *Clin Obstet Gynecol*, 2000;**43**(1):184–197.

40. Guilleminault, C., M.A. Quera-Salva, M. Partinen, and A. Jamieson, Women and the obstructive sleep apnea syndrome. Chest, 1988;**93**(1):104–109.
41. Block, A.J., J.W. Wynne, P.G. Boysen, S. Lindsey, C. Martin, and B. Cantor, Menopause, medroxyprogesterone and breathing during sleep. *Am J Med*, 1981;**70**(3):506–510.
42. Bixler, E.O., A.N. Vgontzas, H.M. Lin, et al., Prevalence of sleep-disordered breathing in women: effects of gender. *Am J Respir Crit Care Med*, 2001;**163**(3 Pt 1):608–613.
43. Carskadon, M.A., H.M. Bearpark, K.M. Sharkey, et al., Effects of menopause and nasal occlusion on breathing during sleep. *Am J Respir Crit Care Med*, 1997;**155**(1):205–210.
44. Dancey, D.R., P.J. Hanly, C. Soong, B. Lee, and V. Hoffstein, Impact of menopause on the prevalence and severity of sleep apnea. *Chest*, 2001;**120**(1):151–155.
45. Sternfeld, B., H. Wang, C.P. Quesenberry Jr., et al., Physical activity and changes in weight and waist circumference in midlife women: findings from the Study of Women's Health Across the Nation. *Am J Epidemiol*, 2004;**160**(9):912–922.
46. Polo-Kantola, P., E. Rauhala, H. Helenius, R. Erkkola, K. Irjala, O. Polo, Breathing during sleep in menopause: a randomized, controlled, crossover trial with estrogen therapy. *Obstet Gynecol*, 2003;**102**(1):68–75.
47. Young, T., L. Finn, D. Austin, and A. Peterson, Menopausal status and sleep-disordered breathing in the Wisconsin Sleep Cohort Study. *Am J Respir Crit Care Med*, 2003;**167**(9):1181–1185.
48. Zhou, X.S., J.A. Rowley, F. Demirovic, M.P. Diamond, and M.S. Badr, Effect of testosterone on the apneic threshold in women during NREM sleep. *J Appl Physiol*, 2003;**94**(1):101–107.
49. Tufano, A., P. Marzo, R. Enrini, L. Morricone, F. Caviezel, and B. Ambrosi, Anthropometric, hormonal and biochemical differences in lean and obese women before and after menopause. *J Endocrinol Invest*, 2004;**27**(7):648–653.
50. Thomas, T., B. Burguera, L.J. Melton 3rd, et al., Relationship of serum leptin levels with body composition and sex steroid and insulin levels in men and women. *Metabolism*, 2000;**49**(10):1278–1284.
51. Keefe, D.L., R. Watson, and F. Naftolin, Hormone replacement therapy may alleviate sleep apnea in menopausal women: a pilot study. *Menopause*, 1999;**6**(3):196–200.
52. Shahar, E., S. Redline, T. Young, et al., Hormone replacement therapy and sleep-disordered breathing. *Am J Respir Crit Care Med*, 2003;**167**(9):1186–1192.
53. Nelson, H.D., L.L. Humphrey, P. Nygren, S.M. Teutsch, and J.D. Allan, Postmenopausal hormone replacement therapy: scientific review. *JAMA*, 2002;**288**(7):872–881.
54. Pickett, C.K., J.G. Regensteiner, W.D. Woodard, D.D. Hagerman, J.V. Weil, nd L.G. Moore, Progestin and estrogen reduce sleep-disordered breathing in postmenopausal women. *J Appl Physiol*, 1989;**66**(4):1656–1661.
55. Manber, R., T.F. Kuo, N. Cataldo, and I.M. Colrain, The effects of hormone replacement therapy on sleep-disordered breathing in postmenopausal women: a pilot study. *Sleep*, 2003;**26**(2):163–168.
56. Doi, Y. and M. Minowa, Gender differences in excessive daytime sleepiness among Japanese workers. *Soc Sci Med*, 2003;**56**(4):883–894.
57. Trinkoff, A.M. and C.L. Storr, Work schedule characteristics and substance use in nurses. *Am J Ind Med*, 1998;**34**(3):266–271.
58. Gopal, M., S. Duntley, M. Uhles, and H. Attarian, The role of obesity in the increased prevalence of obstructive sleep apnea syndrome in patients with polycystic ovarian syndrome. *Sleep Med*, 2002;**3**(5):401–404.
59. Vgontzas, A.N., R.S. Legro, E.O. Bixler, A. Grayev, A. Kales, and G.P. Chrousos, Polycystic ovary syndrome is associated with obstructive sleep apnea and daytime sleepiness: role of insulin resistance. *J Clin Endocrinol Metab*, 2001;**86**(2):517–520.

2

Epidemiology of Sleep Disorders in Women

Hrayr P. Attarian

HISTORICAL PERSPECTIVES

Sleep medicine as a field was not established until the early 1970s after the discovery of obstructive sleep apnea syndrome (OSAS) in Europe in 1965 *(1,2)* and the establishment of the first sleep laboratory at Stanford in 1972. The term *polysomnography* was coined by Dr. Jerome Holland at Stanford, in 1974, to describe the studies that were done during all-night sleep.

In the early years of sleep medicine, sleep centers concentrated on diagnosing and treating OSAS and less frequently narcolepsy. Both conditions were thought rare, in fact OSAS was initially described as a rare disorder of overweight men.

It is now known that OSAS is a very common disorder that affects both men and women (premenopausal women less than postmenopausal women) and can affect both overweight and normal weight people.

Restless legs syndrome (RLS), another well-described sleep disorder, was thought of as being rare until recently as well. RLS is now known to be quite prevalent, especially in women.

In addition, the increased recognition and acceptance of insomnia, a condition more prevalent in women, as a sleep disorder in its own right have established the fact that sleep disorders are quite common and are not gender-specific disorders of the male population.

In this chapter, I discuss the prevalence of the complaint of difficulty sleeping and excessive daytime sleepiness (EDS) in women. I also discuss the gender differences in the prevalence of the two most common sleep syndromes: OSAS and RLS.

INSOMNIA

As several studies looking at different aspects of insomnia have confirmed, insomnia is more prevalent in women. Bixler et al., in 1979, published the results of their survey of 1006 women in the Los Angeles metropolitan area, where they looked at the prevalence of sleep disorders in general. Bixler et al. found a 42.5% prevalence of insomnia. Trouble falling asleep was 14.4% and difficulty with frequent night-

From: *Current Clinical Neurology: Sleep Disorders in Women: A Guide to Practical Management*
Edited by: H. P. Attarian © Humana Press Inc., Totowa, NJ

time awakenings was 22.9%. Women, especially postmenopausal women, were more affected than men *(3)*. Karacan and colleagues also reported a similar prevalence in their community survey, again showing a female preponderance *(4)*. Liljenberg et al. surveyed randomly selected members of the population aged 30 to 65 years from two geographically different rural parts of central Sweden. Difficulty falling asleep was cited by 7.1% of the women and 5.1% of the men and nocturnal awakenings were reported in 8.9% of women and 7.7% of men. Using a stringently defined concept of insomnia as a disorder of initiating sleep (DIS), the prevalence rate of insomnia among women was 1.1% and among men 0.5%. Defining insomnia as a disorder of maintaining sleep (DMS), the prevalence among both women and men was 1.1%. Defining insomnia as a disorder of initiating and maintaining sleep (DIMS), the prevalence rate was 1.7% among women and 1.4% among men. Liljenberg concluded that the reason for the lower prevalence of insomnia in this study was because they used more stringent criteria for the definition of insomnia *(5)*. Morgan et al. surveyed 1023 randomly chosen elderly members of the community in Nottinghamshire, England and discovered subjective insomnia at least *sometimes* in 37.9% of the sample, with women having a higher prevalence than men *(6)*. For example, in Sweden, Liljenberg reported the following in 1988: females significantly more often reported difficulty in falling asleep (7.1% of the women and 5.1% of the men). Among women, 8.9% and among men, 7.7% of individuals reported trouble with nocturnal awakenings. Using a stringently defined concept of insomnia as a DIS, the prevalence rate of insomnia among women was 1.1% and among men 0.5%. Defining insomnia as a DMS, the prevalence among both women and men was 1.1%. Defining insomnia as a DIMS, the prevalence rate was 1.7% among women and 1.4% among men *(5)*. In one Brazilian town, the prevalence of insomnia was 38.9%, being higher among women (45.3%) than men (28.8%) *(7)*. In Hong Kong, females were found to be about 1.6 times at higher risk for insomnia than males *(8)*. In Kuwait, it was found that 14.6% of boys and 20.3% of girls reported difficulty initiating sleep, whereas 8.6% of boys and 15.7% of girls reported difficulty maintaining sleep. Girls had higher mean scores in most of the 12-point insomnia scale items *(9)*. In Germany, the prevalence of severe insomnia was found to be 5% in women vs 3% in men *(10)*. Over the years, multiple other survey-based studies have presented robust data to support the increase prevalence of insomnia in women in different adult population groups in several other countries as well (Netherlands, United Kingdom, India, Japan, and Canada) *(11–17)*.

The National Sleep Foundation started its annual polls in 1995 and every year the polls have demonstrated about 1.5–2/1 female-to-male preponderance of different insomnia complaints. The most recent poll published on the foundation's website on March 29, 2005 polled 1506 adults by phone on a variety of sleep habits. Slightly more than half (51%) of men vs 57% of women complained of any symptom of insomnia at least a few nights a week. Difficulty falling asleep (taking one 30 minutes or longer to fall asleep) was present in 26% of women and only 17% of men. Sleep maintenance issues (awake a lot during the night) were also more common in women (35%) than men 28%. Early morning awakenings were reported in

24% of women and 19% of men. A study in Japan surveyed 555 nurses for symptoms of insomnia. The prevalence of insomnia among shift-working nurses (29.2%) was three to four times higher than that in the general population *(18)*. The same group also discovered increased tobacco use in those with insomnia among a group of 522 female staff nurses *(19)*. Substance use was also reported in a US study among shift-working nurses with insomnia *(20)*. Shift work in women is therefore a significant risk factor for insomnia and subsequent tobacco and alcohol use.

It is therefore clearly established that insomnia is a much more prevalent complaint in women than men. This gender difference seems to be present only in adults. A few studies looking at the prevalence of insomnia in prepubertal children have not demonstrated this gender difference *(21–24)*. This could very well be the result of hormonal changes occurring during the menstrual cycle, during pregnancy, and after menopause. It has been well documented that there is an increase in subjective sleep complaints during the late luteal phase *(25)* and dysmenorrhea is associated with decreased sleep efficiency and worsening daytime functioning *(26)*. Luteal phase is also associated with increased mood problems *(25)*. As a result of both unique hormonal changes and mechanical problems (including backache, urinary frequency, heartburn, fetal movement, and spontaneous awakenings), a significant number of women experience insomnia during pregnancy *(27)*. Insomnia starts becoming prevalent in weeks 23–24 of gestation. By the third trimester, only 1.9% of women fail to experience nocturnal awakenings *(27)*. Despite the complaint of insomnia, partially resulting from napping and partially from "sleeping in," there is an overall increase in total sleep time in pregnancy, despite a reduction in sleep efficiency. A mean increase in sleep duration of 0.7 hours during the first trimester, compared with the prepregnancy period has been reported and a mean increase of more than 30 minutes of total nocturnal sleep time was recorded at 11 to 12 weeks of gestation in 33 women who underwent in-home polysomnography prior to conception and during each trimester of pregnancy *(27)*. Finally, there is a high level of sleep disturbance (occurring in about 42%, according to one study *[28]*) in menopausal women. A total of 521 women were studied in the above-mentioned study and insomnia was associated with higher levels of anxiety, depression, stress, higher systolic and diastolic blood pressures, and greater waist-to-hip ratios. Although cross-sectional analyses indicate that sleep disturbance may be independent of menopausal status, transition into postmenopausal status is associated with deleterious changes in sleep among women not receiving hormone replacement therapy [HRT]; *28*). Interestingly when subjective and objective sleep measures were compared in peri- and postmenopausal women, these women, relative to premenopausal women, were less satisfied with their sleep, but did not have diminished sleep quality measured by polysomnography *(29)*.

HYPERSOMNIA OR EXCESSIVE DAYTIME SLEEPINESS

The complaint of hypersomnia, regardless of cause, is more prevalent in women as well. This has been confirmed repeatedly in different populations around the world. One of the most important studies done in Sweden showed a prevalence of

EDS (23.3% in women and 15.9% in men), despite the fact that women generally reported longer total sleep time. They also looked at psychological status and discovered a higher prevalence of anxiety in women; however, this alone was not enough to explain the more prevalent complaint of EDS *(30)*. A Japanese study showed a prevalence of EDS 13.3% in women and 7.2% in men *(31)*. Similar results of a higher prevalence in women were found in Brazil *(32)*. This gender difference appears to be a phenomenon of the adolescent and postadolescent population. Children have not demonstrated this gender difference in the complaint of EDS in various ethnic groups *(33)*. Even in special groups, such as patients with major depression, EDS was more prevalent in women that men (the study was conducted in matched opposite gender dizygotic twins) *(34)*. In pregnancy, EDS is a common first-trimester complaint that may precede the realization of pregnancy *(27)*.

In conclusion, although prevalence rates of insomnia vary from study to study (depending on the definition of insomnia used) and from one geographical area to another, the female preponderance is always the one constant.

OBSTRUCTIVE SLEEP APNEA SYNDROME

In the landmark study by Young et al. in 1993, published in the *New England Journal of Medicine*, 602 employed men and women 30 to 60 years old were studied. The estimated prevalence of sleep-disordered breathing (SDB) defined as an apnea–hypopnea index [AHI] score of 5 or higher, was found to be 9% for women and 24% for men. They also estimated that 2% of women and 4% of men met the minimal diagnostic criteria for the sleep apnea syndrome (an AHI score of 5 or higher and daytime hypersomnolence). Male sex and obesity were strongly associated with the presence of SDB *(35)*.

Most population-based studies estimate a gender-specific prevalence of two- to threefold greater risk for men compared with women *(36)*, but little progress has been made in understanding the reasons for the risk difference.

The role of sex hormones in OSA pathogenesis has been hypothesized to account for this disparity *(37)*. Clear gender differences in upper airway shape and genioglossal muscle activity during the awake state, in craniofacial morphology, and pattern of fat deposition have been proposed to account for a higher male risk of OSA as well *(38)*. However, no conclusive findings have emerged *(38)*.

In 2001, Bixler et al. further studied the gender difference in the prevalence of OSA and SDB (an AHI score of 10 or higher and daytime hypersomnolence). The overall incidence for women was 1.2% and for men 3.9%. Premenopausal women had a prevalence of 0.6% and postmenopausal women had 1.9%. When they further subdivided postmenopausal women into two groups one on HRT and one not on HRT, they discovered that the prevalence in the first group was only 0.5% vs 2.7% in the second *(39)*. This difference between those with and without HRT (especially estrogen) was also demonstrated in another study in 2003 *(40)*. Age also plays a role on the prevalence of sleep apnea in women. In the same landmark study, Bixler et al. demonstrated that the prevalence in women 20–44 was 0.7%, in women 45–64 it was 1.1%, and in the 65- to 100-year-old age group it was 3.1% *(39)*. Weight also has an impact in increasing the prevalence of OSA in women but not to the degree it does in men. Again, Bixler et al. demonstrated that women with a body mass index (BMI) below 32.3 kg/cm^2 had a prevalence of 0.4% and women with a BMI equal to or more than 32.3 kg/cm^2 had a prevalence of 4.8% *(39)*. This is in concordance with previous studies that have shown the prevalence among obese women (BMI >27.3 kg/m^2) to be 3–7% *(41,42)*. In contrast, the impact of weight in men is much more pronounced. The prevalence for obese men (BMI >27.8 kg/m^2) is 40–76.9% *(41,42)*. Interestingly enough, this male prevalence is what is seen in a group of women with polycystic ovarian syndrome (PCOS). Women with PCOS have hirsutism, obesity, infertility, and enlarged polycystic ovaries. They also have increased androgen production and disordered gonadotropin secretion, it results in chronic anovulation *(43)*. Studies have shown an OSAS prevalence of 17–69.9% (depending on the definition of OSA used) in women with PCOS *(43–45)*.

Pregnancy is another situation where women are at particular risk for OSA *(38)*. Unfortunately, there are very few studies addressing this subject. Twenty-seven percent of otherwise healthy women report snoring in the third trimester *(27)*. Three hundred fifty pregnant women and 110 age-matched nonpregnant women were surveyed at two US Army hospitals. Frequent snoring was reported in 14% of the pregnant women vs 4% of the nonpregnant women *(46)*. Both frequency and loudness of snoring, and episodes of awakening with a choking sensation, appear to increase during pregnancy, with 50% of the women in one study reporting snoring and 14% reporting choking awakenings at 35 to 38 weeks of gestation, vs 37 and 4%, respectively, at 8 to 12 weeks of gestation *(38)*. Another survey of 502 Swedish women at the time of delivery found that 23% reported snoring often or always during the week before delivery, whereas only 4% reported snoring before pregnancy. Most of the time, the snoring increased during the third trimester *(47)*. There is evidence that the impact of pregnancy on snoring resolves within several months after delivery *(38)*.

The high prevalence of snoring and choking awakenings during pregnancy suggests that pregnancy may be associated with OSA; however, there are few data regarding the prevalence of OSA during pregnancy *(38)*. In the largest reported study, polysomnography was performed in 11 snoring women early in the third trimester. All had an AHI less than 5, although all had evidence of increased upper airway resistance characterized by either crescendo respiratory effort or abnormal sustained increases in respiratory effort, occurring more commonly than in control subjects who do not snore *(48)*. The mechanisms underlying the increase in snoring during pregnancy are uncertain, but may include excess weight gain *(38)*, diffuse pharyngeal edema of pregnancy, or the effect of sleep deprivation on pharyngeal dilator muscle activity *(38)*.

In conclusion, OSAS is common in women but not as common as in men. Weight, menopause, age, and endocrine disorders have an impact on increasing the prevalence of OSAS in women.

RESTLESS LEGS SYNDROME

RLS, one of the most common sleep disorders, was first described in 1672. RLS is characterized by uncomfortable, tingling, crawling, burning, prickly limb sensa-

tions associated with an irresistible urge to move the limbs to obtain relief, typically occurring while sedentary or at sleep onset *(49)*. In their series of studies done
in 2003, Hanson et al. found a female-to-male ratio of 2:1 *(49)*. These results were
replicated in the United Kingdom by Van De Vijver et al. in 2004 *(50)*. Similarly,
increased prevalence of RLS in women was found in several other studies *(51,52)*.
Berger et al. looked at the relationship between parity and increased prevalence of
RLS. Nulliparous women had prevalences similar to those among men the risk of
RLS increased gradually for women with one child (odds ratio [OR], 1.98; 95%
confidence interval [CI], 1.25–3.13), two children (OR, 3.04; 95% CI, 2.11–4.40),
and three or more children (OR, 3.57; 95% CI, 2.30–5.55) *(53)*. There was also a
gradually increasing risk of RLS with increasing age that was demonstrated in all
of the above studies *(54)*. Pregnancy also is a significant risk factor. Pregnant
women have at least two or three times higher risk of experiencing RLS than the
general population. These data come from few epidemiological studies finding an
11–27% prevalence of RLS during pregnancy. Women affected by pre-existing RLS
often complain of worsening symptoms during pregnancy. This is usually a benign
form of RLS, with the highest degree of severity in the third trimester and a tendency to disappear around delivery *(55)*.

RLS can also occur with an increasing prevalence in women who had no symptoms prior to pregnancy. Prevalences have been shown to increase from 0%
prepregnancy to 12.5% in the first trimester to 23% by the third trimester *(27)*.

The above studies were all done in the United States and Europe, where the
overall prevalence of RLS is estimated to be 10–12.9% *(56,57)*.

In Asia, the prevalence of RLS is much lower at 3% or less *(58–60)*. Despite the
lower prevalence, the ratio of female to male is high and so is the overall prevalence in pregnancy. One study from India reported a female-to-male ratio of 7:1
(61). A Japanese study targeting pregnant women found the prevalence in this particular group to be 19.9% *(62)*.

This increased prevalence of RLS in women and especially its association with
pregnancy has been thought to be related to reduced iron, ferritin, and/or folate
levels *(27)*.

RLS is much more prevalent in women, especially with pregnancy and menopause, even in ethnic groups where RLS is relatively uncommon.

CONCLUSION

The complaint of both insomnia and hypersomnia is more prevalent in women.
Of the two most common sleep syndromes, OSAS is relatively rare in premenopausal nonpregnant women, whereas its prevalence increases during pregnancy and
menopause.

RLS is much more prevalent in women and that prevalence amplifies as women
get pregnant and when they reach menopause. Interestingly, parity itself increases
the prevalence of RLS in women even after delivery, whereas RLS exacerbations
during pregnancy tend to disappear with delivery.

REFERENCES

1. Gastaut, H., C.A. Tassinari, and B. Duron, [Polygraphic study of diurnal and nocturnal (hypnic and respiratory) episodal manifestations of Pickwick syndrome]. *Rev Neurol* (Paris), 1965;**112**(6):568–579.

2. Jung, R. and W. Kuhlo, Neurophysiological studies of abnormal night sleep and the pickwickian syndrome. *Prog Brain Res*, 1965;**18**:140–159.

3. Bixler, E.O., A. Kales, C.R. Soldatos, J.D. Kales, and S. Healey, Prevalence of sleep disorders in the Los Angeles metropolitan area. *Am J Psychiatry*, 1979;**136**(10):1257–1262.

4. Karacan, I., J.I. Thornby, and R.L. Williams, Sleep disturbance: a community survey In: *Sleep/Wake Disorders: Natural History, Epidemiology and Long Term Evolution* (C. Guilleminault and E. Lugaresi, eds.), Raven: New York, 1983, pp. 37–60.

5. Liljenberg, B., M. Almqvist, J. Hetta, B.E. Roos, and H. Agren, The prevalence of insomnia: the importance of operationally defined criteria. *Ann Clin Res*, 1988;**20**(6):393–398.

6. Morgan, K., H. Dallosso, S. Ebrahim, T. Arie, and P.H. Fentem, Characteristics of subjective insomnia in the elderly living at home. *Age Ageing*, 1988;**17**(1):1–7.

7. Rocha, F.L., E. Uchoa, H.L. Guerra, J.O. Firmo, P.G. Vidigal, and M.F. Lima-Costa, Prevalence of sleep complaints and associated factors in community-dwelling older people in Brazil: the Bambui Health and Ageing Study (BHAS). *Sleep Med*, 2002;**3**(3):231–238.

8. Li, R.H., Y.K. Wing, S.C. Ho, and S.Y. Fong, Gender differences in insomnia—a study in the Hong Kong Chinese population. *J Psychosom Res*, 2002;**53**(1):601–609.

9. Abdel-Khalek, A.M., Prevalence of reported insomnia and its consequences in a survey of 5,044 adolescents in Kuwait. *Sleep*, 2004;**27**(4):726–731.

10. Hajak, G., Epidemiology of severe insomnia and its consequences in Germany. *Eur Arch Psychiatry Clin Neurosci*, 2001;**251**(2):49–56.

11. Brabbins, C., M. Dewey, J. Copeland, et al., Insomnia in the elderly. *Int J Geriatr Psychiatry*, 1993;**8**:473–480.

12. Doi, Y., M. Minowa, M. Okawa, and M. Uchiyama, Prevalence of sleep disturbance and hypnotic medication use in relation to sociodemographic factors in the general Japanese adult population. *J Epidemiol*, 1999;**10**:79–86.

13. Ganguli, M., C.F. Reynolds, and J.E. Gilby, Prevalence and persistence of sleep complaints in a rural older community sample: the MoVIES project. *J Am Geriatr Soc*, 1996;**44**(7):778–784.

14. Kim, K., M. Uchiyama, M. Okawa, et al., Lifestyles and sleep disorders among the Japanese adult population. *Psychiatry Clin Neurosci*, 1999;**53**(2):269–270.

15. Middelkoop, H.A., D.A. Smilde-van den Doel, A.K. Neven, H.A. Kamphuisen and C.P. Springer, Subjective sleep characteristics of 1,485 males and females aged 50–93: effects of sex and age, and factors related to self-evaluated quality of sleep. *J Gerontol A Biol Sci Med Sci*, 1996;**51**(3):M108–M115.

16. Ohayon, M.M., M. Caulet, and C. Guilleminault, How a general population perceives its sleep and how this relates to the complaint of insomnia. *Sleep*, 1997;**20**(9):715–723.

17. Ohayon, M.M., M. Caulet, R.G. Priest, and C. Guilleminault, DSM-IV and ICSD-90 insomnia symptoms and sleep dissatisfaction. *Br J Psychiatry*, 1997;**171**:382–388.

18. Kageyama, T., N. Nishikido, T. Kobayashi, J. Oga, and M. Kawashima, Cross-sectional survey on risk factors for insomnia in Japanese female hospital nurses working rapidly rotating shift systems. *J Hum Ergol* (Tokyo), 2001;**30**(1–2):149–154.

19. Kageyama, T., T. Kobayashi, N. Nishikido, J. Oga, and M. Kawashima, Associations of sleep problems and recent life events with smoking behaviors among female staff nurses in Japanese hospitals. *Ind Health*, 2005;**43**(1):133–141.

20. Trinkoff, A.M. and C.L. Storr, Work schedule characteristics and substance use in nurses. *Am J Ind Med*, 1998;**34**(3):266–271.

21. Morrison, D.N., R. McGee, and W.R. Stanton, Sleep problems in adolescence. *J Am Acad Child Adolesc Psychiatry*, 1992;**31**(1):94–99.

22. Kahn, A., C. Van de Merckt, E. Rebuffat, et al., Sleep problems in healthy preadolescents. *Pediatrics*, 1989;**84**(3):542–546.

23. Fisher, B.E. and A.E. Wilson, Selected sleep disturbances in school children reported by parents: prevalence, interrelationships, behavioral correlates and parental attributions. *Percept Mot Skills*, 1987;**64**(3 Pt 2):1147–1157.

24. Liu, X., Z. Sun, M. Uchiyama, K. Shibui, K. Kim, and M. Okawa, Prevalence and correlates of sleep problems in Chinese schoolchildren. *Sleep*, 2000;**23**(8):1053–1062.

25. Krystal, A.D., Depression and insomnia in women. *Clin Cornerstone*, 2004;**6 Suppl 1B**:S19–S28.

26. Baker, F.C., H.S. Driver, G.G. Rogers, J. Paiker, and D. Mitchell, High nocturnal body temperatures and disturbed sleep in women with primary dysmenorrhea. *Am J Physiol*, 1999;**277**(6 Pt 1):E1013–E1021.

27. Pien, G.W. and R.J. Schwab, Sleep disorders during pregnancy. *Sleep*, 2004;**27**(7):1405–1417.

28. Owens, J.F. and K.A. Matthews, Sleep disturbance in healthy middle-aged women. *Maturitas*, 1998;**30**(1):41–50.

29. Young, T., L. Finn, D. Austin, and A. Peterson, Menopausal status and sleep-disordered breathing in the Wisconsin Sleep Cohort Study. *Am J Respir Crit Care Med*, 2003;**167**(9):1181–1185.

30. Lindberg, E., C. Janson, T. Gislason, E. Bjornsson, J. Hetta, and G. Boman, Sleep disturbances in a young adult population: can gender differences be explained by differences in psychological status? *Sleep*, 1997;**20**(6):381–387.

31. Doi, Y. and M. Minowa, Gender differences in excessive daytime sleepiness among Japanese workers. *Soc Sci Med*, 2003;**56**(4):883–894.

32. Hara, C., F. Lopes Rocha, and M.F. Lima-Costa, Prevalence of excessive daytime sleepiness and associated factors in a Brazilian community: the Bambui study. *Sleep Med*, 2004;**5**(1):31–36.

33. Goodwin, J.L., S.I. Babar, K.L. Kaemingk, et al., Symptoms related to sleep-disordered breathing in white and Hispanic children: the Tucson Children's Assessment of Sleep Apnea Study. *Chest*, 2003;**124**(1):196–203.

34. Khan, A.A., C.O. Gardner, C.A. Prescott, and K.S. Kendler, Gender differences in the symptoms of major depression in opposite-sex dizygotic twin pairs. *Am J Psychiatry*, 2002;**159**(8):1427–1429.

35. Young, T., M. Palta, J. Dempsey, J. Skatrud, S. Weber, and S. Badr, The occurrence of sleep-disordered breathing among middle-aged adults. *N Engl J Med*, 1993;**328**(17):1230–1235.

36. Strohl, K. and S. Redline, Recognition of obstructive sleep apnea. *Am J Respir Crit Care Med*, 1996;**154**:274–289.

37. Krystal, A.D., J. Edinger, W. Wohlgemuth, and G.R. Marsh, Sleep in peri-menopausal and post-menopausal women. *Sleep Med Rev*, 1998;**2**(4):243–253.

38. Young, T., P.E. Peppard, and D.J. Gottlieb, Epidemiology of obstructive sleep apnea: a population health perspective. *Am J Respir Crit Care Med*, 2002;**165**(9):1217–1239.

39. Bixler, E.O., A.N. Vgontzas, H.M. Lin, et al., Prevalence of sleep-disordered breathing in women: effects of gender. *Am J Respir Crit Care Med*, 2001;**163**(3 Pt 1):608–613.

40. Manber, R., T.F. Kuo, N. Cataldo, and I.M. Colrain, The effects of hormone replacement therapy on sleep-disordered breathing in postmenopausal women: a pilot study. *Sleep*, 2003;**26**(2):163–168.

41. Rajala, R., M. Partinen, T. Sane, R. Pelkonen, K. Huikuri, and A.M. Seppalainen, Obstructive sleep apnoea syndrome in morbidly obese patients. *J Intern Med*, 1991;**230**(2):125–129.

42. Vgontzas, A.N., T.L. Tan, E.O. Bixler, L.F. Martin, D. Shubet, and A. Kales, Sleep apnea and sleep disruption in obese patients. *Arch Intern Med*, 1994;**154**(15):1705–1711.

43. Gopal, M., S. Duntly, M. Uhles, and H. Attarian, The role of obesity in the increased prevalence of obstructive sleep apnea syndrome in patients with polycystic ovarian syndrome. *Sleep Med*, 2002;**3**(5):401–404.

44. Fogel, R.B., A. Malhotra, G. Pillar, S.D. Pittman, A. Dunaif, and D.P. White, Increased prevalence of obstructive sleep apnea syndrome in obese women with polycystic ovary syndrome. *J Clin Endocrinol Metab*, 2001;**86**(3):1175–1180.

45. Vgontzas, A.N., R.S. Legro, E.O. Bixler, A. Grayev, A. Kales, and G.P. Chrousos, Polycystic ovary syndrome is associated with obstructive sleep apnea and daytime sleepiness: role of insulin resistance. *J Clin Endocrinol Metab*, 2001;**86**(2):517–520.

46. Loube, D.I., J.S. Poceta, M.C. Morales, M.D. Peacock, and M.M. Mitler, Self-reported snoring in pregnancy. Association with fetal outcome. *Chest*, 1996;**109**(4):885–889.
47. Franklin, K.A., P.A. Holmgren, F. Jonsson, N. Poromaa, H. Stenlund, and E. Svanborg, Snoring, pregnancy-induced hypertension, and growth retardation of the fetus. *Chest*, 2000;**117**(1):137–141.
48. Guilleminault, C., M. Querra-Salva, S. Chowdhuri, and D. Poyares, Normal pregnancy, daytime sleeping, snoring and blood pressure. *Sleep Med*, 2000;**1**(4):289–297.
49. Hanson, M., M. Honour, A. Singleton, et al., Analysis of familial and sporadic restless legs syndrome in age of onset, gender, and severity features. *J Neurol*, 2004;**251**(11):1398–1401.
50. Van De Vijver, D.A., T. Walley, and H. Petri, Epidemiology of restless legs syndrome as diagnosed in UK primary care. *Sleep Med*, 2004;**5**(5):435–440.
51. Ohayon, M.M. and T. Roth, Prevalence of restless legs syndrome and periodic limb movement disorder in the general population. *J Psychosom Res*, 2002;**53**(1):547–554.
52. Nichols, D.A., R.P. Allen, J.H. Grauke, et al., Restless legs syndrome symptoms in primary care: a prevalence study. *Arch Intern Med*, 2003;**163**(19):2323–2329.
53. Berger, K., J. Luedemann, C. Trenkwalder, U. John, and C. Kessler, Sex and the risk of restless legs syndrome in the general population. *Arch Intern Med*, 2004;**164**(2):196–202.
54. Rothdach, A.J., C. Trenkwalder, J. Haberstock, U. Keil, and K. Berger, Prevalence and risk factors of RLS in an elderly population: the MEMO study. Memory and Morbidity in Augsburg Elderly. *Neurology*, 2000;**54**(5):1064–1068.
55. Manconi, M., V. Govoni, A. De Vito, et al., Pregnancy as a risk factor for restless legs syndrome. *Sleep Med*, 2004;**5**(3):305–308.
56. Phillips, B., T. Young, L. Finn, K. Asher, W.A. Hening, and C Purvis, Epidemiology of restless legs symptoms in adults. *Arch Intern Med*, 2000;**160**(14):2137–2141.
57. Hening, W., A.S. Walters, R.P. Allen, J. Montplaisir, A. Myers, and L. Ferini-Strambi, Impact, diagnosis and treatment of restless legs syndrome (RLS) in a primary care population: the REST (RLS epidemiology, symptoms, and treatment) primary care study. *Sleep Med*, 2004;**5**(3):237–246.
58. Sevim, S., O. Dogu, H. Camdeviren, et al., Unexpectedly low prevalence and unusual characteristics of RLS in Mersin, Turkey. *Neurology*, 2003;**61**(11):1562–1569.
59. Bhowmik, D., M. Bhatia, S. Gupta, S.K. Agarwal, S.C. Tiwari, and S.C. Dash, Restless legs syndrome in hemodialysis patients in India: a case controlled study. *Sleep Med*, 2003;**4**(2):143–146.
60. Bhowmik, D., M. Bhatia, S. Tiwari, et al., Low prevalence of restless legs syndrome in patients with advanced chronic renal failure in the Indian population: a case controlled study. *Ren Fail*, 2004;**26**(1):69–72.
61. Kumar, V.G., M. Bhatia, M. Tripathi, A.K. Srivastava, and S. Jain, Restless legs syndrome: diagnosis and treatment. *J Assoc Physicians India*, 2003;**51**:782–783.
62. Suzuki, K., T. Ohida, T. Sone, et al., The prevalence of restless legs syndrome among pregnant women in Japan and the relationship between restless legs syndrome and sleep problems. *Sleep*, 2003;**26**(6):673–677.

3

Workup of Female Patients With Sleep Complaints

A Guide for Mid-Level Health Care Providers

Diana Monaghan

INTRODUCTION

In the primary care setting, fatigue and other sleep complaints are often elicited during the course of history taking for another presenting problem or are mentioned as the practitioner is about to exit the exam room. Women may experience symptoms differently than men do; for example, women with sleep apnea are more likely than men to complain of insomnia, and they may be less aware of observed apneas *(1)*.

Despite the fact that studies show little difference between genders in sleep architecture, women are more likely to have subjective sleep complaints. In fact, sleep complaints are about twice as prevalent in women of all ages as in men *(2)*. Currently, 75% of sleep research has been conducted in males *(3)*.

Evaluation of the patient with sleep complaints includes a thorough history beginning with a sleep screen. Patient's use of caffeine (including hidden sources), nicotine, and alcohol are important considerations. All can disrupt sleep patterns *(4)*. A careful documentation of all medications, including over-the-counter (OTC) medications and herbal product, is required to fully evaluate the patient *(4)*. Antiepileptic medications *(5–7)* and many antidepressants, including selective serotonin reuptake inhibitors (SSRIs), tricyclic antidepressants (TCAs), and noreprinephrine reuptake inhibitors, can either disrupt sleep patterns or cause excessive sleepiness *(8)*. Opiates, muscle relaxants, OTC cold remedies *(9)*, and herbal products, including echinacea *(10)*, valerian *(11)*, and melatonin *(12)*, affect sleep patterns. Patients withdrawing from stimulants *(13)*, including diet aids *(14)*, can experience disrupted sleep. Lifestyle issues should be included in the history along with the patient's daily amount of activity and exercise (or lack thereof).

Most working women report inadequate sleep, but lifestyle factors such as smoking, obesity, and inactivity, as well as relationship issues and mood disturbance, may influence sleep quality more *(15)*.

Shift work, more than any other single factor, disrupts sleep and causes daytime sleepiness *(15)*.The average shift-working woman obtains between 1.5 and 4 hours less sleep per day than her colleagues with routine schedules *(16,17)*. The results

From: *Current Clinical Neurology: Sleep Disorders in Women: A Guide to Practical Management*
Edited by: H. P. Attarian © Humana Press Inc., Totowa, NJ

are often chronic daytime sleepiness and insomnia *(18)*. Shift work also results in an increase in menstrual irregularities *(16)* and a higher risk of infertility, miscarriage, and low birth weight. These women deliver prematurely approx 25% of the time *(19)*.

In order to obtain an accurate sleep history from the patient, the acronym BEARS can be a useful tool *(20)*:

Bedtime
Excessive daytime sleepiness
Awakenings: nighttime and early morning
Regularity and duration of sleep
Snoring

Is the patient going to bed at the same time every night? Is the patient going to bed only when sleepy? Does she have trouble falling asleep? Is the patient having difficulty staying awake at work? Does she feel the need to nap during the day? Often, patients complain of frequent awakenings with difficulty returning to sleep. Patients should be questioned about how much sleep they feel they need, and how much they perceive they get. Weekend sleep patterns should be included. Do they try to "catch up" on the weekend? Also important, does the patient snore, and are there witnessed pauses or gasps? A bed partner is a valuable resource to the health care provider when assessing this last item.

PREMENSTRUAL SYNDROME AND SLEEP

During a woman's lifetime there are several stages and natural conditions that have an impact on sleep and may result in sleep disorders. Among the most common of these is premenstrual syndrome (PMS). Sleep disturbances are frequently linked to PMS symptoms (e.g., bloating, cramping), which begin around the time of menarche and include excessive daytime sleepiness, sleep-onset latency (difficulty falling asleep) and maintenance (difficulty staying asleep), and insomnia *(21,22)*. Many women also experience menstruation-linked periodic hypersomnia, which involves recurrent 6- to 10-day episodic periods of excessive daytime sleepiness *(23)*. Insomnia is addressed further in this chapter and in significant detail in other chapters of this text.

SLEEP AND PREGNANCY

Pregnancy can bring with it a whole host of sleep issues and disorders that can have serious consequences for both fetus and mother. Pregnancy often brings more subjective sleep complaints; especially during the first trimester, during which changes in sleep architecture occur *(24,25)*. Clinically, patients present with fatigue and increased daytime sleepiness. They experience poorer sleep quality and maintenance insomnia. In the third trimester, 97% of women are unable to sleep through the night *(24,25)*. Nasal congestion is common during this time *(24,25)*. Snoring is a frequent occurrence during pregnancy as well and is an important symptom to elicit. Patients may not report snoring unless specifically asked by the practitioner.

Snoring, especially with witnessed pauses and gasps, may signify obstructive sleep apnea (OSA), which must be treated if diagnosed. Almost one-third of women report onset of snoring in pregnancy by the second trimester *(24,25)*. Snoring has been associated with pregnancy-induced hypertension and pre-eclampsia, fetal growth retardation, and decreased Apgar score *(26)*. Growth retardation of the fetus, defined as small for gestational age at birth, occurs in about 7% of infants of snoring mothers vs approx 2.5% of the remaining infants born to nonsnoring mothers *(27)*. Other fetal complications have been observed more often among snorers than nonsnorers *(27)*. OSA generally improves or resolves after childbirth *(28)*.

Obstructive Sleep Apnea: Case Example

A 36-year-old pregnant woman in her third trimester presented to her provider after her husband noted an onset of snoring and witnessed pauses and gasps. The patient herself noted increased fatigue. After the initial interview, the patient was referred to a sleep center and a polysomnogram was ordered. It revealed a respiratory disturbance index (RDI) of 22 per hour. The RDI denotes the number of times a patient stops breathing (apnea) or has a reduction in airflow associated with sleep disturbance and/or desaturation (hypopnea) per hour of sleep. In adults an RDI of 0–5 is normal, 5–19 mild, 20–40 moderate, and more than 40 severe.

During the polysomnogram, the patient's O_2 stats did not fall below 90%. The patient was placed on continuous positive airway pressure (CPAP) during the second part of the study at a pressure of 5 cmH$_2$O, which eliminated both the snoring and the respiratory disturbances. After delivery, a repeat polysomnogram showed resolution of both the snoring, and OSA and CPAP was discontinued.

It is important that even mild OSA be addressed during pregnancy.

Postpartum Sleep

Nearly one-third (30%) of new mothers report disturbed sleep, although this subjective number may represent an underreporting of women affected.

Sleep efficiency (the ratio of time asleep to actual time in bed) during the first 2–4 weeks is lower than in the third trimester of pregnancy *(29)*. First-time mothers' sleep is the most disturbed *(29)*.

Postpartum Depression and Sleep

There are studies reporting depressed mood after childbirth associated with nighttime labor and sleep disruptions during the third trimester.

Sleep–wake patterns correlating with a depressed mood and emotional lability can be found throughout the postpartum period. New mothers must often adopt the sleep patterns of their newborns *(29,30)*.

SLEEP AND MENOPAUSE

For many women, menopause brings sleep disturbances in the form of sleep-onset latency insomnia. About one in five menopausal women reports sleeping less than 6 hours per night *(31,32)*. Sleep maintenance is frequently a significant problem because of the role of nocturnal "hot flashes," and many women experience more frequent arousals/awakenings. OSA is increased in both prevalence and severity in postmenopausal women *(31)*. This may result from changes in fat distribution and the presence of a smaller and stiffer pharynx *(33)*. Hormone replacement therapy (HRT) may improve sleep efficiency and OSA symptoms *(34)*. Insomnia, however, may become conditioned and persist despite HRT *(34)*. Norepinephrine reuptake inhibitors such as venlafaxine and anticonvulsants like gabapentin may be helpful in reducing hot flashes *(35)*.

RESTLESS LEGS SYNDROME/PERIODIC LIMB MOVEMENT DISORDER

During perimenopause and menopause, as with pregnancy and PMS, hormonal changes affect sleeping patterns and may lead to sleep disorders. Two conditions experienced by all three groups are restless legs syndrome (RLS) and the related periodic limb movement disorder (PLMD) *(31,36,37)*. Prevalence in all women is approx 10%, 30% in women older than 65 years, and 26% in pregnant women *(37)*. After delivery, the condition usually resolves *(37)*. RLS causes leg dysthesias ("creeping/crawling"), a feeling that patients may find difficult to describe *(38)*. This is exacerbated by inactivity, relieved by movement, and results in sleep-onset delay. PLMD, a condition characterized by brief, repetitive jerking movements of the lower extremities during stage 1 and 2 sleep, results in arousals and sleep fragmentation. This condition is also known to be more prevalent in menopausal *(36)* and pregnant women *(37)*. It is believed to be more common in PMS as well, but further research is still needed on the subject *(31)*. These conditions have a dopaminergic mechanism *(38)*. Both RLS and PLMD lead to insomnia and daytime sleepiness symptoms.

Diagnostic clues to look for include exacerbation by caffeine, TCAs, SSRIs, and a positive family history *(39)*. For RLS there is also an association with iron-deficiency anemia (check ferritin in all patients), end-stage renal disease, and neurological lesions *(39)*. PLMD requires sleep study confirmation, whereas RLS is a clinical diagnosis *(38)*.

Case Example

A 48-year-old female presented to her primary care physician with a chief complaint of an uncomfortable sensation in her legs, which was alleviated only by moving them. The patient had some medical background, so she researched her symptoms and concluded that she might have a condition known as "restless legs syndrome." Her physician was unfamiliar with the condition and diagnosed her with depression and prescribed fluoxetine as treatment. This medication exacerbated her symptoms. She then self-referred to a sleep center, where she was correctly diagnosed with RLS and successfully treated with a dopamine agonist.

Management includes treating the underlying conditions (anemia, uremia) and, in cases of idiopathic RLS, pharmacological treatment: dopaminergic agents/agonists, opioids, benzodiazepines, anticonvulsants, α-agonists *(38)*. Ropinirole is the only Food and Drug Administration (FDA)-approved drug to treat RLS *(40)*.

INSOMNIA

Although the most common form of insomnia is psychophysiological or primary insomnia, insomnia may be the presenting symptom of any primary sleep disorder. In addition, it may be a part of another medical, psychiatric, or drug-induced condition *(41)*. The latter group is referred to as secondary insomnia. For the purposes of this chapter, we discuss only psychophysiological insomnia.

Psychophysiological, or Conditioned, Insomnia

Psychophysiological insomnia is typically acquired during a period in which other factors (e.g., stress) are at work. After a few days of sleeping poorly, the patient becomes concerned and begins trying harder to get to sleep. The result is arousal and aggravation of the insomnia. Stimuli surrounding bedtime (e.g., the bedroom, the bed itself) may become triggers to arousal *(41)*. Thus, such patients may have severe problems with sleep in their own bedroom but do sleep remarkably well in other locations (e.g., on the livingroom couch, in a motel, in a sleep laboratory) *(41)*. Primary insomnia is much more common in women than in men *(42)*.

Workup

Sleep History

The complaint of daytime sleepiness is generally indicative of another primary sleep disorder, because patients with insomnia are hyposomnolent and often complain bitterly of an inability to take naps *(43)*. They are fatigued but not sleepy *(43)*.

Sleep Logs and Diaries

A sleep log is a graph on which, for 2–3 weeks, the patient records bedtime, approximate sleep time, times and duration of awakenings during the sleep period, final awakening time, and naps taken during the day. Although subjective, this record summarizes the patient's perception of the amount and quality of sleep he or she is getting *(41)*.

Rating Sleep

Sleepiness rating scales (used primarily in sleep labs to assess daytime sleepiness) include the Epworth Sleepiness Scale and the Stanford Sleepiness Scale. Patients with primary insomnia score very low on these scales—lower than healthy controls *(44)*.

Case Example

A 38-year-old woman who had a lifetime history of being a light sleeper and was easily disturbed by noises presented for treatment of insomnia. Her problem centered around sleep maintenance. She was able to fall asleep, but woke during the night and had difficulty returning to sleep and staying asleep. This occurred 4–5 nights a week. This pattern developed 10 years previously when, at age 28, as a new mother she awoke frequently to nurse her newborn son. She had tried many OTC sleep aids, which made her feel groggy the next day. Sleep diaries showed that, depending on the week, she was averaging 6.5 hours of sleep per night with fragmented sleep through the weekdays and sleeping in on the weekends. Her treatment included sleep hygiene, behavioral therapy, and a sleep regime with a restricted sleep schedule in which she went to bed no later than midnight and got up at 6:30 every morning (6.5 hours) for 3 weeks, including weekends. Thirty minutes of sleep was added to the schedule every 3 weeks until 8 hours of sleep per night was achieved. She was prescribed a nonbenzodiazepine hypnotic from the start, which, upon reaching her sleep goal, was gradually tapered over 2–3 months.

Management Principles

The first and foremost intervention should be to identify and treat the underlying causes. Second and equally important is to educate patients on sleep hygiene guidelines *(45)*:

> Go to bed only when sleepy.
> Use the bed only for sleeping.
> Do not read, watch television, or eat in bed.
> If unable to sleep, get up and move to another room.
> Stay up until you are definitely sleepy and then return to bed.
> Set the alarm and get up at the same time every morning, regardless of how much you have slept through the night.
> Do not nap.
> Do not engage in stimulating activity just before bed.
> Do not exercise just before going to bed.
> Avoid caffeine in the afternoon.
> Do not drink alcohol close to bedtime
> Eliminate clocks in the bedroom.
> Schedule a period to review stressful events of the day before bedtime.
> Practice quiescent tasks that occupy the mind to promote relaxation and sleep.

The best management for primary insomnia is a combination of hypnotic medication and behavioral methods *(46–48)*. Although current FDA guidelines recommend most hypnotic medications only for short-term use, studies have shown that the risk of tolerance, addiction, dependence, and rebound insomnia are low, especially with the newer nonbenzodiazepines *(46,49–51)*. Hypnotics that have clinically proven efficacy include (a) the newer nonbenzodiazepine hypnotics zolpidem *(46,52,53)*, zaleplon *(54,55)*, and eszopiclone (the only one approved by the FDA for long-term use) *(56)*, (b) the benzodiazepines, (c) and low-dose trazodone, which has been shown to be effective only in depressed patients *(57)*.

Among the OTC medications, valerian root has also been shown to be effective in the treatment of primary insomnia *(58–60)*. OTC hypnotics that contain primarily antihistamines are rarely indicated because of a poor side-effect profile *(51,61)* and are of unproven value as hypnotics *(62)*. Melatonin is of proven efficacy in the treatment of insomnia associated with circadian rhythm abnormalities and in schizophrenia *(63)*, but not in psychophysiological insomnia *(64)*. There is a paucity of data on the efficacy of the other antidepressants in the treatment of insomnia. In addition, the risk of serious adverse effects with these medications is well documented *(46)*.

Behavioral methods include sleep restriction consolidation, sleep hygiene education, relaxation therapy, stimulus control therapy *(42)*, and correcting distorted perception of sleep *(65)* and are usually performed by a trained behavioral sleep specialist. Both behavioral and pharmacological treatments are equally effective in the short-term treatment of insomnia *(66)*. Cognitive behavior therapy also facilitates supervised tapering and discontinuation of benzodiazepines in older adults with chronic insomnia *(67)* and prevents relapse *(68)*. Preliminary data suggest that phototherapy with full-spectrum light may be effective in treating insomnia *(69,70)*.

CONCLUSION

Sleep disorders are more prevalent in women than previously thought. Health care providers, in general, have less awareness of these disorders in women because of a number of factors, including gender bias and slightly different symptomatology. If undiagnosed, these disorders can be deleterious. Sleep-related health questions should be asked as part of routine medical evaluation, and when in doubt, patients should be referred to a local sleep center for further evaluation and treatment.

REFERENCES

1. Shepertycky, M., K. Banno, and M. Kryger, Differences between men and women in the clinical presentation of patients diagnosed with obstructive sleep apnea syndrome. *Sleep*, 2005;**28**(3):309–314.
2. *National Sleep Disorders Research Plan*, 2nd ed. Bethesda, MD: National Center on Sleep Disorders Research, U.S. Department of Health and Human Services, National Institutes of Health, National Heart, Lung and Blood Institute, 2003:152.
3. Driver, H., J. Cachon, L. Dableh, et al., Gender representation in sleep research. *J Sleep Res*, 1999;**8**(2):157–159.
4. Attarian, H., Psychophysiological insomnia. In: *Clinical Handbook of Insomnia* (H. Attarian, ed.), Totowa, NJ: Humana Press, 2004:67–80.
5. Sadler, M., Lamotrigine associated with insomnia. *Epilepsia*,1999;**40**(3):322–325.
6. Leppik, I.E., Felbamate. *Epilepsia*, 1995;**36**(Suppl 2):S66–S72.
7. Salinsky, M.C., B.S. Oken, and L.M. Binder, Assessment of drowsiness in epilepsy patients receiving chronic antiepileptic drug therapy. *Epilepsia*, 1996;**37**(2):181–187.
8. Wilson, S. and S. Argyropoulos, Antidepressants and sleep: a qualitative review of the literature. *Drugs*, 2005;**65**(7):927–947.
9. Wellington, K. and B. Jarvis, Cetirizine/pseudoephedrine. *Drugs*, 2001;**61**(15):2231–2242.
10. Yale, S.H. and K. Liu, Echinacea purpurea therapy for the treatment of the common cold: a randomized, double-blind, placebo-controlled clinical trial. *Arch Intern Med*, 2004;**164**(11):1237–1241.
11. Stevinson, C. and E. Ernst, Valerian for insomnia: a systematic review of randomized clinical trials. *Sleep Med*, 2000;**1**(2):91–99.
12. Wesensten, N.J., T.J. Balkin, R.M. Reichardt, M.A. Kautz, G.A. Saviolakis, and G. Belenky, Daytime sleep and performance following a zolpidem and melatonin cocktail. *Sleep*, 2005;**28**(1):93–103.
13. Williamson, S., M. Gossop, B. Powis, P. Griffiths, J. Fountain, and J. Strang, Adverse effects of stimulant drugs in a community sample of drug users. *Drug Alcohol Depend*, 1997;**44**(2–3):87–94.
14. Waters, W.F., R.A. Magill, G.A. Bray, et al., A comparison of tyrosine against placebo, phentermine, caffeine, and D-amphetamine during sleep deprivation. *Nutr Neurosci*, 2003;**6**(4):221–235.
15. Lee, K.A., Self-reported sleep disturbances in employed women. *Sleep*, 1992;**15**(6):493–498.

16. Labyak, S., S. Lava, F. Turek, and P. Zee, Effects of shiftwork on sleep and menstrual function in nurses. *Health Care Women Int*, 2002;**23**(6–7):703–714.
17. Rotenberg, L., L.F. Portela, and R.A. Duarte, Gender and sleep in nightworkers: a quantitative analysis of sleep in days off. *J Hum Ergol* (Tokyo), 2001;**30**(1–2):333–338.
18. Garbarino, S., L. Nobili, M. Beelke, V. Balestra, A. Cordelli, and F. Ferrillo, Sleep disorders and daytime sleepiness in state police shiftworkers. *Arch Environ Health*, 2002;**57**(2):167–173.
19. Mozurkewich, E.L., B. Luke, M. Avni, and F.M. Wolf, Working conditions and adverse pregnancy outcome: a meta-analysis. *Obstet Gynecol*, 2000;**95**(4):623–635.
20. Owens, J.A. and V. Dalzell, Use of the 'BEARS' sleep screening tool in a pediatric residents' continuity clinic: a pilot study. *Sleep Med*, 2005;**6**(1):63–69.
21. Freeman, E.W., M.D. Sammel, P.J. Rinaudo, and L. Sheng, Premenstrual syndrome as a predictor of menopausal symptoms. *Obstet Gynecol*, 2004;**103**(5 Pt 1):960–966.
22. Hart, W.G. and J.W. Russell, A prospective comparison study of premenstrual symptoms. *Med J Aust*, 1986;**144**(9):466–468.
23. Bamford, C.R., Menstrual-associated sleep disorder: an unusual hypersomniac variant associated with both menstruation and amenorrhea with a possible link to prolactin and metoclopramide. *Sleep*, 1993;**16**(5):484–486.
24. Pien, G.W. and R.J. Schwab, Sleep disorders during pregnancy. *Sleep*, 2004;**27**(7):1405–1417.
25. Sharma, S. and R. Franco, Sleep and its disorders in pregnancy. *Wisconsin Med J*, 2004;**103**(5):48–52.
26. Izci, B., S.E. Martin, K.C. Dundas, W.A. Liston, A.A. Calder, and N.J. Douglas, Sleep complaints: snoring and daytime sleepiness in pregnant and pre-eclamptic women. *Sleep Med*, 2005;**6**(2):163–169.
27. Franklin, K.A., P.A. Holmgren, F. Jonsson, N. Poromaa, H. Stenlund, and E. Svanborg, Snoring, pregnancy-induced hypertension, and growth retardation of the fetus. *Chest*, 2000;**117**(1):137–141.
28. Edwards, N., et al., Severity of sleep-disordered breathing improves following parturition. *Sleep*, 2005;**28**(6):737–741.
29. Wolfson, A.R., S.J.Crowley, U. Anwer, and J.L. Bassett, Changes in sleep patterns and depressive symptoms in first-time mothers: last trimester to 1-year postpartum. *Behav Sleep Med*, 2003;**1**(1):54–67.
30. Lee, K.A., Alterations in sleep during pregnancy and postpartum: a review of 30 years of research. *Sleep Med Rev*, 1998;**2**(4):231–242.
31. Moline, M.L., L. Broch, and R. Zak, Sleep in women across the life cycle from adulthood through menopause. *Sleep Med Rev*, 2003;**7**(2):155–177.
32. Owens, J.F. and K.A. Matthews, Sleep disturbance in healthy middle-aged women. *Maturitas*, 1998;**30**(1):41–50.
33. Mohsenin, V., Effects of gender on upper airway collapsibility and severity of obstructive sleep apnea. *Sleep Med*, 2003;**4**(6):523–529.
34. Saletu-Zyhlarz, G., P. Anderer, G. Gruber, et al., Insomnia related to postmenopausal syndrome and hormone replacement therapy: sleep laboratory studies on baseline differences between patients and controls and double-blind, placebo-controlled investigations on the effects of a novel estrogen-progestogen combination (Climodien, Lafamme) versus estrogen alone. *J Sleep Res*, 2003;**12**(3):239–254.
35. Shanafelt, T.D., D.L. Barton, A.A. Adjei, and C.L. Loprinzi, Pathophysiology and treatment of hot flashes. *Mayo Clin Proc*, 2002;**77**(11):1207–1218.
36. Jones, C.R. and L. Czajkowski, Evaluation and management of insomnia in menopause. *Clin Obstet Gynecol*, 2000;**43**(1):184–197.
37. Manconi, M., V. Govoni, A. De Vito, et al., Restless legs syndrome and pregnancy. *Neurology*, 2004;**63**(6):1065–1069.
38. Hening, W.A., R.P. Allen, C.J. Earley, D.L. Picchietti, and M.H. Silber, An update on the dopaminergic treatment of restless legs syndrome and periodic limb movement disorder. *Sleep*, 2004;**27**(3):560–583.

39. Kavanagh, D., S. Siddiqui, and C.C. Geddes, Restless legs syndrome in patients on dialysis. *Am J Kidney Dis*, 2004;**43**(5):763–771.

40. Bliwise, D.L., A. Freeman, C.D. Ingram, D.B. Rye, S. Chakravorty, and R.L. Watts, Randomized, double-blind, placebo-controlled, short-term trial of ropinirole in restless legs syndrome. *Sleep Med*, 2005;**6**(2):141–147.

41. Attarian, H.P., Helping patients who say they cannot sleep. Practical ways to evaluate and treat insomnia. *Postgrad Med*, 2000;**107**(3):127–130, 133–137, 140–142.

42. Attarian, H.P., Practical approaches to insomnia. *Primary Care Reports*, 2001;**20**(7):171–178.

43. Bonnet, M.H. and D.L. Arand, Level of arousal and the ability to maintain wakefulness. *J Sleep Res*, 1999;**8**(4):247–254.

44. Johns, M.W., A new method for measuring daytime sleepiness: the Epworth sleepiness scale. *Sleep*, 1991;**14**(6):540–545.

45. Attarian, H.P., Sleep hygiene. In: *Clinical Handbook of Insomnia* (H.P. Attarian, ed.), Totowa, NJ: Humana Press, 2004:99–106.

46. Attarian, H.P., Psychophysiological insomnia. In: *Medlink Neurology* (S. Gilman, ed.), San Diego: 2005.

47. Hajak, G., B. Bandelow, J. Zulley, and D. Pittrow, "As needed" pharmacotherapy combined with stimulus control treatment in chronic insomnia—assessment of a novel intervention strategy in a primary care setting. *Ann Clin Psychiatry*, 2002;**14**(1):1–7.

48. Vgontzas, A.N. and A. Kales, Sleep and its disorders. *Annu Rev Med*, 1999;**50**:387–400.

49. Doghramji, K., The need for flexibility in dosing of hypnotic agents. *Sleep*, 2000;**23**(Suppl 1):S16–S22.

50. Schenck, C.H. and M.W. Mahowald, Long-term, nightly benzodiazepine treatment of injurious parasomnias and other disorders of disrupted nocturnal sleep in 170 adults. *Am J Med*, 1996;**100**(3):333–337.

51. Walsh, J.K. and P.K. Schweitzer, Ten-year trends in the pharmacological treatment of insomnia. *Sleep*, 1999;**22**(3):371–375.

52. Darcourt, G., D. Pringuey, D.E. Salliere, and J. Lavoisy, The safety and tolerability of zolpidem—an update. *J Psychopharmacol*, 1999;**13**(1):81–93.

53. Holm, K.J. and K.L. Goa, Zolpidem: an update of its pharmacology, therapeutic efficacy and tolerability in the treatment of insomnia. *Drugs*, 2000;**59**(4):865–889.

54. Elie, R., E. Ruther, I. Farr, G. Emilien, and E. Salinas, Sleep latency is shortened during 4 weeks of treatment with zaleplon, a novel nonbenzodiazepine hypnotic. Zaleplon Clinical Study Group. *J Clin Psychiatry*, 1999;**60**(8):536–544.

55. Hedner, J., R. Yaeche, G. Emilien, I. Farr, and E. Salinas, Zaleplon shortens subjective sleep latency and improves subjective sleep quality in elderly patients with insomnia. The Zaleplon Clinical Investigator Study Group. *Int J Geriatr Psychiatry*, 2000;**15**(8):704–712.

56. Krystal, A.D., J.K. Walsh, E. Laska, et al., Sustained efficacy of eszopiclone over 6 months of nightly treatment: results of a randomized, double-blind, placebo-controlled study in adults with chronic insomnia. *Sleep*, 2003;**26**(7):793–799.

57. Mendelson, W.B., A review of the evidence for the efficacy and safety of trazodone in insomnia. *J Clin Psychiatry*, 2005;**66**(4):469–476.

58. Dominguez, R.A., R.L. Bravo-Valverde, B.R. Kaplowitz, and J.M. Cott, Valerian as a hypnotic for Hispanic patients. *Cultur Divers Ethnic Minor Psychol*, 2000;**6**(1):84–92.

59. Dorn, M., [Efficacy and tolerability of Baldrian versus oxazepam in non-organic and non-psychiatric insomniacs: a randomised, double-blind, clinical, comparative study]. *Forsch Komplementarmed Klass Naturheilkd*, 2000;**7**(2)79–84.

60. Poyares, D.R., C. Guilleminault, M.M. Ohayon, and S. Tufik, Can valerian improve the sleep of insomniacs after benzodiazepine withdrawal? *Prog Neuropsychopharmacol Biol Psychiatry*, 2002;**26**(3):539–545.

61. Weiler, J.M., J.R. Bloomfield, G.G. Woodworth, et al., Effects of fexofenadine, diphenhydramine, and alcohol on driving performance. A randomized, placebo-controlled trial in the Iowa driving simulator. *Ann Intern Med*, 2000;**132**(5):354–363.

62. Sproule, B.A., U.E. Busto, C. Buckle, N. Herrmann, and S. Bowles, The use of non-prescription sleep products in the elderly. *Int J Geriatr Psychiatry*, 1999;**14**(10):851–857.
63. Shamir, E., M. Laudon, Y. Barak, et al., Melatonin improves sleep quality of patients with chronic schizophrenia. *J Clin Psychiatry*, 2000;**61**(5):373–377.
64. Zisapel, N., The use of melatonin for the treatment of insomnia. *Biol Signals Recept*, 1999;**8**(1–2):84–89.
65. Tang, N.K. and A.G. Harvey, Correcting distorted perception of sleep in insomnia: a novel behavioural experiment? *Behav Res Ther*, 2004;**42**(1):27–39.
66. Smith, M.T., M.L. Perlis, A. Park, et al., Comparative meta-analysis of pharmacotherapy and behavior therapy for persistent insomnia. *Am J Psychiatry*, 2002;**159**(1):5–11.
67. Morin, C.M., C. Bastien, B. Guay, M. Radouco-Thomas, J. Leblanc, and A. Vallieres, Randomized clinical trial of supervised tapering and cognitive behavior therapy to facilitate benzodiazepine discontinuation in older adults with chronic insomnia. *Am J Psychiatry*, 2004;**161**(2):332–342.
68. Morin, C.M., L. Belanger, C. Bastien, and A. Vallieres, Long-term outcome after discontinuation of benzodiazepines for insomnia: a survival analysis of relapse. *Behav Res Ther*, 2005;**43**(1):1–14.
69. Kirisoglu, C. and C. Guilleminault, Twenty minutes versus forty-five minutes morning bright light treatment on sleep onset insomnia in elderly subjects. *J Psychosom Res*, 2004;**56**(5):537–542.
70. Lack, L., H. Wright, K. Kemp, and S. Gibbon, The treatment of early-morning awakening insomnia with 2 evenings of bright light. *Sleep*, 2005;**28**(5):616–623.

4

The Impact of Life Cycle on Sleep in Women

Margaret Moline, Lauren Broch, and Rochelle Zak

INTRODUCTION

Across the life cycle of women, the quality and quantity of sleep can be markedly affected by both internal (e.g., hormonal changes and vasomotor symptoms) and external (e.g., financial, marital, and child-care responsibilities) factors. This chapter outlines some of the major phases of the life cycle that have been associated with sleep problems in women. Very little systematic, large-scale research has been performed in any of the areas reviewed here, and, once identified, sleep problems are generally best addressed using standard therapeutic approaches. However, in the case of pregnant and lactating women, the welfare of the fetus or child must be considered in the treatment decision. This chapter is organized into sections that address sleep problems associated with the menstrual cycle, pregnancy, postpartum, and perimenopause.

Anecdotal reports recommend treatment that addresses specific physical discomforts experienced by women during many of these phases (e.g., analgesics for premenstrual pain, pregnancy pillows for backache, hormone replacement therapy [HRT] for hot flashes). The importance of developing standard treatment recommendations is stressed, especially because the development of chronic insomnia has been linked to precipitating events. Additionally, primary sleep disorders (e.g., sleep apnea, restless legs syndrome [RLS]) have been shown to increase during pregnancy and menopause, but treatment recommendations may be contraindicated for pregnant women. Thus, it may be necessary to develop unique therapeutic strategies for women.

SLEEP DISRUPTION RELATED TO THE MENSTRUAL CYCLE

Studies of the influence of menstrual cycle phase on sleep began in 1966 with a paper by Williams et al. (1). The literature since that time has been limited and contradictory, in part because numerous methodological issues make designing studies in this area a challenge. Lee and Shaver (2) discussed many of these methodological factors, including (a) defining menstrual phases, in that menstrual cycles

From: *Current Clinical Neurology: Sleep Disorders in Women: A Guide to Practical Management*
Edited by: H. P. Attarian © Humana Press Inc., Totowa, NJ

are not uniform in length among women or between consecutive cycles; (b) documenting the timing of ovulation, demarcating follicular from luteal phase; (c) the wide age range in the perimenopausal interval; (d) oral contraceptives use; and (e) life situations. For example, the sleep of a woman with normal menstrual cycles and young children at home may differ from that of a woman without children *(3)*. This may translate into differences observed in the laboratory between "normal" cohorts and clinical populations studied in treatment trials. In addition, many studies of women across the menstrual cycle have included only small numbers of subjects *(3,4)*.

The International Classification of Sleep Disorders (ICSD) lists several sleep disorders related to the menstrual cycle: menstrual-associated sleep disorder. These include premenstrual insomnia, premenstrual hypersomnia, and menopausal insomnia. The rationale for the latter category is not clear, because by definition, menopausal women have no menstrual cycles. Schenck and Mahowald *(5)* recommended adding another disorder, premenstrual parasomnia, to the category based on their clinical observations.

Despite the inclusion of premenstrual insomnia in the ICSD, Manber and Armitage *(4)* discussed the lack of research on this entity. In apparently the only research study focusing on this issue, Manber's group *(6)* used sleep logs and actigraphy to study women with psychophysiological insomnia across the menstrual cycle. They found that daily irregularity in the insomnia pattern outweighed any menstrual cycle effect. A case report *(7)* documented a phase delay in core temperature in association with premenstrual insomnia. More research will be required to validate this diagnosis.

Menstrual cycle influences on sleep have been reported in survey studies of women and women with premenstrual syndrome (PMS) *(8)*. A recent paper suggests that the perception of sleep quality declines premenstrually and in the early follicular phase without an impact on sleep continuity *(9)*.

PMS is a common problem characterized by mood and/or physical symptoms that appear regularly in the luteal phase and remit during or shortly after the onset of menses. Severe, predominantly mood and anxiety symptoms that markedly impact a woman's ability to function at home or the workplace or in her relationships with others can lead to an additional diagnosis, premenstrual dysphoric disorder (PMDD). Sleep complaints, either insomnia or hypersomnia, comprise 1 of the 11 symptoms listed in the fourth edition of the *Diagnostic and Statistical Manual* (DSM-IV) for PMDD, 5 of which must be considered positive for the diagnosis to be given.

Women with PMS and PMDD report sleep-related complaints including "insomnia, hypersomnia, tiredness or fatigue, disturbing dreams or nightmares, lethargy, and inability to concentrate" *(10)*. Because PMDD may be a variant of an affective disorder, and because patients with major depression have well-characterized sleep abnormalities, the sleep of women with premenstrual conditions was compared with women with major depression. It has been suggested that women with PMDD may have underlying circadian rhythm abnormalities in temperature *(11,12)*, in melatonin *(13,14)*, or in the coupling of rhythms *(15)*, which could impact sleep.

Survey studies *(16,17)* suggest that the late luteal phase may be associated with more frequent subjective sleep disturbances, including restless sleep, sleep disturbances, unpleasant dreams, and unrefreshing sleep. There has been limited research using polysomnography across the menstrual cycle *(13,14,16–22)*. Several of these groups reported no major reproducible differences in sleep architecture in women with PMS/PMDD compared to control women or in the control women themselves *(23)*. Thus, it appears that there are no clear menstrual cycle changes in sleep architecture and that the sleep of women with PMS does not share the key features of sleep of depressed women.

However, women do complain of difficulty sleeping in the premenstrual phase. No definitive clinical trials have specifically addressed the treatment of women with premenstrual insomnia *(24)*. Thus, the management of disrupted sleep in this population should be similar to the treatment of sleeping problems at other times. Consideration should also be given to addressing physical symptoms such as pain, headache, and bloating, which could make the patient uncomfortable. Limiting caffeine and salt intake and consuming frequent small meals have been suggested as behavioral measures to relieve the common premenstrual symptoms of insomnia, bloating, and food craving, respectively *(25)*. Although there are few supporting data for these recommendations, they may be helpful in mitigating difficulty falling asleep caused by caffeine or acid reflux, for example. Regular aerobic exercise has some research support as a treatment for some symptoms of PMS *(25)*, but exercise should be avoided too close to bedtime *(26)*.

Treatments for PMS/PMDD, such as selective serotonin reuptake inhibitors, may also be effective in reducing sleep complaints, although their specificity in addressing insomnia (or hypersomnia) *per se* has not been reported to date *(24)*.

Another important disorder related to the menstrual cycle that may impact sleep is dysmenorrhea. Dysmenorrhea refers to severe pain associated with menstruation. It can also include painful cramping before the onset of menstrual flow. Dysmenorrhea is common, but apparently only one paper on this population has been published in the sleep literature *(27)*. Subjects with dysmenorrhea reported more subjective fatigue than control subjects. Given that pain can contribute to insomnia *(28)*, therapeutic interventions for dysmenorrhea may ameliorate the sleep complaints, a question that should be addressed in controlled research studies.

Several reports describe hypersomnia episodes that were temporally linked to the menstrual cycle *(29–31)*. However, no definitive clinical trials have specifically addressed the treatment of women with premenstrual hypersomnia.

As mentioned above, premenstrual parasomnia is not currently listed in the ICSD. Schenck and Mahowald *(5)* described two female patients, each of whom had experienced sleep terrors and injurious sleepwalking that were linked to the premenstrual phase. With treatment—one by self-hypnosis and the other by self-hypnosis and medication—symptoms were decreased. To date, however, no definitive clinical trials have specifically addressed the treatment of women with premenstrual parasomnia. However, if the behaviors occurring during the episodes are dangerous, benzodiazepine medication (the standard treatment for parasomnias) might be considered. Clinicians who encounter female patients past menarche with complaints of parasomnias will hopefully inquire about the temporal association of symptoms with menstrual cycle events to help establish the clinical validity of this diagnosis.

SLEEP PROBLEMS DURING PREGNANCY

Although pregnancy, childbirth, and postpartum can be fulfilling and exhilarating experiences for women, these periods are also fraught with considerable sleep disruption. Reports of altered sleep during pregnancy range from 13 to 80% in the first trimester and increase to 66–97% by the third trimester *(32,33)*. The marked rise in gonadal steroid hormones during the first trimester and the added physical discomfort associated with the growing fetus during the second and third trimesters are obvious reasons for sleep disturbance. The recent addition of the diagnosis of pregnancy-associated sleep disorder in the ICSD validates sleep difficulties during pregnancy. However, as Santiago and colleagues point out *(34)*, physicians may presume that a sleep problem is a result of normal physiological changes during pregnancy and overlook the possibility of a primary sleep disorder such as sleep apnea or RLS.

Sleep research during pregnancy has been limited by varying data collection procedures, small and often nonrepresentative samples, poorly controlled studies, pooled data that may obscure individual variation, cross-sectional designs, and studies that are descriptive rather than hypothesis-driven. Unfortunately, few generalizations exist beyond women's almost universal complaints of disrupted sleep and fatigue during the first trimester, varying degrees of a grace period in the second trimester, and substantial sleep disruption during the third trimester and postpartum. As Lee *(35)* discusses in a comprehensive review of the literature, research on sleep during childbearing has received little attention since the pioneering work of Karacan and colleagues in the 1960s *(36)*. Furthermore, little to no research exists on possible treatments for sleep disruption and safe, effective treatment of primary sleep disorders during pregnancy and postpartum.

Subjective studies during pregnancy *(32,33)* find that the most common reasons cited for altered sleep vary according to the trimester. In the first trimester, women complain of nausea and vomiting, urinary frequency, backaches, and feeling uncomfortable and fatigued. By the second and third trimesters, fetal movements, heartburn, cramps or tingling in the legs, and shortness of breath are also reported. In addition to physical discomfort, women also report that emotional concerns such as dreams about the fetus and anxiety over the eminent change in lifestyle play a role in their insomnia. A most provocative finding in Mindell and Jacobson's study *(33)* was that despite the fact that virtually all women at the end of pregnancy reported poor sleep, only one-third of women believed that they had a current sleep problem. The authors suggest that pregnant women may resign themselves to poor sleep because they believe it is an expected and perhaps untreatable part of pregnancy.

Both subjective and objective studies largely concur in showing that early in pregnancy, most women become sleepier, and their nighttime sleep may become more disrupted. Mean sleep durations average around 7 and 8 hours, and total sleep time (TST) increases roughly 1 hour per day when compared to prepregnancy levels. As the pregnancy progresses, however, sleep becomes more fragmented, with a resulting decrease in TST back to prepregnancy levels and lower by the end of pregnancy. Studies of the sleep architecture of the pregnant woman demonstrate increased stage 1 sleep (light sleep) and reduction in rapid eye-movement sleep. Although findings regarding slow-wave sleep are equivocal *(35)*, objective sleep studies confirm the universal complaints of disrupted sleep, particularly as the pregnancy progresses, in showing increased wake after sleep onset.

To compensate for disrupted nighttime sleep and the soporific effects of rising hormones, pregnant women alter their sleep habits by sleeping later, especially on weekends, and napping more often. Studies agree that the most commonly endorsed complaints are of physical discomfort, but reported prevalences of sleep problems can vary widely and depend to some degree on the format of the survey studies (e.g., self-report, questionnaires, sleep logs, Likert scales). Although hormonal and physical changes contribute profoundly to sleepiness and sleep disruption, age, parity, and history of mood disorders can affect sleep as well. Alterations in sleep and wake schedules, anxiety, and primary sleep disorders also contribute to an unknown extent.

The treatment of sleep problems during pregnancy consists primarily of addressing the specific physical discomfort experienced by the woman (e.g., backache, nausea, urinary frequency). Anecdotal reports from pregnant women suggest that certain interventions such as a reduction in spicy foods and caffeine, sleeping elevated and taking antacids for heartburn, a reduction of fluid intake in the evenings to decrease nocturia, pregnancy pillows and side-sleeping positions for back discomfort may improve a pregnant woman's sleep. Stress-related insomnia during pregnancy has not been studied, but general recommendations include meditation, stress-management therapies, and psychotherapy to relieve anxiety and depression, which may be associated with pregnancy.

In studies of nonpregnant women and men, it has been shown that alterations and irregular sleep schedules such as napping or sleeping later in response to sleep disruption may result in the development of poor sleep hygiene and conditioned anxiety about the sleep process, which in turn may contribute to a more chronic form of insomnia in some women. However, there are no behavioral studies showing that poor sleep hygiene in pregnant women results in a more lasting insomnia or, on the other hand, that good sleep hygiene treatment benefits the pregnant woman. The most obvious reason for the lack of behavioral treatment studies in pregnant women is the possible deleterious effects of pharmacotherapy on the developing fetus as well as the false belief that sleep problems during pregnancy are inevitable and, also, untreatable.

For similar concerns regarding the developing fetus, little research exists regarding sleep aids. In one of the earliest survey studies *(32)*, 12% of pregnant women reported using sleep aids. It is likely that fewer women now take sleep medication, since medication recommendations during pregnancy have become more stringent. A Medline search of literature between 1966 and 2000 *(37)* revealed that the currently available literature is insufficient to determine whether the potential benefits of benzodiazepines to the mother outweigh the potential risks to the fetus. In fact, recommendations regarding the use of OTC or prescription sleep aids during pregnancy extrapolate mainly from the relatively few studies done during in nursing mothers.

A case series *(38)* showed that a nursing infant's exposure to its mother's use of benzodiazepines was relatively limited. In particular, the review reported that it appears to be safe to take diazepam during pregnancy. On the other hand, the review cites case reports of sedation, poor feeding, and respiratory distress in nursing infants, particularly with diazepam use. However, when data have been pooled, the findings suggest a low incidence of adverse events, particularly with low dosages of benzodiazepines. General guidelines for physicians treating pregnant women are as follows: (a) determine if the medication is necessary; (b) choose the safest drug available (e.g., diazepam, lorazepam, clonazepam); (c) use the lowest dosage for the shortest duration; and (d) avoid the first trimester, if possible *(37,39)*.

SLEEP DISORDERS DURING PREGNANCY

Given the changes in pulmonary mechanics during pregnancy, the incidence of sleep-disordered breathing (SDB) during pregnancy has become a topic of interest. Whereas progesterone, a respiratory stimulant, may play a protective role, there are at least theoretical concerns that narrowed upper airways coupled with increased body habitus may result in compromised breathing during sleep in pregnancy. It is well known that snoring increases during pregnancy, especially during the third trimester, with estimated frequencies increasing from 4% in the nonpregnant woman to ranges of 14–23% during pregnancy *(40,41)*. These findings are potentially important because snoring during pregnancy has been linked to maternal hypertension and is a risk factor for pre-eclampsia and fetal growth retardation *(41,42)*. In one case report, a 25-year-old woman in her third trimester (37 weeks) being evaluated and treated for pre-eclampsia overnight was also confirmed to have sleep apnea, with maternal oxygen desaturations and concurrent fetal heart rate decelerations *(43)*. She then delivered an infant who was small for gestational age.

Unfortunately, definitive conclusions are lacking regarding the incidence of snoring and SDB owing to the absence of large prospective, longitudinal studies. However, the data suggest that sleep apnea is more likely to develop in pregnant women who have a preexisting tendency toward SDB and worsen in those women who already have sleep apnea *(44)*. A recent study by Shepertycky et al. *(45)* suggested that sleep apnea may present differently in women because women recently diagnosed with sleep apnea were found to be more likely to have signs and symptoms of hypothyroidism, depression, and insomnia than were men with sleep apnea.

Nasal continuous positive airway pressure (CPAP) has been used effectively in a number of pregnant women and was found to reduce nocturnal blood pressure increments in women with pre-eclampsia *(41)*. In a study by Guilleminault et al. *(46)*, pregnant women diagnosed with SDB either early in or prepregnancy and treated with nasal CPAP with repeat titrations at 6 months gestational age (GA) had full-term pregnancies and delivered healthy-sized infants. At least half of the pregnant women needed CPAP pressure readjustment at 6 months GA.

Future research should (a) assess for upper airway resistance syndrome, a more subtle form of SDB, by utilizing more sophisticated breathing equipment and (b) investigate the possible relationship of SDB with maternal and fetal complications.

In addition to sleep apnea, RLS increases during pregnancy, particularly during the final trimester, and then decreases after delivery *(33,35)*. The International RLS Study Group defines RLS as (a) an urge to move one's legs, usually accompanied by an unpleasant or uncomfortable sensation in the legs that is (b) worse when at rest and during the evening and nighttime and (c) partially or totally relieved by movement. RLS can result in difficulty falling and staying asleep. Lee's group *(47)* found that the prevalence increased from 0% of the 30 women preconception to 13% in the first trimester, 18% in the second, and 23% by the third trimester. Only one subject continued to have restless legs after delivery. When compared to those without complaints, the women with restless legs had lower ferritin levels (<50 μg/ dL) and significantly lower folate levels before and during pregnancy. They suggest that these findings support the role of iron and folate in the etiology of RLS during pregnancy. Indeed, Botez and Lambert *(48)* found that the prevalence in RLS in pregnant women taking vitamins with folate (9%) was lower than those taking supplements without folate (80%).

Most dopaminergic agents used to treat idiopathic RLS fall into category C (uncertain safety in pregnancy—animal studies show an adverse effect, no human studies) with the exception of pergolide, which is in category B (presumed safety based on animal studies) *(49)*. However, there are no published studies using pergolide in pregnant women with RLS. Conservative treatments for RLS include avoidance of caffeinated beverages and nicotine, restriction of carbohydrate-rich foods, treatment of anemia (if present), calf stretches, massage, warm or cold compresses, and vitamin supplementation with folate. Also, over-the-counter sleep aids that contain diphenhydramine and other antihistamines should be avoided because they can worsen RLS symptoms. Given the precipitous increase in RLS in pregnancy, research should be undertaken to address other possible nutritional approaches to this problem.

SLEEP PROBLEMS DURING POSTPARTUM

The postpartum period, which is associated with considerable sleep disruption, begins with delivery and ends for most women approximately 6–12 months later when the infant is sleeping through the night. The postpartum distress that most women experience (estimates range from 35 to 80%) occurs 3–5 days after birth. The more serious form of postpartum depression may require antidepressant treatment 2–4 weeks after delivery. Ten to 15% develop postpartum depression, of whom only one-third has a prior history of affective disorder *(50)*.

Although postpartum sleep loss is both intuitive and well documented, interpretation of the small number of objective and subjective sleep studies has been challenging. First, data-collection procedures have varied widely, especially those used in earlier studies in which the mother's sleep was studied without the infant present. More recent postpartum sleep studies have been conducted in a naturalistic setting with the infant at home or in the hospital room. Second, there is great variability in prior sleep deprivation and sleep–wake patterns. Finally, other important variables (e.g., parity, length of labor, time of day, type of delivery, feeding method, postpartum day studied) are often not considered.

Sleep patterns during pregnancy not only have short-term effects but have also been shown to affect such variables as labor, delivery, and postpartum depression. Lee and Gay *(51)* found that women who slept less than 6 hours during late pregnancy had longer labors and were 4.5 times more likely to have cesarean sections than pregnant women who slept more than 6 hours. These findings led the authors *(51)* to recommend that physicians and other health care providers not only discuss sleep quantity and quality with their pregnant patients, but also emphasize to patients that they are, in a sense, "sleeping for two."

Sleep patterns in pregnancy may also predict postpartum depressive symptoms, as shown by Wolfson and colleagues *(52)*. In this study, women with depressive symptoms 2–4 weeks postpartum were more likely to nap and have increased TSTs during the third trimester. However, there was no difference in TST between depressed and nondepressed women postpartum. Wolfson et al. suggest that women with increased TST during pregnancy have more difficulty tolerating postpartum sleep deprivation, which may result in depression.

Although the most common reason cited for maternal awakenings in postpartum studies is the infant's sleep and feeding schedule *(53,54)*, there is considerable discrepancy in the average TSTs (range 4–7.5 hours) reported owing to small sample sizes and the variability of sleep during the first few postpartum weeks *(55,56)*. There is some suggestion that slow-wave sleep is somewhat preserved due to the effects of chronic sleep deprivation *(55)*. Like during pregnancy, women compensate for lost nighttime sleep by sleeping on a more irregular schedule and napping to some extent while the infant naps *(57)*, although the ability to nap is affected by parity. Gay and Lee *(58)* compared new mothers and new fathers using wrist actigraphy and found that while both partners' sleep was more disrupted than during the third trimester of pregnancy, new moms slept less at night but new dads had less TST when compared to their partners' sleep postpartum. Beyond the obvious sleep disruptions caused by the infant, recent studies suggest a myriad of other factors (e.g., emotional and physical health of mother, parity, methods of birth and feeding, infant's sleep–wake rhythm, co-sleeping) that further affect postpartum sleep.

In a polysomnographic study investigating parity, Waters and Lee *(59)* found that although both first-time mothers and mothers with children at home did not differ in TSTs during the third trimester, first-time mothers had a decrease in sleep efficiency from the third trimester to 1 month postpartum, whereas multipara's sleep efficiency remained relatively stable. A most provocative finding in the Waters and Lee study is that new mothers had more fatigue than experienced mothers, yet scored lower on a measure of participation in household chores. The authors propose that the differences in sleep and fatigue found in novice and experienced mothers reflect the new challenges in maternal role acquisition in the primigravida group. They also suggest that the process of integrating and achieving competence in mothering behaviors together with sleep deprivation may put new mothers at risk of developing postpartum depression.

Feeding method may also impact the sleep of mothers with infant children, although this subject has not been well studied *(60)*. Quillin's study *(60)* showed that those mothers who breast-fed had more awakenings within the first month postpartum and tended to sleep less during the night than women who bottle-fed. However, in another study *(61)*, lactation was associated with a significant increase in slow-wave sleep in women who breast-fed when compared to women who bottle-fed. Mosko and colleagues *(62)* conducted laboratory polysomnography on bed-sharing and solitary-sleeping breast-feeding Latino infant–mother pairs. Although they found differences in arousals and a small decrease in slow-wave sleep in the bed-sharing condition, there was no difference in overall nocturnal wakefulness and TSTs between the two conditions.

Although all of the above-mentioned variables affect mother's and baby's sleep, studies show that ultimately mother's sleep will improve along with baby's development. Subjective and objective studies conducted in new mothers and their infants show that by around 3 months, the infants' sleep and wake patterns become more regular and, in turn, the mothers' sleep becomes more continuous *(54,63)*. In a study conducted in England, 50% of the babies were found to sleep through the night by 8 weeks and 75% by 3 months *(63)*. Factors that affected sleeping through the night at an earlier age were greater birth weight, female gender, younger mothers with less stress, co-sleeping less than 2 hours or not at all, no central heating, and the baby not sharing a room with a sibling. Although many infants sleep through the night by 1 year, Ferber *(64)* reports that bothersome nocturnal awakenings continue to occur in 23–33% of 1- and 2-year-old children in the United States.

Recommendations for new mothers include the old adage "sleep when you can," which essentially means sleeping on an irregular schedule to conform to the infant's erratic pattern of sleeping. And although this type of schedule has not been formally researched, anecdotal reports suggest that it may help to stave off severe sleep deprivation for many women. However, the long-term effects of an irregular sleep–wake regimen have been associated with insomnia in other populations *(24)*. Establishing a clear circadian pattern (day–night difference) in the child's bedroom will also facilitate adjustment to night sleeping. Commonly used behavioral interventions such as controlled crying and systematic ignoring have also been shown to decrease infant sleep problems in randomized controlled trials *(65)*. In addition, education regarding normal sleep cycles and maintaining regular bedtime routines and schedules and consistent nap schedules can help establish a more predictable sleep–wake rhythm in the baby *(66)*.

In cases where the effects of sleep deprivation and insomnia are affecting the new mother's general welfare and ability to take care of her infant, sleep aids are sometimes warranted. Generally accepted guidelines *(39)* regarding medication during lactation include (a) establish the risk/benefit ratio to determine if the medication is necessary, (b) choose the safest drug available (e.g., safe when administered directly to infants, short-half life and high molecular weight, low milk:plasma ratio, high protein binding in maternal serum, ionized in maternal plasma, and less lipophilic), and (c) consult with the pediatrician when possible. Also, the mother should take the medication after breast-feeding and/or right before the infant's longest sleep period and arrange monitoring of the infant's serum drug levels if the medication is possibly injurious to the infant.

As already mentioned, the Medline review article *(37)* conducted a search of the terms "benzodiazepines," "diazepam," "chlordiazepoxide," "clonazepam," "lorazepam," and "alprazolam" and found 118 articles. After the data for each medication were summarized, it was found that diazepam was not recommended during lactation due to potential effects of lethargy, sedation, and weight loss in infants. Chlordiazepoxide and lorazepam were found to be safe during lactation.

A case series *(38)* measuring infants' serum levels of psychotropic medication and active metabolites from mothers taking psychotropic medications showed that medications were not detected in infant serum when mothers had taken these agents solely during the postpartum period. Also, mothers did not report any difficulties with their infants.

It is obvious that postpartum sleep in new mothers is seriously disrupted, likely as a result of a multitude of factors, including parenting approaches, infant sleep–wake schedule, bed-sharing, parity, breast-feeding, how and where an infant is readied for sleep, the tenor of the parents' interaction with the child, and general household demeanor. The parents' general physical and emotional health, cumulative sleep deprivation, and their ability to bounce back from severe sleep disruption must also be considered.

Future research should investigate effective treatments for irregular sleep–wake schedules in infants. Many of the factors affecting the infant and mother's sleep are likely amenable to intervention that benefits the mother without compromising the infant. Yet, like research on sleep during pregnancy, there are few evidence-based data on which to base treatment recommendations for postpartum sleep disruption. Because sleep deprivation has been linked to postpartum depression in some women, the importance of finding workable treatment alternatives in this population is important.

SLEEP PROBLEMS DURING PERIMENOPAUSE

There is an increased prevalence of insomnia in postmenopausal women, with estimates of complaints of insomnia in peri- and postmenopausal women ranging from 44% *(67)* to 61% *(68)*. Four major causes have been proposed to account for poor sleep in perimenopausal women: (a) sleep disruption associated with hot flashes, (b) increased incidence of obstructive sleep apnea, (c) mood disorders, and (d) inadequate sleep hygiene leading to a chronic insomnia.

Not surprisingly, the focus of therapeutic interventions is on HRT, as well as on standard treatments for these four disorders. The results of the Women's Health Initiative (WHI) *(69)* have now put into question the safe use of HRT as a treatment option for menopausal women. Like the conclusions reported here, the implications of the WHI apply only to the particular hormone preparation used in that study, which was oral conjugated equine estrogen and medroxyprogesterone. There are theoretical reasons, at least, to suspect that transdermally delivered estradiol and oral progesterone may not necessarily have the same adverse events. Because some women choose to remain on HRT and long-term safety and efficacy data on the newer HRT formulations may at some point become available, it is reasonable to discuss the role of this therapy in treating sleep disorders in menopausal women.

Hot flashes are one of the oldest reported causes of sleep disruption. However, the debate continues as to whether or not they actually are associated with sleep disruptions. On polysomnography, some authors found an association of hot flashes with nocturnal awakenings *(70)* and decreased sleep efficiency *(71,72)*. More recent studies, some involving the same authors, have found no correlation between the presence of hot flashes and polysomnographic measures of poor sleep *(73,74)*. It is suggested that one of the methodological problems with the older studies is that they did not screen for concomitant sleep disorders or drug use as possible causes of sleep disruption *(74)*.

Not only is the role of hot flashes in perimenopausal insomnia unclear, so is the efficacy of HRT in treating this problem. Two papers analyzing the effect of oral synthetic estrogen on objectively determined hot flashes and sleep found improvements in both *(70,76)*. In contrast, another study analyzing the combination of estrogen and progesterone *(77)* found no difference in objective hot flashes between treatment and placebo.

Not only do the objective studies disagree, but those studies looking at patient self-reports of hot flashes also conflict. Two double-blind crossover studies, one with transdermal estrogen *(78)* and one with oral synthetic estrogen *(79)*, found a decrease in subjectively reported hot flashes. On the other hand, a double-blind placebo-controlled study using oral synthetic estrogen *(76)* did not find a greater decrease in subjectively reported hot flashes in the treatment the two groups.

Clearly there are objective and subjective data that both support and refute a role of HRT in treating hot flashes. Nonetheless, if a woman is complaining of hot flashes, particularly at night, it would seem prudent to treat these symptoms using a form of HRT or some other treatment. Hot flash frequencies vary directly with temperature. Sleeping in a cool environment can decrease the frequency of hot flashes *(80,81)*, so one could also advise women with hot flashes to lower the temperature in the bedroom.

SDB is another proposed cause of poor sleep in perimenopausal women. The incidence of SDB increases with menopause. After controlling for age, body mass index, and several lifestyle factors *(82)*, postmenopausal women were 2.6 times more likely than premenopausal women to have SDB. Proposed mechanisms for this apparent increase have included a change in the distribution of body fat with an increase in the waist-to-hip circumference ratio *(83)* and a decrease in sex hormones, in general *(84)*, and progesterone, a known respiratory stimulant, in particular *(4)*.

The literature on HRT and SDB is divided into cross-sectional analyses and prospective clinical trials. The majority of the results from the large cross-sectional studies favor a positive effect of HRT (either estrogen or estrogen plus progesterone) on SDB, with two showing statistically significant decreases in the prevalence of SDB among women using HRT compared with those not *(85,86)*. One study found somewhat decreased odds of having SDB with HRT use *(82)*. Thus, epidemiological data suggest a therapeutic effect of HRT.

The prospective drug trials have shown an effect in mild but not in moderate or more severe obstructive sleep apnea. A pilot study using the newer, more physiological forms of HRT (transdermal estradiol with oral progesterone) in postmenopausal women with mild to low-moderate SDB found an effect with estrogen that disappeared with the addition of progesterone *(87)*. Treatment did not normalize the apnea–hypopnea index (AHI), leaving residual mild SDB. However, the study was both of short duration and small sample size. Another pilot study using estradiol and a synthetic progestin (trimegeston) demonstrated normalization of the AHI in subjects with mild obstructive sleep apnea *(88)*. These studies suggest that HRT may be effective in treating mild sleep apnea.

The results of using HRT to treat moderate or more severe SDB are not as promising. One study of HRT use in women with high to moderate SDB found a statistically significant improvement with HRT but not resolution of the SDB *(89)*. A second study similarly looked at subjects with moderate to severe SDB before and after HRT *(90)* and found no overall improvement with HRT. These findings, however, are neither surprising nor disappointing, in that the gold standard of treatment for moderate to severe SDB is nasal CPAP.

Mood disturbances can affect sleep. Both depression and anxiety can be associated with less refreshing and more fragmented sleep *(91)*. It is unclear if the hormonal changes of menopause, *per se*, can account for depression and anxiety in this population *(92)* or if the depression and anxiety that can be associated with menopause represent unresolved grief *(93)*, a response to life circumstances *(94)*, or relate to the presence of hot flashes *(93)*. Nonetheless, for some patients psychotherapy was necessary to treat insomnia despite diminution of hot flashes with HRT (using transdermal estradiol and a progestin) *(95)*. There are many more studies that looked at using HRT (either estrogen alone or estrogen plus progestin) to treat perimenopausal depression. Not surprisingly, some found efficacy *(96)* and others did not *(73,97)*. Thus, it is important to consider a mood disorder when a woman is complaining of poor sleep in association with menopause.

As with all cases of insomnia, one should look for a precipitating cause that then has perpetuating factors, generally the result of inadequate sleep hygiene. In an excellent review of this topic, Krystal and colleagues *(93)* proposed a primary insomnia of menopause in which a precipitating factor (sometimes hot flashes) resolves, after which perpetuating factors (elements of inadequate sleep hygiene) then intervene, maintaining the insomnia. Clearly, the treatment for this would be the standard insomnia therapies—patient education about principles of good sleep hygiene, sleep restriction, and relaxation techniques, among others.

Other nonpharmacological therapies for menopause-related insomnia that have been investigated include stretching and exercise. A recent study looking at the efficacy of stretching vs exercise on symptoms of insomnia in a group of postmenopausal women not using HRT found that stretching was more effective than exercise. An effect was seen with exercise in the morning for more than 3 hours per week *(98)*.

In addition to treating specific causes of insomnia, many studies look at using HRT to treat sleep complaints in general. As for the efficacy of HRT in treating hot flashes, there are conflicting data on the efficacy of HRT in treating disturbed sleep during menopause. Literature from the 1970s documented improved polysomnographic sleep parameters with oral synthetic estrogens *(97,99)*. More recent studies using transdermal estrogen *(78,100)* and one using oral conjugated estrogen and an oral progestin *(77)* showed no objective polysomnographic improvements. In the two studies using transdermal estrogen, however, the subjects noted a subjective improvement in their sleep. Another trial suggests that progesterone (vs a synthetic progestin) may be necessary to see a beneficial effect of estrogen on sleep *(75)*. Again, a subjective improvement was noted even in the group in which there was no objective improvement. Therefore, there are data that support a therapeutic effect of HRT on sleep as well as data that suggest a subjective improvement of HRT on sleep without an objective correlate.

In summary, when evaluating a menopausal woman with sleep complaints, the clinician should take a thorough sleep history to look for symptoms that would suggest the primary sleep disorders, having a higher suspicion for SDB than one might in younger women, and treat them as usual (e.g., nasal CPAP for moderate or severe SDB), while recognizing the important but as-yet-unresolved question about the efficacy of HRT for mild SDB. Then, one should assess whether or not the patient is experiencing hot flashes—even if she is unaware of them occurring at night—and treat these appropriately. Depression and anxiety should be included in the differential diagnoses and treated. One should look for an initiating event (hot flashes, personal trauma) that has since dissipated or been treated, but that resulted in an irregular sleep–wake schedule or other elements of inadequate sleep hygiene (e.g., increased caffeine consumption, napping) and treat these problems. Finally, one can recommend a program of stretching to increase relaxation and, ideally, promote more restful sleep and consider the use of HRT.

REFERENCES

1. Williams, R.L., H.W. Agnew, and W.B. Webb, Sleep patterns in the young adult female: an EEG study. *Electroenceph Clin Neurophysiol*, 1966;**20**:264–266.
2. Lee, K. and J. Shaver, Women as subjects in sleep studies: methodological issues. *Sleep Res*, 1985;**14**:271.
3. Leibenluft, E., P.L. Fiero, and D.R. Rubinow, Effects of the menstrual cycle on dependent variables in mood disorder research. *Arch Gen Psychiatry*, 1994;**51**:761–781.
4. Manber, R., and R. Armitage, Sex, steroids and sleep: a review. *Sleep*, 1999;**22**:540–545.
5. Schenck, C.H. and M.W. Mahowald, Two cases of premenstrual sleep terrors and injurious sleepwalking. *J Psychosom Obstet Gynecol*, 1995;**16**:79–84.
6. Manber, R., R. Bootzin, and K. Bradley, Menstrual cycle effects on sleep of female insomniacs. *Sleep Res*, 1997;**26**:248.
7. Suzuki, H., M. Uchiyama, K. Shibui, et al., Long-term rectal temperature measurements in a patient with menstrual-associated sleep disorder. *Psychiatr Clin Neurosci*, 2002,**56**:475–478.
8. Miller, E.H., Sleep disorders and women. Women and Insomnia. *Clin Cornerstone*, 2004;**6**(S1B):1–17.
9. Baker, F.C. and H.S. Driver, Self-reported sleep across the menstrual cycle in young, healthy women. *J Psychosom Res*, 2004;**56**:239–243.

10. Mauri, M., Sleep and the reproductive cycle: a review. *Health Care Women Int*, 1990;**11**:409–421.

11. Severino, S.K., D.R. Wagner, M.L. Moline, S.W. Hurt, C.P. Pollak, and S. Zendell, High nocturnal temperature in premenstrual syndrome and late luteal phase dysphoric disorder. *Am J Psychiatry*, 991;**148**:1329–1335.

12. Parry, B.L., B. LeVeau, N. Mostofi, et al., Temperature circadian rhythms during the menstrual cycle and sleep deprivation in premenstrual dysphoric disorder and normal comparison subjects. *J Biol Rhythms*, 1997;**12**:34–46.

13. Parry, B.L., S.L. Berga, D.F. Kripke, et al., Altered waveform of plasma nocturnal melatonin secretion in premenstrual depression *Arch Gen Psychiatry*, 1990;**47**:1139–1146.

14. Parry, B.L, S.L. Berga, N. Mostofi, M.R. Klauber, and A. Resnick, Plasma melatonin circadian rhythms during the menstrual cycle and after light therapy in premenstrual dysphoric disorder and normal control subjects. *J Biol Rhythms*, 1997;**12**:47–64.

15. Shinohara, K., M. Uchiyama, M. Okawa, et al., Menstrual changes in sleep, rectal temperature and melatonin rhythms in a subject with premenstrual syndrome. *Neurosci Lett*, 2000;**281**:159–162.

16. Sheldrake, P. and M. Cormack, Variations in menstrual cycle symptom reporting. *J Psychosom Res*, 1976;**20**:169–177.

17. Mauri, M., R.L. Reid, and A.W. MacLean, Sleep in the premenstrual phase: a self-report study of PMS patients and normal controls. *Acta Psychiatr Scand*, 1988;**78**:82–86.

18. Driver H.S., D. Dijk, E. Werth, K. Biedermann, and A.A. Borbely, Sleep and the sleep electroencephalogram across the menstrual cycle in young healthy women. *J Clin Endocrinol Metab*, 1996,**81**:728–735.

19. Hartmann, E. Dreaming sleep (the D-state) and the menstrual cycle. *J Nerv Ment Dis*, 1966;**143**:406–416.

20. Chuong, C.J., S.R. Kim, O. Taskin, and I. Karacan, Sleep pattern changes in menstrual cycles of women with premenstrual syndrome: a preliminary study. *Am J Obstet Gynecol Online*, 1997;**177**:

21. Lee, K.A., J.F. Shaver, E.C. Giblin, and N.F. Woods, Sleep patterns related to menstrual cycle phase and premenstrual affective symptoms. *Sleep*, 1990;**13**:403–409.

22. Parry, B.L. W.B. Mendelson, W.C. Duncan, D.A. Sack, and T.A. Wehr, Longitudinal sleep EEG, temperature and activity measurements across the menstrual cycle in patients with premenstrual depression and age-matched controls. *Psych Res*, 1989;**30**:285–303.

23. Dzaja, A., S. Arber, J. Hislop, et al., Women's sleep in health and disease. *J Psychiatr Res*, 2005;**39**:55–76.

24. Krystal, A.D., Insomnia in women. *Clin Cornerstone*, 2004;**5**:41–50.

25. Moline, M.L. and S.M. Zendell, Evaluating and managing PMS. *MedScape Women's Health*, 2000;**5**:http://www.medscape.com/Medscape/WomensHealth/journal/2000/v05.n02/wh3025.moli/wh3025.moli-01.html

26. Lee-Chiong, T.L., Manifestations and classification of sleep disorders. In: *Sleep Medicine* (T.L. Lee-Chiong, M.J. Sateia, and M.A. Carskadon, eds.), Philadelphia: Hanely & Belfus, 2002:131.

27. Baker, F.C., H.A. Driver, G.G. Rogers, J. Paiker, and D. Mitchell, High nocturnal body temperatures and disturbed sleep in women with primary dysmenorrhea. *Am J Physiol*, 1999;**40**:E1013–E1021.

28. Sateia, M.J., Epidemiology, consequences and evaluation of insomnia. In: Lee-Chiong T.L., Sateia M.J., Carskadon MA. *Sleep Medicine*. Philadephehia: Hanely & Belfus, 2002:131.

29. Billiard, M., C. Guilleminault, and W. Dement, A menstruation-linked periodic hypersomnia. *Neurology*, 1975;**25**:436–443.

30. Sachs, C., H.E. Persson, and K. Hagenfeldt, Menstruation-related periodic hypersomnia: a case study with successful treatment. *Neurology*, 1982;**32**:376–1379.

31. Bamford, C.R., Menstrual-associated sleep disorder: an unusual hypersomniac variant associated with both menstruation and amenorrhea with a possible link to prolactin and metoclopramide. *Sleep*, 1993;**16**:484–486.

32. Schweiger, M.S., Sleep disturbances in pregnancy. *Am J Obstet Gynecol*, 1972;**114**:879–882.

33. Mindell, J.A. and B.J. Jacobson, Sleep disturbances during pregnancy. *J Obstet Gynecol Neonatal Nurs*, 2000;**29**:590–597.

34. Santiago, J.R., M.S. Nolledo, W. Kinzler, and T.V. Santiago, Sleep and sleep disorders in pregnancy. *Ann Intern Med*, 2001;**134**:396–408.

35. Lee, K.A., Alterations in sleep during pregnancy and postpartum: a review of 30 years of research. *Sleep Med Rev*, 1998;**2**:231–242.

36. Karacan, I., W. Heine, H.W. Agnew, et al., Characteristics of sleep patterns during late preganancy and the postpartum periods. *Am J Obstet Gynecol*, 1968;**101**:579–586.

37. Iqbal, M.M., T. Sobhan, and T. Ryals, Effects of commonly used benzodiazepines on the fetus, the neonate, and the nursing infant. *Psych Services*, 2002;**53**(1):39–49.

38. Birnbaum, C.S., L.S. Cohen, and J.W. Bailey, Serum concentrations of antidepressants and benzodiazepines in nursing infants: a case series. *Pediatrics*, 1999;**104**(1):e11.

39. Della-Giustina, K. and G. Chow, Medications in pregnancy and lactation. *Emerg Med Clin North Am*, 2003;**21**(3):585–613.

40. Loube, D.I., J.S. Poceta, M.C. Morales, M.D. Peacock, and M.M. Mitler, Self-reported snoring in pregnancy and association with fetal outcome. *Chest*, 1996;**109**:885–889.

41. Franklin, K.A., P.A. Homgren, F. Jonsson, N. Poromaa, H. Stenlund, and E.Svanborg, Snoring, pregnancy-inducted hypertension, and growth retardation of the fetus. *Chest*, 2000;**117**:137–141.

42. Izci, B., S.E. Martin, K.C. Dundas, W.A. Liston, A.A. Calder, and N.J. Douglas, Sleep complaints: snoring and daytime sleepiness in pregnant and pre-eclamptic women. *Sleep Med*, 2005;**6**:163–169.

43. Rousch, S.F. and L. Bell, Obstructive sleep apnea in pregnancy. *J Am Board Fam Pract*, 2004;**17**(4):292–294.

44. Edwards, N., P.G. Middleton, D.M. Blyton, and C.E. Sullivan, Sleep disordered breathing and pregnancy. *Thorax*, 2002;**57**:555–558.

45. Shepertycky, M.R., K. Banno, and M.H. Kryger, Differences between men and women in the clinical presentation of patients diagnosed with obstructive sleep apnea syndrome. *Sleep*, 2005;**28**(3):309–314.

46. Guilleminault, C., M. Kreutzer, and J.L. Chang, Pregnancy, sleep disordered breathing and treatment with nasal continuous positive airway pressure. *Sleep Med*, 2004;**5**:43–51.

47. Lee, K.A., M.E. Zaffke, and K. Barette-Beebe, Restless legs syndrome and sleep disturbance during pregnancy: the role of folate and iron. *J Women's Health Gender-Based Med*, 2001;**10**(4):335–341.

48. Botez, M.I. and B. Lambert, Folate deficiency and restless legs syndrome in pregnancy (letter). *NEJM*, 1977;**297**:670.

49. Happe, S. and C. Trenkwalder, Role of dopamine receptor agonists in the treatment of restless legs syndrome. *CNS Drugs*, 2004;**18**(1):27–36.

50. Coble, P.A., C.F. Reynolds, D.J. Kupfer, et al., Childbearing in women with and without a history of affective disorder. 1. Psychiatric symptomatology. *Compr Psychiatr*, 1994;**35**:205–214.

51. Lee, K.A. and C.L. Gay, Sleep in late pregnancy predicts length of labor and type of delivery. *Am J Obstet Gynecol*, 2004;**191**:2041–2046.

52. Wolfson, A.R., S.J. Crowley, U. Anwer, and J.L. Bassett, Changes in sleep patterns and depressive symptoms in first-time mothers: last trimester to 1-year postpartum. *Behav Sleep Med*, 2003;**1**:54–67.

53. Campbell, I., Postpartum sleep patterns of mother-baby pairs. *Midwifery*, 1986;**2**:193–201.

54. Shinkoda, H., K. Matsumoto, and Y.M. Park, Changes in sleep-wake cycle during the period from late pregnancy to puerperium identified through the wrist actigraph and sleep logs. *Psychiatry Clin Neurosci*, 1999;**53**:133–135.

55. Zaffke, M.E. and K.A. Lee, Sleep architecture in a postpartum sample: a comparative analysis. *Sleep Res*, 1992;**21**:327.

56. Lee, K.A., G. McEnany, and M.E. Zaffke, REM sleep and mood state in childbearing women:sleepy or weepy? *Sleep*, 2000;**23**(7):877–885.

57. Bassett, J.L., J.M. Giovanni, K.L. Peterson, et al., Sleep and mood from the last trimester of pregnancy through four months postpartum. *Sleep Res*, 1999;**22**(Suppl):S245–S246.

58. Gay, C.L., K.A. Lee, and S.Y. Lee, Sleep patterns and fatigue in new mothers and fathers. *Bio Res Nurs*, 2004;**5**(4):311–318.
59. Waters, M.A. and K.A. Lee, Differences between primigravidae and multigravidae mothers in sleep disturbances, fatigue, and functional status. *J Nurse Midwifery*, 1996;**41**:364–367.
60. Quillin, S.I.M., Infant and mother sleep patterns during 4th postpartum week. *Issues Compr Ped Nurs*, 1997;**20**:115–123.
61. Blyton, D.M., C.E. Sullivan, and N. Edwards, Lactation is associated with an increase in slow-wave sleep in women. *J Sleep Res*, 2002;**11**:297–303.
62. Mosko, S., C. Richard, and J. McKenna, Maternal sleep and arousals during bedsharing with infants. *Sleep*, 1997;**20**:142–150.
63. Adams, S.M., D.R. Jones, A. Esmail, and E.A. Mitchell, What affects the age of first sleeping through the night? *J Paediatr Child Health*, 2004;**40**:96–101.
64. Ferber, R., Sleeplessness in children. In: *Principles and Practice of Sleep Medicine in the Child* (R. Ferber and M. Kryger, eds.). Philadelphia: W. B. Saunders, 1995:79–89.
65. Leeson, R., J. Barbour, D. Romaniuk, and R. Warr, Management of infant sleep problems in a residential unit. *Child Care Health Dev*, 1994;**20**:89–100.
66. Hiscock, H. and M. Wake, Randomised controlled trial of behavioural infant sleep intervention to improve infant sleep and maternal mood. *Br Med J*, 2002;**324**:1–6.
67. Brugge, K.L., D.F. Kripke, S. Ancoli-Israel, and L. Garfinkel, The association of menopausal status and age with sleep disorders. *Sleep Res*, 1989;**18**:208.
68. Kripke, D.F., R. Brunner, R. Freeman, et al. Sleep complaints of postmenopausal women. *Sleep* (submitted).
69. Writing Group for the Women's Health Initiative Investigators. Risks and benefits of estrogen plus progestin in healthy postmenopausal women. *JAMA*, 2002;**288**(3):321–333.
70. Erlik, Y., I.V. Tataryn, D.R. Meldrum, P. Lomax, J.G. Bajorek, and H.L.Judd, Association of waking episodes with menopausal hot flushes. *JAMA*, 1981;**245**:1741–1744.
71. Woodward, S. and R. Freedman, The thermoregulatory effects of menopausal hot flashes on sleep. *Sleep*, 1994;**17**:497–501.
72. Shaver, J., E. Giblin, M. Lentz, et al., Sleep patterns and stability in perimenopausal women. *Sleep*, 1988;**11**:556–561.
73. Polo-Kantola, P., R. Erkkola, K. Irjala, et al., Climacteric symptoms and sleep quality. *Obstet Gynecol*, 1999;**94**:219–224.
74. Freedman, R.R. and T.A. Roehrs, Lack of sleep disturbances from menopausal hot flashes. *Fertil Steril*, 2004;**82**:138–144.
75. Montplaisir, J., J. Lorrain, D. Petit, and R. Denesle, Differential effects of two regimens of hormone replacement therapy on sleep in postmenopausal women. *Sleep Res*, 1997;**26**:119.
76. Scharf, M.B., M.D. McDannold, R. Stover, N. Zaretsky, and D.V. Berkowitz, Effects of estrogen replacement therapy on rates of cyclic alternating patterns and hot-flush events during sleep in postmenopausal women: a pilot study. *Clin Ther*, 1997;**19**:304–311.
77. Purdie, D.W., J.A.C. Empson, C. Crichton, and L. MacDonald, Hormone replacement therapy, sleep quality and psychological well-being. *Br J Obstet Gynecol*, 1995;**102**:735–739.
78. Polo-Kantola, P., R. Erkkola, K. Irjala, et al., Effect of short-term transdermal estrogen replacement therapy on sleep: a randomized, double-blind crossover trial in postmenopausal women. *Fertil Steril*, 1999;**71**:873–880.
79. Schiff, I., Q. Regestein, D. Tulchinsky, and K.J. Ryan, Effects of estrogens on sleep and psychological state of hypogonadal women. *JAMA*, 1979;**242**:2405–247.
80. Woodward, S., C.L. Arfken, D.W. Ditri, et al., Ambient temperature effects on sleep and mood in menopausal women. *Sleep*, 1999;**22**:S224–S225.
81. Kronenberg, F., Menopausal hot flashes: randomness or rhythmicity. *Chaos*, 1991;**1**:271–278.
82. Young, T., L. Finn, D. Austin, and A. Peterson, Menopausal status and sleep-disordered breathing in the Wisconsin Sleep Cohort Study. *Am J Respir Crit Care Med*, 2003;**167**:1181–1185.
83. Young, T., Analytic epidemiology studies of sleep disordered breathing—what explains the gender difference in sleep disordered breathing? *Sleep*, 1993;**16**:S1–S2.

84. Dancey, D.R., P.J. Hanly, C. Soong, B. Lee, and V. Hoffstein, Impact of menopause on the prevalence and severity of sleep apnea. *Chest*, 2001;**120**:151–155.
85. Bixler, E.O., A.N. Vgontzas, H.M. Lin, et al., Prevalence of sleep-disordered breathing in women: effects of gender. *Am J Respir Crit Care Med*, 2001;**163**:608–613.
86. Shahar, E., S. Redline, T. Young, et al., Hormone replacement therapy and sleep-disordered breathing. *Am J Respir Crit Care Med*, 2003;**167**:1186–1192.
87. Manber, R., T.F. Kuo, N. Cataldo, et al., The effects of hormone replacement therapy on sleep-disordered breathing in postmenopausal women: a pilot study. *Sleep*, 2003;**26**:163–18.
88. Wesstroem, J., J. Ulfberg, and S. Nilsson, Sleep apnea and hormone replacement therapy: a pilot study and a literature review. *Acta Obstet Gynecol Scand*, 2005;**84**:54–57.
89. Keefe, D.L., R. Watson, and F. Naftolin, Hormone replacement therapy may alleviate sleep apnea in menopausal women: a pilot study. *Menopause*, 1999;**6**:196–200.
90. Cistulli, P.A., D.J. Barnes, R.R. Grunstein, and C.E. Sullivan, Effect of short-term hormone replacement in the treatment of obstructive sleep apnoea in postmenopausal women. *Thorax*, 1994;**49**:699–702.
91. Thorpy, M., *The International Classification of Sleep Disorders*, revised. Rochester, MD: Davies Printing Company, 1997:223,227.
92. Belchetz, P.E., Drug therapy: hormonal treatment of postmenopausal women. *NEJM*, 1994;**330**:1062–1071.
93. Krystal, A.D., J. Ediger, W. Wohlgemuth, et al., Sleep in perimenopausal and postmenopausal women. *Sleep Med Rev*, 1998;**2**:243–253.
94. Shaver, J.L.F. and S.N. Zenk, Sleep disturbance in menopause. *J Women Health Gender Med*, 2000;**9**:109–118.
95. Anarte, M.T., J.L. Cuadros, and J. Herrera, Hormonal and psychological treatment: therapeutic alternative for menopausal women? *Maturitas*, 1998;**19**:203–213.
96. Rudolph, I., E. Palombo-Kinne, B. Kirsch, et al., Influence of a continuous combined HRT (2 mg estradiol valerate and 2 mg dienogest) on postmenopausal depression. *Climacteric*, 2004;**7**:301–311.
97. Thomson, J. and I. Oswald, Effect of oestrogen on the sleep, mood, and anxiety of monopausal women. *Br Med J*, 1977;**2**:1317–1319.
98. Tworoger, S.S., Y. Yasui, M.V. Vitiello, et al., Effects of a yearlong moderate-intensity exercise and a stretching intervention on sleep quality in postmenopausal women. *Sleep*, 2003;**26**:830–836.
99. Schiff, I., Q. Regestein, D. Tulchinsky, and K.J. Ryan, Effects of estrogens on sleep and psychological state of hypogonadal women. *JAMA*, 1979;**242**:2405–2407.
100. Antonijevic, I.A., G.K. Stalla, and A. Steiger, Modulation of the sleep electroencephalogram by estrogen replacement in postmenopausal women. *Am J Obstet Gynecol*, 2000;**182**:277–282.

5

Normal Reproductive and Endocrine Life Stages and Their Impact on Different Sleep Disorders

Rochelle Goldberg

INTRODUCTION

Sleep disorders affect people at all stages of life. For women, sleep complaints may vary by hormonal status as well as endocrine life stage. Certain broad perceptions about sleep and sleep disorders are supported by population surveys *(1)*. Elderly women seem to have more insomnia complaints, women develop sleep problems with pregnancy and menopause *(1–3)*, and sleep-disordered breathing (SDB) increases in the postmenopausal population *(4)*. Despite these perceptions, study findings may be inconclusive or contradictory. In earlier research, gender-specific aspects are not distinguished within the study populations. Other older studies of women do not identify hormonal condition or cycle status. Formal research in these areas and the differing effects of hormonal status on sleep disorders is a more recent focus of the sleep community. This chapter provides an overview of the current perceptions of the effects of life stage and reproductive status on sleep disorders in women from menarche through menopause.

MENARCHE AND THE MENSTRUAL CYCLE

Daytime sleepiness increases with puberty and adolescence. Carskadon *(5)* evaluated children for changes in nocturnal sleep and daytime sleepiness. Children were grouped by Tanner stage, and those in later stages *(3–5)* showed significant reductions in slow-wave sleep time as well as a greater degree of daytime sleepiness. The increase in daytime sleepiness was not the result of abbreviated sleep time at night, but was clearly associated with maturation to Tanner stage 3. The results support that children in early adolescence are sleepier than during their prepubertal state. This has important implications for learning and school performance. The additional sleep loss related to earlier school start times and other circadian issues may compromise daytime function at this life stage *(6)*.

In addition to the increase in sleepiness, puberty is also associated with changes in upper airway morphology that may potentiate SDB. In a study of 226 adoles-

From: *Current Clinical Neurology: Sleep Disorders in Women: A Guide to Practical Management*
Edited by: H. P. Attarian © Humana Press Inc., Totowa, NJ

cents *(7)*, ages 11–19 years, symptoms of SDB were identified using a questionnaire. Subjects underwent home polygraphy, including respiratory monitoring with actigraphy. Although postpubertal males showed a significantly higher frequency of snoring and increased respiratory disturbance index (RDI) compared with their prepubertal counterparts, females did not. Gender differences in RDI were normalized when adjusted for waist-to-hip index. The authors suggest that female sex hormones may exert a protective effect on the pathogenetic factors associated with SDB. This is also consistent with the potential role of hormone status in increased SDB in later life stages.

Sleep complaints in young adult women may vary across the menstrual cycle. The International Classification of Sleep Disorders identifies menstrual-related hypersomnia as a subset of recurrent hypersomnia *(8)*. It is characterized by complaints of sleepiness prior to or during menses. Symptoms are denied otherwise during the menstrual cycle. Despite these designations and broad anecdotal observations, there is little beyond case reports to support these diagnoses.

Estrogen is associated with reduced sleep latency and fewer awakenings and an overall increase in total sleep time (TST). Thus, during the luteal phase of the menstrual cycle, when estrogen is low, sleep fragmentation occurs. Progesterone acts as a γ-aminobutyric acid agonist, thereby favoring sleep stability. The hormone peaks during the midluteal phase and drops sharply at the onset of menses, with observed increases in arousals from sleep. Thus, normal hormonal changes through the menstrual cycle may favor sleep stability midcycle and sleep fragmentation during menses *(9)*. These changes may be associated with reports of insomnia or hypersomnolence. Although several studies show subjectively longer sleep durations, but more fragmented sleep premenstrually *(10–12)*, these results are not supported by other studies *(13,14)*.

In addition to the normal cyclical hormonal role in sleep complaints, premenstrual syndrome (PMS) and premenstrual dysphoric disorder (PMDD) are associated with a complaint of insomnia. Some earlier studies report more frequent sleep complaints in women with PMS symptoms *(15,16)*. Another study that included objective sleep parameters *(17)* and involved women with PMDD and a control group found similar changes in sleep. Significant differences were found across the cycle in sleep electroencephalogram (EEG) for the two groups. Other reports fail to identify differences in sleep characteristics despite subjective complaints *(18,19)*. In addition, a more recent study of healthy and depressed women suggests that the effect of oral contraceptives on sleep EEG may be different in these groups and may complicate conclusions in other studies if oral contraceptive use is not acknowledged *(20)*. Overall, studies in women with PMS/PMDD are inconsistent in their findings, with varied methodology and endpoints and small numbers of subjects making objective conclusions a challenge.

PREGNANCY

Sleep disturbance as a feature of normal pregnancy is well known. This association is illustrated in the widespread use of thalidomide as a sleep-conducive agent with subsequent findings of its teratogenicity. The International Classification of Sleep Disorders *(8)* includes pregnancy-associated sleep disorder as a subset of insomnia resulting from a medical condition. The features of the disorder include poor sleep quality that occurs especially in the third trimester. Symptoms resolve postpartum. Polysomnographic findings are consistent with subjective complaints including sleep fragmentation or extended sleep duration and reduced sleep latency on the multiple sleep latency test.

Hormonal and other physiological changes throughout pregnancy may contribute to other specific sleep problems. In addition, the effect of normal pregnancy on the incidence and prevalence of sleep disorders has been widely studied.

Insomnia

Insomnia is a common pregnancy-related sleep complaint. The frequency of nocturnal awakenings prior to and during each trimester of pregnancy was evaluated by both sleep diary and polysomnography *(21)*. The reasons for awakenings were identified, some of which had not been noted prior to the pregnancy. A 1.4-fold increase in awakenings during the first two trimesters and a 2-fold increase for the third trimester occurred compared to baseline. Most notable was the increase in nocturnal urination (51.4% of first-trimester awakenings and similar in third trimester). Other described sources of awakenings included nausea, fetal movement, joint pains, and general discomforts.

Sleep patterns and sleep disturbance were evaluated in a questionnaire study at four data points during pregnancy *(22)*. Each subject responded only once, so individual changes throughout pregnancy are not identified. As in the prior study, nighttime waking was a common finding. By the fourth-quarter measure (third trimester), 97.3% of women were waking at night. The frequency of nocturnal awakenings increased across the data points, as did the duration of awakenings. In addition, third-trimester women tended to wake earlier in the morning than was reported at earlier points. The complaint of insomnia, expressed as difficulty falling asleep, staying asleep, and waking too early, was common. Restless sleep occurred at most data points, with the highest occurrence (91.9%) in the last quarter. A full one-third of the women identified themselves as having a sleep problem.

Similar findings were shown for 100 patients questioned about their sleep during late third-trimester pregnancy *(2)*. Altered sleep (referenced by nocturnal awakenings from heartburn, discomfort, and cramps) was reported in 68%, most commonly in the third trimester. Longer sleep times were described in 19%. Insomnia complaints were evidenced by sedative hypnotic use in 12 patients, all of whom denied use of sleep agents prior to the pregnancy.

Restless Legs Syndrome

Restless legs syndrome (RLS) is a clinical diagnosis characterized by an unpleasant sensation in the lower extremities accompanied by an irresistible urge to move the legs. Symptoms typically occur in sedentary situations and tend to be associated with difficulty initiating sleep *(23)*. The prevalence in the general population ranges from 2 to 5% *(24)* and up to 20% in the elderly *(25)*. Although most studies in pregnancy indicate increased RLS complaints, frequencies vary. The variability, in part, relates to the lack of standardization of diagnostic methodology as well as symptom frequency (weekly vs monthly).

Using the four standard criteria, Manconi and Ferini-Strambi *(26)* found a prevalence of 27% of RLS in an interview study of 606 pregnant women. Preexisting RLS occurred in 10% of all women, whereas 17% noted onset of RLS during pregnancy with postpartum resolution of symptoms. Although the symptoms were not severe, they contributed to increased sleep latency and decreased TST *(27)*. A lower prevalence (19.9%) was identified in a national questionnaire study in Japan that included 16,528 subjects *(28)*. The difference in these studies may well result from the less rigorous, nonstandard style of questioning in the latter study. The Japanese group found an association of sleep complaints associated with RLS with current smoking, use of alcohol or medication for sleep, and longer duration of pregnancy. Both RLS and periodic limb movement disorder occurred in 22% of Mindell's study subjects and were associated with sleep onset and maintenance complaints *(22)*.

The epidemiological study by Marconi *(27)* also evaluated the association of iron deficiency and RLS. Although mild, the decreases in plasma iron and hemoglobin were significant. In another study, Lee *(29)* explored the relationship of serum ferritin and folate. Patients with RLS (overall prevalence 23%) had low ferritin and folate at preconception and throughout pregnancy. These findings are consistent with the role of iron metabolism in RLS pathogenesis *(30)*. The substantially greater iron and folate requirements during pregnancy suggest a possible mechanism for the increase of RLS in pregnancy.

Conclusions regarding RLS in pregnancy include an increased risk (two to three times higher than in nonpregnant women). For women with preexisting RLS, symptoms worsen during pregnancy. The third trimester is the time of greatest symptom frequency and severity. Pregnancy-related RLS (which resolves postpartum) is likely to recur with future pregnancies. An association of relative iron and folate deficiency may underlie the increased risk for RLS in pregnancy.

Sleep-Disordered Breathing

The hormonal and physiological changes occurring during pregnancy affecting upper airway function and respiration have the potential to exacerbate SDB. However, other changes during pregnancy may be seen to be protective. These are summarized in Table 1 *(31)*.

Findings in various studies of SDB in pregnancy are mixed in their conclusions. Schutte *(32)* noted third-trimester snoring in 27% of normal pregnant women. In another study of self-reported snoring *(33)*, 14% of women in their second or third trimesters snored compared to 4% of control nonpregnant premenopausal women ($p < 0.05$). Self-reported apnea was similar between these groups. There were no differences in daytime sleepiness or mean birthweight and Apgar scores for infants born of snoring mothers. Furthermore, snoring prevalence decreased by 3 months postpartum, returning to prepregnancy levels *(34)*. In contrast, Franklin et al. *(35)*

Table 1
Changes During Pregnancy That May Influence
the Development of Sleep-Disordered Breathing

Changes that increase risk of sleep apnea	Changes that decrease risk of sleep apnea
Gestational weight gain	Increased minute ventilation
Nasopharyngeal edema	Preference for lateral sleep posture
Decreased functional reserve capacity	Decreased REM sleep time
Increased arousals from sleep	

REM, rapid eye movement. (From ref. *31.*)

found higher rates of gestational hypertension, pre-eclampsia, and small-for-gestational-age (SGA) infants in habitual snorers than in nonsnorers. In obese pregnant women compared with nonobese pregnant controls, a significantly higher apnea–hypopnea index (AHI) was found (1.7 vs 0.2 events per hour of sleep; $p < 0.05$) *(36)* at 12 weeks gestation. Increases in snoring and AHI in the obese group occurred at 30 weeks gestation. Gestation length and fetal outcomes (birthweights) were comparable between groups. One obese mother had an AHI of more than 10 events per hour of sleep on the second study and developed pre-eclampsia. Respiratory events normalized in this woman when measured 6 months postpartum. In a study of multiple pregnancies *(37)*, a single polysomnogram conducted at 30–36 weeks gestation found no evidence of obstructive sleep apnea (OSA), although episodes of increased airway resistance were found in four subjects.

Sleep-Disordered Breathing and Positive Airway Pressure

In two case reports *(38,39)* of sleep apnea during pregnancy, both mothers continued to have severe OSA postpartum, although neither study had prepregnancy sleep data. Both mothers were successfully treated with nasal continuous positive airway pressure (nCPAP) for the duration of the pregnancy. Both had induced labor, one with a normal infant, and the other with a SGA infant. In contrast, in a study of 11 women with pre-eclampsia, all subjects had evidence of increased upper airway resistance. Treatment with an auto-titrating positive airway pressure unit resulted in reversal of flow limitation and prevented the nocturnal blood pressure increments noted previously *(40)*.

Snoring and sleep apnea symptoms should be acknowledged in pregnancy. Obese women most likely have an increased risk for the development of sleep apnea during pregnancy. SDB may predispose to pre-eclampsia and should be considered in patients presenting with this condition. Treatment with positive airway pressure is a viable and effective option and may reduce fetal risk.

MENOPAUSE

Insomnia

Increased sleep disturbance is frequently observed during menopause. Sleep fragmentation and nonrestorative sleep are common complaints. The role of hormonal changes is naturally questioned. Vasomotor symptoms (flashes and sweating) are observed in 68–85% of women *(3,41)* and may often be reported in conjunction with nocturnal awakenings. Sleep disturbance may also occur in the absence of these features.

Young et al. *(42)* evaluated subjective and objective sleep quality in 589 postmenopausal women. Subjective sleep complaints were common and significantly more serious than in premenopausal controls. Perimenopausal and postmenopausal women had twice the odds of reporting sleep dissatisfaction. In the subset of women with vasomotor complaints, there was a significant difference in reports of sleep dissatisfaction and sleep-related hot flashes. The objective sleep findings, however, did not support the subject complaints. By polysomnography, postmenopausal women had better sleep quality with higher TST, better sleep efficiency, and greater percentage of slow-wave sleep. In a subgroup with sleep apnea with increased severity of respiratory events, both pre- and postmenopausal women had compromised sleep architecture. However, sleep fragmentation was more prominent in the premenopausal subjects at all levels. Similarly, hormone replacement therapy (HRT) was not found to have favorable effects on objective measures of sleep. In fact, sleep architecture measures, including sleep onset, sleep efficiency, and duration and depth of sleep, were all better in the postmenopausal group without HRT.

Subjective sleep complaints however, may respond more favorably to HRT *(43)*. Subjects taking HRT reported improvement in falling asleep, less restlessness, and fewer nocturnal awakenings. They were also less tired during the day. Although improvements were most striking in those with severe vasomotor symptoms, insomnia complaints were also favorably affected by HRT in those without vasomotor symptoms.

Although study findings on this topic are varied, the differences may relate to the dichotomy of subjective and objective sleep features. Treatment considerations for insomnia in the postmenopausal woman must therefore address goals of subjective sleep response, while weighing the risk of treatment against more equivocal objective findings.

Restless Legs Syndrome in Menopause and Beyond

Berger et al. *(44)* found an overall increased prevalence of RLS with age using standard International Restless Legs Syndrome Study Group (IRLSSG) criteria *(23)*. The study included men and women and did not identify hormonal status for the women subjects. However, the increase in RLS for women 50–59 years old (19.4%) showed a more significant change compared to the younger groups (approx 10% for women 30–39 and 40–49 years old). This empirically suggests that RLS may be a more common feature in peri- and postmenopausal women. There was no attempt to determine incidence within the groups. A Swedish study *(45)* of RLS in women aged 18–64 years (mean age 45 years) found a prevalence of 11.4% (16 women), 14 of whom were older than 34 years. Hormonal status was not identified.

The prevalence in elderly women is noteworthy, however, reported in 27% of women older than 65 years in a National Sleep Foundation poll *(1)*. Patients with late-onset (>45 years old—could most of these women be postmenopausal?) RLS may have a more rapid course than the often-described waxing and waning characteristics reported in younger age groups *(46)*. Another study *(47)*, using IRLSSG criteria, found a similar frequency of RLS in elderly women. An overall 13.7% prevalence was identified for women older than 65 years. Percentages were similar for the three age groups (65–69, 70–74, and ≥75 years).

These studies are consistent in showing an increased prevalence of RLS with age in women. Further increases in the perimenopausal age subgroup in one of the studies may suggest hormonal link. Differences in clinical behavior of RLS in late-onset groups are also suggestive.

Sleep-Disordered Breathing

A number of protective factors have been proposed to explain the observed differences in sleep apnea prevalence in men and women. Physiological changes, particularly relating to sex hormones coincident with menopause, may help explain observed differences in the prevalence of SDB in postmenopausal women.

Premenopausal women, in contrast to men, have gynecoid rather than android fat distribution, less fat deposition in the neck *(48)*, stiffer upper airway *(49)*, more active genioglossal electromyograms *(50)*, and better immediate load compensation favoring pharyngeal patency *(51)*. The role of progesterone as a respiratory stimulant and the decreased levels of this hormone with menopause have been implicated in the increased prevalence of sleep apnea in postmenopausal women.

Popovic and White *(52)* looked at upper airway muscle activity, represented by genioglossus muscle activity (EMG_{gg}) in pre- and postmenopausal women (Fig. 1). Progesterone levels were significantly different between three groups (premenopausal women in the follicular phase, luteal phase, and postmenopausal women). Significantly reduced peak phasic EMG_{gg} was found between the luteal phase and postmenopausal women. The expiratory tonic EMG_{gg} was highest in the luteal phase and significantly lower in the postmenopausal women. The observed differences did not, however, correspond to measurable changes in upper airway resistance. The authors found a positive correlation between inspiratory peak phasic EMG_{gg} and blood progesterone levels. Similarly, increases in EMG_{gg} occurred in the postmenopausal women following a 2-week course of HRT.

Bixler et al.'s *(53)* findings show an increase in sleep apnea with menopause. Women were grouped as premenopausal, postmenopausal without HRT, and postmenopausal with HRT. The age-specific prevalence of SDB was 0.7% in the 20- to 44-year age group, 1.1% in the 45- to 64-year age group, and 3.1% in those older than 65 years. The peak prevalence occurred in the 64- to 69-year age group. The body mass index (BMI)-specific prevalence for symptomatic patients with AHI of more than 10 events per hour of sleep was 0.4% vs 4.8% for nonobese and obese, respectively ($p = 0.0001$). Menopausal status favored SDB (0.6% vs 1.9% in pre- and postmenopausal women; $p = 0.04$), whereas HRT subjects had a prevalence similar to that of premenopausal subjects (0.5% vs 0.6%). Obesity may facilitate SDB in this group as well. All of the premenopausal and postmenopausal HRT

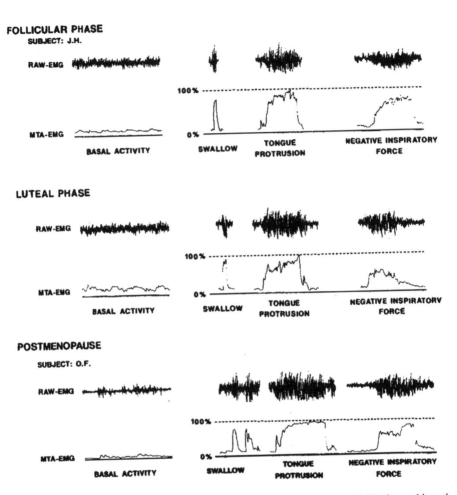

Fig. 1. Genioglossal electromyography in premenopausal women in follicular and luteal phases of cycle and postmenopausal women. (From ref. *52.*)

subjects with SDB were obese, and only 49.4% of postmenopausal without HRT were obese.

In a study of obese subjects, Resta et al. *(54)* found significant differences in anthropometric parameters and sleep apnea in pre- and postmenopausal women. Neck circumference, percentage of predicted normal neck circumference, waist-to-hip ratio, RDI, and prevalence of SDB were higher ($p < 0.001$ for each parameter). In the postmenopausal group, the BMI (40.5 vs 44.5 kg/m^2) was significant as well ($p < 0.01$).

Millman et al. *(55)* found an association of SDB and body fat distribution. Unlike the previous studies, there were no group differences in AHI, S$_a$O$_2$, BMI, or skinfold and circumference measures in the 12 premenopausal and 13 postmenopausal women. The women with SDB had higher BMIs and body fat (assessed by skinfold sum) than the general population. The AHI corresponded best with the sum of subscapular and triceps skinfolds.

Menopause as an independent risk factor for SDB was assessed in a study by Young et al. *(56)* (Fig. 2). SDB prevalence was higher across menopausal groups (pre- compared with peri-, peri-/post-, and postmenopause). This difference persisted when controlled for age and BMI. There were no further increases in SDB for subjects beyond 5 years of menopause, suggesting a latent period for the development of the disorder. In this study, a small protective effect of HRT was noted. Dancy et al. *(4)* also found an increase in SDB in the postmenopausal population that persisted after controlling for BMI and neck circumference, again suggesting a risk inherent in the menopausal state.

Despite observed differences in the above studies, studies of HRT on upper airway responsiveness have failed to identify a mechanism. Polo-Kantola et al. *(57)* found an increase in upper airway resistance in postmenopausal subjects. Unopposed estrogen replacement therapy (ERT) in a 3-month placebo-controlled design had a small effect on those subjects' sleep apnea, although this was a small percentage of the study population. The majority of subjects had increased upper airway resistance and did not show a response to ERT alone. Cistulli et al. *(58)* found no overall improvement in the clinical severity of SDB in a group of women with moderately severe sleep apnea when given HRT. There was, however, a small improvement in the rapid eye-movement apnea index with HRT. Women underwent short-term HRT (50 days) with estrogen alone or an estrogen/progesterone combination. In contrast, Pickett et al.'s *(59)* population showed a decrease in respiratory events following a 1-week crossover study of combined HRT vs placebo. These subjects did not have SDB; the response showed a decrease in baseline episodes of 15 per night per subject, reduced to 3 per night per subject. There were no observable differences in objective sleep quality or subjective reports.

These studies suggest an increased risk of OSA during the transition to menopause. The risk appears to be independent of BMI, neck circumference, and age. The role of HRT in modifying upper airway mechanics, SDB episodes, and related sleep characteristics is unclear.

CONCLUSION

Women describe sleep complaints and sleep disorders at all ages. Differences in hormonal state or endocrine life stage may be seen to modify the risk for specific sleep problems. Study results for population prevalence, risks, and mechanisms of common sleep disorders are often mixed or inconclusive. However, more exacting study designs are now beginning to better define these populations. Studies that respect not only gender and age, but differences in cyclical hormonal effects and those hormonal and demographic changes associated with pregnancy and menopause should ultimately lead to a better understanding of mechanisms and clinical risks.

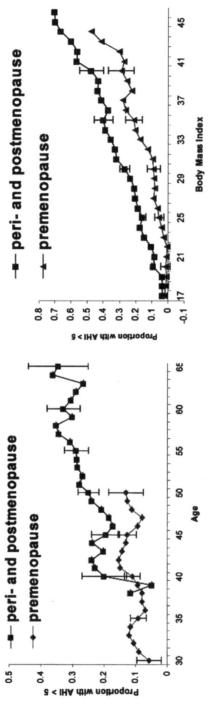

Fig. 2. Prevalence of SDB indicated by AHI >5 for premenopausal women and perimenopausal women plus postmenopausal women by age (left) and by body mass index (BMI) (right). (From ref. 56.)

REFERENCES

1. National Sleep Foundation. Sleep in America Poll 2002. Accessed at www.sleepfoundation.org, 2002 Sleep in American Poll.
2. Schweiger, M.S., Sleep disturbance in pregnancy: a subjective survey. *Am J Obstet Gynecol*, 1972;**114**(7);879–882.
3. Anderson, E., S. Hamburger, J.H. Liu, and R.W. Rebar, Characteristics of menopausal women seeking assistance. *Am J Obstet Gynecol*, 1987;**156**:428–433.
4. Dancy, D.R., P.J. Hanly, C. Soong, B. Lee, and V. Hoffstein, Impact of menopause on the prevalence and severity of sleep apnea. *Chest*, 2001;**120**(1):151–155.
5. Carskadon, M.A., K. Harvey, P.Duke, T.F. Anders, I.F. Litt, and W.C. Dement, Pubertal changes in daytime sleepiness. *Sleep*, 1980;**2**(4):453–460.
6. Dexter, D., J. Bijwadia, D. Schilling, and G. Applebaugh, Sleep, sleepiness and school start times: a preliminary study. *WMJ*, 2003;**102**(1):44–46.
7. Fuentes-Pradera, M.A., A. Sanchez-Armengol, F. Capote-Gil, et al., Effects of sex on sleep-disordered breathing in adolescents. *Eur Respir J*, 2004;**23**:250–254.
8. *International Classification of Sleep Disorders* (2nd ed.). Westchester IL: American Academy of Sleep Medicine, 2005.
9. Driver, H.S., D.J. Dijk, E. Werth, K. Biedermann, and A. Borbely, Sleep and the sleep EEG across the menstrual cycle in young healthy women. *J Clin Endocrinol Metab*, 1996;**81**:728–735.
10. Lee, K.A., J.F. Shaver, E.C. Giblin, and N.F. Woods, Sleep patterns related to menstrual cycle phase and premenstrual affective syndrome. *Sleep*, 1990;**13**(5):403–409.
11. Patkai, P., G. Johannson, and B. Post, Mood, alertness and sympathetic-adrenal medullary activity during the menstrual cycle. *Psychosom Med*, 1974;**36**:503–512.
12. Ishizuka, Y., A. Usui, K. Shirasishi, et al., A subjective evaluation of sleep during the menstrual cycle. *Sleep Res*, 1989;**18**:421.
13. Ho, A., Sex hormones and the sleep of women. *Sleep Res*, 1972;**1**:184.
14. Williams, D.L., and A.W. MacLean, Relationship between the menstrual cycle and the sleep of young women. *Sleep Res*, 1980;**9**:129.
15. Hartmann, E., Dreaming sleep (the D-state) and the menstrual cycle. *J Nerv Ment Dis*, 1966;**143**:406–416.
16. Sheldrake, P. and M. Cormack, Variations in menstrual cycle symptom reporting. *J Psychosom Res*, 1976;**20**:169–177.
17. Parry, B.L., N. Mostofi, B. LeVeau, et al., Sleep EEG studies during early and late partial sleep deprivation in premenstrual dysphoric disorder and normal controls. *Psych Res*, 1999;**85**:127–143.
18. Mauri, M., R.L. Reid, and A.W. Maclean, Sleep in the premenstrual phase: a self report study of PMS patients and normal controls. *Acta Psychiatr Scand*, 1988;**78**:82–86.
19. Chuong, C.J., S.R. Kim, O. Taskin, and I. Karacan, Sleep pattern changes in menstrual cycles of women with premenstrual syndrome: a preliminary study. *Am J Obstet Gynecol Online*, 1997;177.
20. Burdick, R.S., R. Hoffman, and R. Armitage, Short note: oral contraceptives and sleep in healthy and depressed women. *Sleep*, 2002;**25**(3):347–349.
21. Baratte-Beebe, K.R. and K. Lee, Sources of midsleep awakenings in childbearing women. *Clin Nurs Res*, 1999;**8**(4):386–397.
22. Mindell, J.A. and B.J. Jacobson, Sleep disturbances during pregnancy. *J Obstet, Gynecol, Neonatal Nurs*, 2000;**29**(6):590–597.
23. Hening, W., R. Allen, C. Earley, C. Kushida, D. Picchietti, and M. Silber, The treatment of restless legs syndrome and periodic limb movement disorder. *Sleep*, 1999;**22**(7):970–999.
24. Ekbom, K.A., Restless legs. In: *Handbook of Clinical Neurology* (P.J. Vinken and G.W. Bruyn, eds.). Amsterdam: North Holland Publishing Company 1970:311–320.
25. Coleman, R.M., L.E. Miles, C.C. Guilleminault, V.P. Zarcone, J. van den Hoed, and W.C. Dement, Sleep-wake disorders in the elderly: polysomnographic analysis. *J Am Geriatr Soc*, 1981;**29**:289–296.
26. Manconi, M. and L. Ferini-Strambi, Restless legs syndrome among pregnant women. *Sleep*, 2004;**27**(2):250.

27. Manconi, M., V.,Govoni, E. Cesnik, et al., Epidemiology of the restless legs syndrome in a population of 606 pregnant women. *Sleep*, 2003;**26**:A330.
28. Suzuki, K., T. Ohida, T. Sone, et al., The prevalence of restless legs syndrome among pregnant women in Japan and the relationship between restless legs syndrome and sleep problems. *Sleep*, 2003;**26**(6):673–677.
29. Lee, K.A., M.E. Zaffke, and K. Baratte-Beebe, Restless legs syndrome and sleep disturbance during pregnancy: the role of folate and iron. *J Wom Health Gender-Based Med*, 2001;**10**(1):335–341.
30. Early, C.J., J.R. Connor, J.L. Beard, E.A. Malecki, D.K. Epstein, and R.P. Allen, Abnormalities in CSF concentrations of ferritin and transferring in restless legs syndrome. *Neurology*, 2000;**54**:1698.
31. Pien, G.W. and R.J. Schwabe, Sleep disorders during pregnancy. *Sleep*, 2004;**27**(7):1405–1417.
32. Schutte,S., A. Del Conte, K. Doghramji, et al., Snoring during pregnancy and its impact on fetal outcome. *Sleep Res*, 1994;**24**:199.
33. Loube, D.I., S. Poceta, M.C. Morales, M.D. Peacock, and M.M. Mitler, Self-reported snoring in pregnancy: association with fetal outcome. *Chest*, 1996;**109**:885–889.
34. Hedman, C., T. Pohjasvaara, U.Tolonen, et al., Effects of pregnancy on mother's sleep. *Sleep Med*, 2002;**3**:37–42.
35. Franklin, K.A., P.A. Holmgren, F. Jonsson, et al., Snoring, pregnancy-induced hypertension, and growth retardation of the fetus. *Chest*, 2000;**117**:137–141.
36. Maasilta, P., A. Bachour, K. Teramo, O. Polo, and L.A. Laitinen, Sleep-related disordered breathing during pregnancy in obese women. *Chest*, 2001;**120**:1448–1454.
37. Nikkola, E., U. Ekblad, K. Ekholm, H. Mikola, and O. Polo, Sleep in multiple pregnancy: breathing patterns, oxygenation and periodic leg movements. *Am J Obstet Gynecol*, 1996;**174**:1622–1625.
38. Charbonneau, M., T. Falcone, M. Cosio, R.D. Levy, Obstructive sleep apnea during pregnancy: therapy and implications for fetal health. *Am Rev Respir Dis*, 1991;**144**:461–463.
39. Kowall, J., G. Clark, G. Nino-Murcia, and N. Powell, Precipitation of obstructive sleep apnea during pregnancy. *Obstet Gynecol*, 1989;**74**:453–455.
40. Edwards, N., D.M. Blyton, T. Krjavaninen, G.J. Kesby, and C.E. Sullivan, Nasal continuous positive airway pressure reduces sleep-induced blood pressure increments in preeclampsia. *Am J Respir Crit Care Med*, 2000;**162**:252–257.
41. Brincat, M. and J.W.W. Studd, Menopause: a multisystem disease. *Ballieres Clin Obstet Gynaecol*, 1988;**2**:289–316.
42. Young, T., D. Rabago, A. Zgierska, D. Austin, and L. Finn, Objective and subjective sleep quality in premenopausal, perimenopausal and postmenopausal women: the Wisconsin Sleep Cohort Study. *Sleep*, 2003;**26**(6):667–672.
43. Anderer, P., H.V. Semlistch, B. Saletu, et al., Effects of hormone replacement therapy on perceptual and cognitive event-related potentials in menopausal insomnia. *Pyschoneuroendocrinology*, 2003;**28**:419–445.
44. Berger, K., J. Luedemann, C. Trenkwalder, U. John, and C. Kessler, Sex and the risk of restless legs syndrome in the general population. *Arch Intern Med*, 2004;**164**:196–202.
45. Ulfberg, J., B. Nystrom, N. Carter, and C. Edling, Restless legs syndrome among working-aged women. *Eur Neurol*, 2001;**46**:17–19.
46. Allen, R.P. and C.J. Earley, Defining the phenotype of the restless legs syndrome using age of symptom onset. *Sleep Med*, 2000;**1**:11–19.
47. Rothdack, A.J., C. Trenkwalder, J. Haberstock, U. Keil, and K. Berger, Prevalence and risk factors of RLS in an elderly population: the MEMO study. *Neurology*, 2000;**54**:1064–1068.
48. Ledoux, M., J. Lambert, B.A. Reeder, and J.P. Depres, Canadian Heart Health Surveys Research Group. Correlation between cardiovascular risk factors and simple anthropometric measures. *Can Med Assoc J*, 1997;**157**(1 Suppl):S46–S53.
49. Rubinstein, I., V. Hoffstein, and T.D. Bradley, Lung volume-related changes in the pharyngeal area of obese females with and without obstructive sleep apnea. *Eur Respir J*, 1989;**2**:344–351.
50. Popovic, R.M. and D.P. White, Influence of gender on waking genioglossal electromyogram and upper airway resistance. *Am J Respir Crit Care Med*, 1995;**152**:725–731.

51. Rowley, J.A., X. Zhou, I. Vergine, et al., Influence of gender on upper airway mechanics: upper airway resistance on P_{crit}. *J Appl Physiol*, 2001;**91**(5):2248–2254.
52. Popovic, R.M. and D.P. White, Upper airway muscle activity in normal women: influence of hormonal status. *J Appl Physiol*, 1998;**84**(3):1055–1062.
53. Bixler, E.O., A.N. Vgontzas, H. Lin, et al. Prevalence of sleep-disordered breathing in women: effects of gender. *Am J Respir Crit Care Med*, 2001;**163**:608–613.
54. Resta, O., G. Caratozzolo, N. Pannacciulli, et al., Gender, age and menopause effects on the prevalence and the characteristics of obstructive sleep apnea in obesity. *Eur J Clin Invest*, 2003;**33**(12):1084–1089.
55. Millman, R.P., C.C. Carlisle, S.T. McGarvey, S.E. Eveloff, and P.D. Levinson, Body fat distribution and sleep apnea severity in women. *Chest*, 1995;**107**:362–366.
56. Young, T., L. Finn, D. Austin, and A. Peterson, Menopausal status and sleep-disordered breathing in the Wisconsin Sleep Cohort Study. *Am J Respir Crit Care Med*, 2003;**167**:1181–1185.
57. Polo-Kantola, P., E. Rauhala, H. Helenius, R. Erkkola, K. Irjala, and O. Polo, Breathing during sleep in menopause: a randomized, controlled, crossover trial with estrogen therapy. *Obstet Gynecol*, 2003;**102**:68–75.
58. Cistulli, P.A., D.J. Barnes, R.R. Grunstein, and C.E. Sullivan, Effect of short term hormone replacement in the treatment of obstructive sleep apnoea in postmenopausal women. *Thorax*, 1994;**49**:699–702.
59. Pickett, C.K., J.G. Regensteiner, W.D. Woodard, D.D. Hagerman, J.V. Weil, and L.G. Moore, Progestin and estrogen reduce sleep-disordered breathing in postmenopausal women. *J Appl Physiol*, 1989;**66**(4):1656–1661.

II Adolescents

6

Delayed Sleep Phase Syndrome in Adolescents

John Garcia

INTRODUCTION

To some degree, delayed sleep phase syndrome (DSPS) is present in most, if not all adolescents. It is thought to be a normal biological developmental phase. Thorpy et al. *(1)* first described its common presence in teenagers in 1988, and, in 1993, Carskadon et al. *(2)* first linked it to the biological process of puberty. The relationship was more significant in girls than in boys.

The International Classification of Sleep Disorders describes DSPS as a disorder in which the major sleep episode is delayed in relation to the desired clock time, resulting in complaints of sleep-onset insomnia and/or difficulty in awakening at the desired time. Symptoms must be present for at least 1 month, and other explanations to account for excessive daytime sleepiness (EDS) must be excluded *(3)*. This chapter briefly summarizes the basic science regarding circadian rhythm disorders. I review clinical research regarding DSPS as well as available interventions. Treatment options and future directions are also discussed.

THE BASIC SCIENCE SURROUNDING CIRCADIAN RHYTHM CONTROL

Light is the most powerful entraining agent of the circadian system. Retinal cells mediate the effects of light to the suprachiasmatic nucleus (SCN) in the hypothalamus through the chemical mediator melanopsin. Activated by melanopsin, the SCN increases its uptake of glucose, leading to the expression of genes, including *per*, *clock*, and *tim*. Cytochromes in the cells of the SCN also play a role in the expression of *per*, *clock*, and *tim*. Oscillations generated by rhythms in gene and protein expression create long feedback loops (Fig.1). These long feedback loops ultimately regulate the release of hormones, such as melatonin in the pineal gland, and numerous peripheral circadian rhythms of the body, including thyroid-stimulating hormone release, cortisol secretion, and core body temperature control *(4)*.

The above process creates the oscillating sleep propensity or circadian rhythm known as process C. The two-process model proposed by Borbely in 1982 describes

From: *Current Clinical Neurology: Sleep Disorders in Women: A Guide to Practical Management*
Edited by: H. P. Attarian © Humana Press Inc., Totowa, NJ

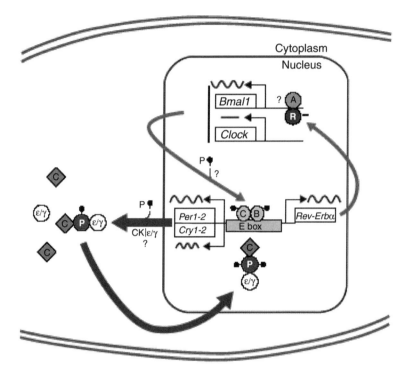

Fig. 1. Mammalian circadian clockwork model.

a balanced model whereby process C is affected by the sleep homeostasis process also known as process S *(5)*. Process S describes how sleep propensity increases as duration of wakefulness accumulates and dissipates during sleep (Fig. 2). The interaction of processes S and C leads to the manifest sleep–wake cycle.

CLINICAL RESEARCH

Teens have an increased incidence of circadian rhythm disorders, particularly DSPS. The incidence of DSPS in teens is 7% *(6)*, 10 times that found in middle-aged adults *(7)*. Contrary to popular belief, a physiological imperative to delayed sleep is seen in teens in general but, more strikingly, in teens with DSPS, who have delayed release of melatonin *(8)*. This biological imperative contradicts the conventional wisdom that rationalizes teen sleep patterns as being a consequence of social pressures.

Recent research has also revealed alterations in the sleep homeostasis process in teens with DSPS. In one study, patients with DSPS did not exhibit recovery sleep during the subjective day despite sleep deprivation. The authors suggest, therefore, that DSPS may involve problems related to the homeostatic regulation of sleep after sleep deprivation *(9)*.

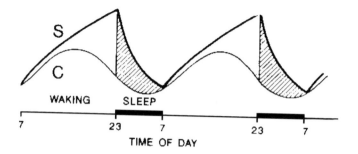

Fig. 2. A two-process model of sleep regulation showing that DSPS may involve problems related to the homeostatic regulation of sleep.

CASE HISTORY

Erica is a 15-year-old female who presents with a several-year history of difficulty falling asleep. Her parents complain that they have difficulty waking her in the morning. In fact, over the past 5 months she has missed 35 days of school because her parents were physically unable to get her out of bed. Truancy officers are threatening remedial action. A 24-hour history reveals that although she goes to bed at 11 PM, she often does not fall asleep until between 1 and 4 AM (Fig. 3). She denies feeling anxious while lying in bed. She does not have leg restlessness, nor does she complain of pain anywhere in her body preventing sleep onset. Once asleep, she remains so without arousals. Her parents begin calling her at 7 AM. After several calls they will try and rouse her from bed physically. Often they are unable to awaken her. On weekends, holidays, and days she does not go to school, she awakens between noon and 2 PM. During summer vacation when she sleeps ad lib, she does not complain of EDS. During the school year she shares that most days she falls asleep in her first three classes.

TREATMENT

Treatment of circadian rhythm disorders falls into three categories: phototherapy, chronotherapy, and pharmacotherapy. The motivation of the teen should be assessed. Regular use of the interventions discussed here requires discipline. The teen must be involved in the implementation. If resistance is encountered, searching for a cause such as depression should be pursued. In fact, if depression is present, treating it simultaneously is necessary *(10)*.

Phototherapy involves increasing morning light and decreasing evening light *(11)*. In North America, increasing morning light may mean using a "light box." It is important to purchase a light box that delivers 10,000 lux *(12,13)*. The ultraviolet light filter should be in place. Patients may also benefit from avoidance of exposure to bright light in the evening *(14)*.

Chronotherapy involves the timing of wakefulness and sleep to minimize EDS. A general review of sleep hygiene is recommended. Specifically, wake time on the

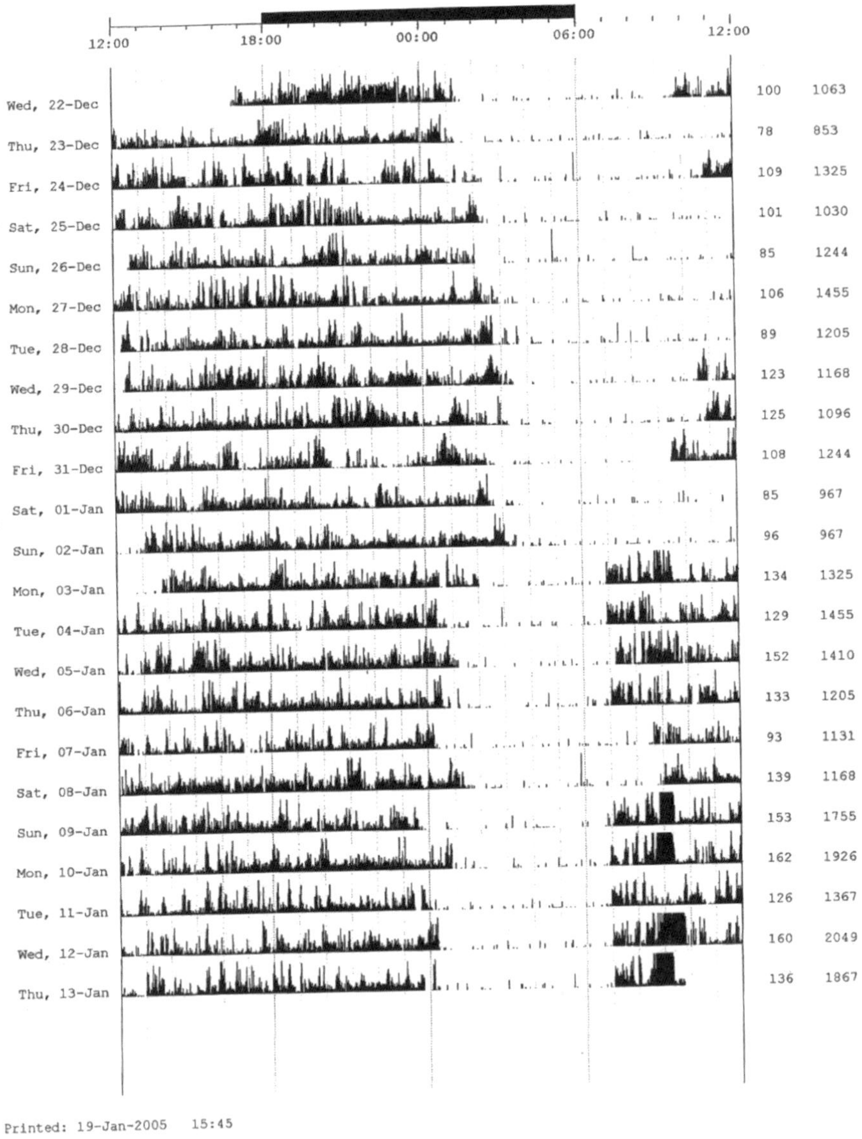

Fig. 3. Actigraphy showing the subject's delayed sleep phase.

weekends should not be more than 2 hours later than wake time during the weekdays. Sometimes daytime napping can be included as long as it does not further delay the sleep-onset time.

The physician can act as an advocate for teens. Standard high school early morning start times are not in alignment with the physiological sleep–wake patterns of teens in general and are grossly incompatible and may be academically devastating for teens with DSPS. Writing a letter advocating a 9 AM or later school start time is certainly not unreasonable.

Some physicians recommend phase advancement, during which the wake and bedtimes are 15 minutes earlier each day until the target wake time is achieved *(15)*. Other physicians promote phase delay *(16,17)*. Progressive phase delay involves delaying the bedtime and wake time 2–3 hours each day until the target sleep-onset and wake times are achieved. Phase delay is generally reserved for more severely affected DSPS patients.

Pharmacotherapy is limited to sedative/hypnotics and melatonin. Sedative/hypnotics may be used in addition to phototherapy and chronotherapy. Many teens with DSPS have sleep-onset insomnia despite being significantly sleep deprived. A short-acting sedative/hypnotic such as zaleplon, a nonbenzodiazepine hypnotic agent, may be prescribed for several weeks *(18)*. The short duration of action of zaleplon decreases the likelihood of morning lethargy.

Several studies have shown that melatonin advances the sleep phase of patients with DSPS *(19,20)*. In early studies, 5 mg of melatonin were given 5 hours before the mean group sleep-onset time. The majority of patients reported a small advance in sleep phase *(21)*. Recent studies in blind individuals with circadian rhythm disorders have revealed that small doses (0.5 mg) of melatonin were effective *(22,23)*. It remains to be seen whether similar low-dose therapy could be effective in the treatment of DSPS. The National Sleep Foundation has warned against using melatonin in patients with immune disorders and lymphoproliferative disorders and patients who take corticosteroids or other immunosuppressants *(3)*. The use of melatonin in children remains controversial because its effects in the developing brain and body are not known. Melatonin is not approved by the US Food and Drug Administration *(24)*.

It must be admitted that many teens are not successful in the implementation of the interventions described here. Because there is known heterogeneity of genetic mutations manifesting as advanced sleep phase syndrome *(25)*, it is reasonable to assume that genetic variability will be found in DSPS. Furthermore, it is likely that some mutations are more amenable to treatment than others. Rather than blaming the patient, this should lead the physician to recommend adaptation of the external environment. One strategy is the integration of school officials and truancy officers in the creation of a plan that helps the teen to graduate. This may mean advocating for evening classes with credits that apply to graduation.

FUTURE DIRECTIONS

Challenges for future research include determining the degree of contribution of homeostatic vs circadian processes in children with DSPS. Carskadon is currently studying the homeostatic contribution to DSPS by a method she calls forced desynchrony *(26)*, which imposes a 20-hour day on individuals involved in the study for 2 weeks. The hypothesis is that the homeostatic process will be revealed as the available sleep time is shifted away from the circadian phase. The field also needs to improve the objective verification of this diagnosis instead of relying only on self-report information. This could best be done using actigraphy. Guidelines for the clinical use of actigraphy in the evaluation of circadian rhythm disorders, including DSPS, are available *(27)*. Finally, conducting treatment research aimed at determining efficacy, effectiveness, and mechanism or mechanisms of action is necessary *(14)*. The field is eagerly awaiting an effective chronobiotic agent.

REFERENCES

1. Thorpy, M.J., E. Korman, A.J. Spielman, and P.B. Glovinsky, Delayed sleep phase syndrome in adolescents. *J Adolesc Health Care*, 1988;**9**(1):22–27.
2. Carskadon M.A., C. Vieira, and C. Acebo, Association between puberty and delayed phase preference. *Sleep*, 1993;**16**(3):258–262.
3. Touitou, Y., Human aging and melatonin: clinical relevance. *Exp Gerontol*, 2001;**36**(7):1083–1100.
4. Dijk, D. and S. Lockley, Integration of human sleep-wake regulation and circadian rhythmicity. *J Appl Physiol*, 2002;**92**:852–862.
5. Borbely, A., A two process model of sleep regulation. *Hum Neurobiol*, 1982;**1**:195–204.
6. Pealy R. and P. Bovinski, Prevalence of delayed sleep phase syndrome among adolescents. *Sleep Res*, 1998;**17**:362.
7. Ando K. and S. Ancoli-Israiel, Estimated prevalence of delayed and advanced sleep phase syndromes. *Sleep Res*, 1995;**24**:509.
8. Shibui, K., M. Uchiyama, and M. Okawa, Melatonin rhythms in delayed sleep phase syndrome. *J Biol Rhythms*, 1999;**14**(1):72–76.
9. Uchiyama, M., M. Okawa, K. Shibui, et al., Poor recovery sleep after sleep deprivation in delayed sleep phase syndrome. *Psychiatry Clin Neurosci*, 1999;**53**(2):195–197.
10. Shirayama, M., Y. Shirayama, H. Iida, et al., The psychological aspects of patients with delayed sleep phase syndrome (DSPS). *Sleep Med*, 2003; **4**(5):427–433.
11. Rosenthal, N., J.R. Joseph-Vanderpool, A.A. Levendosky, et al., Phase-shifting effects of bright morning light as treatment for delayed sleep phase syndrome. *Sleep*, 1990;**13**(4):354–361.
12. Khalsa, S., M.E. Jewett, C. Cajochen, and C.A. Czeisler, A phase response curve to single bright light pulses in human subjects. *J Physiol*, 2003;**549**(Pt 3):945–952.
13. Chesson, A. L. Jr., M. Littner, D. Davila, et al., Practice parameters for the use of light therapy in the treatment of sleep disorders. Standards of Practice Committee, American Academy of Sleep Medicine. *Sleep*, 1999;**22**:641–660.
14. Wyatt, J., Delayed sleep phase syndrome: pathophysiology and treatment options. *Sleep*, 2004;**27**(6):1195–1203.
15. Regestein, Q., Treating insomnia: a practical guide for managing chronic sleeplessness. *Compr Psychiatry*, 1975;**17**(4):517–526.
16. Czeisler, C., G.G. Richardson, R.M. Coleman, et al., Chronotherapy: resetting the circadian clocks of patients with delayed sleep phase insomnia. *Sleep*, 1981;**4**(1):1–21.
17. Weitzman, E., C.A. Czeisler, R.M. Coleman, et al., Delayed sleep phase syndrome. A chronobiological disorder with sleep-onset insomnia. *Arch Gen Psychiatry*, 1981;**38**(7):737–746.
18. Pelayo, R.M.,W. Chen,S. Monzon, and Guilleminault, C. Pediatric sleep pharmacology: you want to give my kid sleeping pills? *Pediatr Clin North Am*, 2004;**51**(1):117–134.
19. Kamei, Y., T. Hayakawa, J. Urata, et al., Melatonin treatment for circadian rhythm sleep disorders. *Psychiatry Clin Neurosci*, 2000;**54**(3):381–382.
20. Smits, M., J.E. Nagtegaal, J. van der Heijden, A.M. Coenen, and G.A. Kerkhof, Melatonin for chronic sleep onset insomnia in children: a randomized placebo-controlled trial. *J Child Neurol*, 2001;**16**(2):86–92.
21. Dagan, Y., I. Yovel, D. Hallis, H. Eisenstin, and I. Raichik, Evaluating the role of melatonin in the long-term treatment of delayed sleep phase syndrome. *Chronobiol Int*, 1998;**15**(2):181–190.
22. Lewy, A.J., J. Emens, R.L. Sack, B.P. Hasler, and R.A. Bernert, Zeitgeber hierarchy in humans: resetting the circadian phase positions of blind people using melatonin. *Chronobiol Int*, 2003;**20**(5):837–852.

23. Hack, L.M., S.W. Lockley, J. Arendt, and D.J. Skene, The effects of low-dose 0.5 mg melatonin on the free-running circadian rhythms of blind subjects. *J Biol Rhythms*, 2003;**18**(5):430–429.

24. Wagner, J., M. Wagner, and W. Hening, Beyond benzodiazepines: alternative pharmacologic agents for the treatment of insomnia. *Ann Pharmacother*, 1998;**32**(6):680–691.

25. Satoh, K., K. Mishima, Y. Inoue, T. Ebisawa, and T. Shimizu, Two pedigrees of familial advanced sleep phase syndrome in Japan. *Sleep*, 2003;**26**(4):416–417.

26. Carskadon, M., Forced desynchrony as a means of assessing circadian and sleep/wake homeostatic, 2004; www.hhs.gov/ohrp/panels/407-01pnl/grantapp.pdf.

27. Littner, M., C.A. Kushida, W.M. Anderson, et al., and the Standards of Practice Committee of the American Academy of Sleep Medicine. Practice parameters for the role of actigraphy in the study of sleep and circadian rhythms: an update for 2002. *Sleep*, 2003;**26**(3):337–341.

7

Defining, Assessing, and Treating Adolescent Insomnia and Related Sleep Problems

Amy R. Wolfson, Alison Quinn, and Anna Vannucci

INTRODUCTION

As parents, teachers, coaches, health care providers, and teenagers themselves know, adolescence is filled with significant physical, cognitive, emotional, and social change. Sleep is a crucial and often ignored aspect of adolescents' lives as it changes and influences factors in their overall development, as well as in their daily lives. The quality and quantity of adolescents' sleep significantly influences their ability to think, behave, and feel in school, on the playing field, at work, as well as in a variety of other situations. Over the last two decades, laboratory data have demonstrated that adolescents have an increased need for sleep and experience a phase delay during puberty *(1–5)*. Despite this need, survey and field studies indicate that as early as sixth grade, adolescents obtain less sleep, report increased morning drowsiness, and have more spontaneous daytime naps than do younger children *(6–8)*. School schedules, work and extracurricular hours, and other environmental constraints are not beneficial to adolescents' sleep schedules and requirements *(2,4,7,9)*. In fact, teenagers develop a sleep debt by getting a minimal amount of sleep on school nights and making up for this by sleeping longer on the weekends *(7)*. Sleep debt results in frequent absences or tardiness from school, sleepiness and emotional lability, attention difficulties, and academic struggles *(7,10–13)*. Other adolescents may develop sleep disorders such as insomnia, phase-delay disorder, sleep apnea, or other sleep problems that also impair ability to function during the day. Recently, the National Institutes of Health recognized adolescents and young adults (12–25 years) as a population at high risk for problem sleepiness based on "evidence that the prevalence of problem sleepiness is high and increasing with particularly serious consequences" *(14)*. This chapter focuses on insomnia and phase-delay disorders in adolescents.

SLEEP NEED AND SCHEDULE CHANGES DURING ADOLESCENCE

Numerous surveys and actigraphy studies have shown that female and male adolescents usually obtain much less sleep than elementary school-age children: 10 hours during middle childhood, 8 hours in middle school, and less than 7 hours by

From: *Current Clinical Neurology: Sleep Disorders in Women: A Guide to Practical Management*
Edited by: H. P. Attarian © Humana Press Inc., Totowa, NJ

the end of high school *(7,8,10,15–17)*. Adolescents tend to stay up increasingly later over the middle and high school years, get up extremely early for school, and, as a result, get less sleep over the course of adolescence *(7,8,10,18)*.

Although surveys and actigraphy studies document that teenagers are getting less sleep over the middle and high school years, laboratory studies have demonstrated that adolescents require at least as much sleep as they did when they were in elementary school *(2,5,8,10,19)*. A 6-year longitudinal summer laboratory study by Carskadon and colleagues found the opportunity for sleep constant at 10 hours in children who were 10, 11, or 12 years old at their first three-night assessment *(2)*. They hypothesized that the youngsters would sleep fewer hours as they grew older, reaching an adult sleep length of 7.5–8 hours by their late teens. This landmark study, however, demonstrated that sleep quantity remained constant at approx 9.2 hours across all pubertal stages; sleep need is not reduced during adolescence.

Female and male adolescents also tend to delay the timing of sleep by staying up later at night and sleeping in later in the morning than children *(3)*. For example, on weekends and during vacations, adolescents tend to fall asleep and wake up later and obtain more sleep in comparison with school days. Studies have clearly demonstrated that this phase shift is attributed to psychosocial factors and to biological changes that take place during puberty along with psychosocial factors *(2,20,21)*.

Furthermore, weekend sleep times average 30 minutes to 1 hour more than school-night sleep times in pre- and young adolescents, and this difference increases to 1.5–2 hours in older teenagers *(4,8,16)*. Researchers and clinicians often interpret these data as suggesting that teenagers do not get enough sleep on school nights and then extend sleep on weekend nights to pay back a sleep debt. Lengthening sleep, however, does not eliminate difficulties. Adolescents with very irregular weekly sleep schedules report more behavior and academic problems, daytime sleepiness, and depressed mood *(7)*. The most obvious explanation for the adolescent sleep debt appears to be a pattern of insufficient school-night sleep resulting from a combination of early school start times, poor sleep hygiene practices, late afternoon/ evening activities and employment responsibilities, academic and social pressures, and a physiological sleep requirement that does not decrease with puberty *(4,5,10,22)*.

Overall, remarkably few studies report significant gender differences in adolescents' sleep duration and/or bed and rise times. Some studies find that female middle and high school-age teenagers wake up slightly earlier than their male peers *(7,23)*. Clinicians and researchers speculate that adolescent girls may be getting up earlier to prepare for school or to assist with family responsibilities. In terms of sleep latency, both middle and high school-age adolescent girls are more likely to report difficulty falling asleep in comparison with boys; however, this gender difference is likely explained by girls' higher pubertal status *(24)*. Later in this chapter, gender differences in the prevalence of insomnia sre discussed further.

Undoubtedly, research has shown that the amount of sleep acquired by both younger (middle school) and older adolescents (high school) often does not meet their actual sleep needs. This sleep deprivation negatively impacts adolescents' academic performance, emotional and behavioral well-being, and health and safety.

Yet, some adolescents' sleep is even more problematic because of insomnia and/or delayed sleep phase syndrome (DSPS; *25,26*).

DEFINING AND DIFFERENTIATING INSOMNIA AND DSPS

Far less is known about insomnia in adolescents in comparison with adults. However, increasingly more clinicians are reporting, diagnosing, and treating insomnia and phase-delay disorders among adolescents *(25,26)*. According to the fourth edition of the *Diagnostic and Statistical Manual of Mental Disorders* (DSM-IV), insomnia is defined as "a subjective complaint of difficulty falling or staying asleep or poor sleep quality. Types of insomnia include: initial insomnia—difficulty in falling asleep; middle insomnia—awakening in the middle of the night followed by eventually falling back to sleep, but with difficulty; and terminal insomnia—awakening before one's usual waking time and being unable to return to sleep" *(27)*.

The DSM-IV also notes that insomnia often causes clinically significant distress or impairment in social, occupational (e.g., school), or other important areas of daytime functioning *(27)*. In assessing adolescents, it is often difficult to distinguish insomnia from DSPS. DSPS, also called phase lag syndrome, is a circadian rhythm sleep disorder *(28–30)*. However, unlike jet lag and the effects of shift work, DSPS is a persistent condition. DSPS results from a desynchronization between the adolescent's internal biological clock and the external environment. Unlike jet lag, this desynchronization is not activated by travel or change in external environment. Rather, the adolescent's propensity to fall asleep is simply more "delayed" in relation to that of the average adolescent. Subsequently, a teenager with DSPS is desynchronized with the routine that governs most of his or her life. Adolescents with DSPS or their parents may initially refer to their symptoms as insomnia. For the most part, adolescents with DSPS are able to fall asleep and maintain sleep; however, their bed and rise times are even more delayed than their peers' already late sleep–wake schedules. DSPS makes it hard to wake up in the morning when simultaneously indulging in a late night sleep routine.

Recently, Mindell surveyed nearly 300 college students to tease apart the occurrence of sleep-onset insomnia and DSPS. About 18% of the students met the criteria for insomnia, 25% had DSPS, and nearly 10% had DSPS, although they described themselves as having insomnia. In all likelihood, then, about 35% of these students were dealing with DSPS, whereas 18% had "true" insomnia *(26)*.

INSOMNIA DURING ADOLESCENCE

Chronic insomnia affects nearly 10–15% of the adult population *(31)*. In recent years, a few studies have investigated the prevalence of insomnia in adolescents. Ohayon and Roberts estimated the prevalence of DSM-IV insomnia to be 4% and the incidence of phase-delay disorder 1% for 15- to 18-year-olds; approx 25% reported insomnia symptoms during the previous 30 days *(32)*. In an earlier study, Morrison and colleagues used DSM-III to evaluate 15-year-old adolescents and estimated that approx 15% experienced insomnia *(33)*. More recently, Roberts and colleagues reported that nearly 18% of adolescents 11–17 years of age had experienced nonrestorative sleep nearly every day in the previous month *(34)*. Generally, adolescents report more difficulty initiating sleep than maintaining sleep. Yet, because studies (and likely individual clinicians) have relied on various diagnostic criteria, it is often unclear whether the adolescent is experiencing insomnia or more of a phase-delay disorder. Both DSPS and insomnia may cause problem sleepiness and difficulty functioning during the day for adolescents. In recent years, Roberts and colleagues have found that insomnia and related sleep problems have adverse consequences for the future functioning of adolescents. In particular, insomnia symptoms such as nonrestorative sleep, difficulty initiating sleep, and daytime sleepiness are associated with self-esteem difficulties, interpersonal relationship problems, symptoms of depression, somatic complaints, and academic difficulties *(34–36)*.

Female Adolescents and Insomnia

It is common knowledge that 1.5–2 times more women than men report insomnia *(37)*. However, it is not entirely understood why women (and, possibly, adolescent girls) are diagnosed with insomnia more often than men. Although some studies find gender differences in the incidence of insomnia among teenagers, others do not. For example, in a self-report study of more than 5000 ninth graders, 15% of females vs 9% of males reported symptoms of insomnia *(35)*. In particular, high school-age females tend to report less restorative sleep, poorer sleep quality, more difficulty initiating and maintaining sleep, and greater use of medications for sleep and/or to counteract daytime sleepiness *(35,38)*. In a structured interview study of just over 1000 adolescents and their parents, girls reported a greater prevalence of insomnia than boys (20 vs 14%) *(39)*. Pubertal development was associated with increased risk of insomnia among girls but not boys, and the median age of onset of insomnia was 11 *(38,39)*. Of the adolescents with lifetime insomnia, 94% reported experiencing insomnia symptoms twice a week for a month or more during the past 12 months and 85% did so within the past month. About 32% of adolescents with lifetime insomnia also had another DSM-IV psychiatric disorder *(39)*. Similarly, Yang and colleagues surveyed slightly more than 800 Chinese adolescents and found that about 15% of their sample had insomnia *(40)*. Girls in this study had slightly more trouble falling asleep than boys (17 vs 12%). There were no differences between older (15–18 years) and younger (12–14 years) adolescents. It appears that increasingly more studies are finding that the increased insomnia or problems in initiating and maintaining sleep seen in adult women may begin in early adolescence *(41)*.

Associations between hormone levels and sleep are complex. Studies have shown that hormonal changes in the menstrual cycle can and do interfere with sleep for an average 2–3 days per monthly cycle for some healthy, young women; however, young, recently menstruating females are less likely to report sleep changes as a result of menstruation *(37)*. Effectively minimal research, however, has been conducted on menstruation and sleep in adolescents. For healthy young women, the interference with sleep is largely a result of a bloated feeling, but clearly contributed to by other factors. The most marked disturbance occurs during the first few days of menstruation. As progesterone levels fall toward the end of the menstrual cycle, sleep is disrupted. Adolescent and young adult females may experience some difficulty falling asleep or insomnia-like symptoms during this time period. Johnson and colleagues also found that girls were 2.5 times more likely to experience insomnia after their first period than prior to the onset of menses *(39)*.

The premenstrual period is also associated with poor sleep; insomnia is common, but sometimes hypersomnia or increased daytime sleepiness is reported *(42,43)*. In a recent study *(43)*, Baker and Driver found that young women (mean age 21 years) reported poorer sleep quality over the 3 premenstrual days and 4 days during menstruation in comparison to the mid-follicular and early/mid-luteal phases. Total sleep time, sleep-onset latency, number/duration of wakings, and morning vigilance were not affected by the menstrual cycle. These researchers conclude that young women (immediately postadolescence) perceive some changes in sleep quality over the menstrual cycle, but sleep quantity and continuity does not change *(43)*. Undoubtedly, more studies are required to understand the association between menstrual cycle-related insomnia, particularly in adolescents.

Insomnia difficulties may be particularly problematic for adolescents experiencing premenstrual syndrome (PMS); however, few studies have evaluated PMS in adolescents because symptoms typically begin after puberty, between the ages of 25 and 35 *(44)*. Similar to the adult female population, it is estimated that about 5–13% of adolescent females experience severe PMS *(44,45)*. Sleep disturbances such as insomnia have been documented in adult women with PMS; however, researchers have not focused on adolescent females. The most common sleep-related problems reported by women with PMS are as follows: sleep-onset and maintenance insomnia, hypersomnia, difficulty waking in the morning, and daytime sleepiness *(37)*.

Adolescent females are also more likely to experience depression and anxiety, which could increase the prevalence of insomnia *(46)*. One study found that prior insomnia was associated with a twofold increased risk of subsequent onset of depression, whereas prior depression was similarly associated with subsequent onset of insomnia. Depression and insomnia are discussed later in this chapter.

Etiology: Precipitating and Perpetuating Factors

The "causes" or predisposing, precipitating, and/or perpetuating factors that contribute to insomnia for adolescents are varied and not well researched. Some researchers and clinicians categorize the so-called causes as physiological, psychological, and behavioral *(26)*. Physiological precipitating factors include an underlying or preexisting sleep disorder such as sleep-disordered breathing and restless legs syndrome (RLS) and periodic limb movements in sleep. Sometimes sleep-disordered breathing difficulties result in difficulties maintaining sleep, whereas RLS symptoms (e.g., uncomfortable, sometimes painful, sensations in the extremities at bedtime) often make it difficult for the adolescent to fall asleep at night. Use of over-the-counter and/or prescription medications (e.g., medications for attention deficit hyperactivity disorder and/or depression), caffeine use, alcohol and drug abuse, and other medical problems may also contribute to insomnia symptoms *(37,47)*.

Psychological precipitants include depression, anxiety, and other emotional difficulties. Insomnia may be secondary or coexist with depression, or sleeplessness may contribute to the development of depression. Symptoms of major depressive disorder include insomnia (75% of cases) and hypersomnia (25%). Insomnia symptoms usually include difficulty falling asleep and a subjective sense of not having slept deeply all night. Early morning awakenings are less prevalent in adolescents than in adults with depression. Recently, clinicians and researchers have seen increasingly more adolescents with overlapping phase-delay disorders and/or other sleep–wake schedule disorders with depression. Studies suggest that depressed adolescents may have difficulty falling asleep and maintaining sleep, are unable to get up or refuse to go to school, sleep until late in the day, complain of daytime tiredness, and, over time, shift to increasingly more delayed sleep–wake schedules *(48–50)*. Moreover, beginning in middle school or even elementary school, young adolescents' worries, concerns, and questions can interfere with falling asleep as well as difficulty falling back to sleep during the night. Anxiety disorders such as generalized anxiety disorder, panic disorder, and others also contribute to insomnia.

Finally, behavioral and environmental factors contribute to the development and/or perpetuation of insomnia and insomnia-like symptoms. Irregular school–weekend night schedules, long, spontaneous daytime naps, and erratic bedtime routines may individually or together lead to longer sleep latencies and eventually insomnia for some adolescents. Furthermore, extensive television and computer use is often associated with sleep problems during childhood and adolescence. Studies find that children and adolescents who watch 3 or more hours of television daily are at risk for sleep difficulties (e.g., later bed and rise times, less time in bed, increased sleepiness) and other behavioral problems *(51–53)*. Computer game playing and internet use also negatively impact sleep hygiene behaviors *(52,53)*.

Assessment and Treatment

Assessment of insomnia in adolescents involves several steps. Initially, a personal and family sleep history is recommended. This initial history taking may involve an interview as well as a written questionnaire. Parents may be more or less involved depending on the age and maturity of the adolescent. Moreover, the parents'/guardians' perceptions of the sleep problems may be quite different from those of the teenager, and, therefore, it will be helpful to gather independent information from both the adolescent and his or her parents. Areas that should be addressed include bedtime, bedtime routines, television viewing, nap history, caffeine and alcohol intake, and medication (prescription and over-the-counter) use *(26)*. Nighttime behaviors need to be evaluated, including sleep latency and sleep onset, behaviors during the night, and the number and duration of night awakenings. Questions about morning activities are also important, such as wake time, time in bed after awakening, and level of sleepiness. Additionally, any unusual occurrences, such as night terrors, seizures, enuresis, respiratory disturbances, and abnormal arousals, should be discussed and/or recorded. Clinicians should also inquire about symptoms of anxiety and depression, which often result in a lack of sleep and possibly insomnia. The initial interview should also inquire about significant life events or stressors, as they may also be related to sleep disturbances that may lead to insomnia (e.g., death in the family, school failure, social problems, significant change in family economic status, etc.).

Second, use of a daily sleep–wake diary will add to the assessment process. Sleep–wake diaries record subjective evaluations of bedtimes, sleep-onset latencies, number of nighttime awakenings, rise times, total sleep times, and the number and duration of naps. The sleep diary should be kept for a minimum of 2 weeks to obtain an accurate evaluation of sleep habits. Stores suggests that parents of younger adolescents also report their child's sleep patterns to reveal any discrepancies between the perceptions of the child's subjective evaluation and the parents' perceptions *(25)*. Furthermore, if there is a suspicion that the insomnia may have a physiological root and/or to assess other possible sleep disorders (e.g., sleep apnea), polysomnography can confirm sleep–wake diary and interview data.

Third, it may be helpful for clinicians to assess pubertal status for both female and male patients. One noninvasive scale is the Pubertal Development Scale *(3,54)*, which classifies children according to the following pubertal development stages: prepubertal, early pubertal, midpubertal, late pubertal, and postpubertal. Respondents (adolescent and/or parent) answer questions about growth in height, growth of body hair, skin changes, such as pimples, voice and facial hair changes (for boys), and breast and menstruation development (for girls). Additionally, when females present with complaints of premenstrual-related insomnia symptoms, use of a premenstrual daily symptom diary is recommended *(44)*. Often it is helpful to have the adolescent female keep the premenstrual diary for several consecutive months so that cycle-to-cycle variability may be observed.

Some clinicians and researchers recommend that the choice of treatment be based on the underlying "causes" of the particular symptoms of insomnia. However, Morin, one of the leading experts on insomnia, along with others in the field, has clearly demonstrated that regardless of the initial "cause" or event that precipitates insomnia, it is maintained through learned behaviors and cognitions that promote sleeplessness *(55)*. Cognitive–behavioral therapy (CBT) for insomnia has three courses of action: behavioral, cognitive, and educational. Over the last two decades, numerous studies have demonstrated that CBT is effective for 70–80% of adults, including young adults *(55–57)*, in comparison with pharmacotherapy. CBT is most effective in reducing sleep-onset latency symptoms and increasing sleep efficiency. Unfortunately, few studies have evaluated the efficacy of CBT approaches for adolescents. The authors of this chapter recommend CBT as a first-line intervention for treating adolescents with insomnia; however, further treatment outcome research is needed.

The handful of studies that have looked at treatment efficacy for adolescent insomnia had small sample sizes and/or relied on a single-case design *(26)*. In particular, two case studies successfully utilized relaxation training and reduction of parental attention *(58,59)*, and another study treated three adolescents with a combination of relaxation training and biofeedback *(60)*.

Cognitive–behavioral strategies generally include sleep hygiene, and, as Mindell points out, treatment plans for adolescents should include education about the specific components *(26)*. Sleep hygiene includes the following: comfortable, dark, and quiet sleep environment; consistent bedtime and waking routines, including weekends; avoiding excessive hunger but also large amounts of food close to bed-time; passing up naps in the late afternoon and early evening; steering clear of stimulating activities 1 hour before bedtime, such a television watching, telephone conversations, computer activities, or exercising; and eliminating caffeine 4–6 hours before bedtime *(61)*.

In the next section, the CBT techniques that are most efficacious for insomnia are outlined *(see* Table 1). Relaxation therapy (e.g., relaxation training, progressive muscle relaxation, meditation, etc.) helps the adolescent slow her or his racing thoughts and relaxes muscles so that she or he experiences a more restful, calm sleep. Specific techniques are effective in decreasing anxiety and body tension *(37)*. Stimulus control techniques consist of a set of procedures designed to curtail sleep-incompatible behaviors and regulate the sleep–wake schedule. Stimulus control therapy is meant to help the adolescent recondition her- or himself to associate bed and bedtime with sleep as opposed to other activities (e.g., studying, talking on the cell phone, using a laptop computer in bed). Also, adolescents learn to maximize cues that are associated with feeling sleepy and falling asleep and to decrease the cues associated with staying awake. Sleep restriction is another highly recommended behavioral treatment for insomnia *(62)*. This approach involves limiting the amount of time spent in bed, because some adolescents with insomnia tend to spend too much time in bed unsuccessfully trying to sleep. The allowed time in bed is increased or decreased by 15–20 minutes (or kept stable) for a given week depending on whether the adolescent's sleep efficiency that week increases, decreases, or stays the same. (The sleep restriction steps are outlined in Table 1.) Many teenagers have numerous misconceptions about sleep that actually interfere with their ability to fall asleep or to maintain sleep. Cognitive therapy helps the adolescent get rid of false beliefs and assumptions (e.g., misconceptions about causes of insomnia, faulty ideas about sleep promotion habits, etc.) and replace them with appropriate and more helpful interpretations *(37)*.

Finally, medications may also be helpful. A number of medications have been shown to be effective for adults; however, further research must be conducted to evaluate the effects of medications on adolescents and children. Hypnotics — members of the benzodiazepine family — are commonly used in treatment. Short-term use is stressed to avoid dependency. Tricyclic drugs have been suggested for sleep problems that involve arousal (e.g., difficulty initiating sleep) *(25)*. In one study, Kallepalli and colleagues assessed the efficacy of trazodone vs fluoxetine for insomnia in 60 adolescents with depression. Trazodone relieved insomnia symptoms faster than fluoxetine (2.5 vs 5.1 days) *(63)*. It is the view of these authors that medications for insomnia are a final treatment option only.

DELAYED SLEEP PHASE SYNDROME: A STRIKINGLY ADOLESCENT PROBLEM

DSPS is especially troublesome for adolescents. There are a number of recent reviews of DSPS and other circadian rhythm disorders *(64–66)*. DSPS is mani-fested by sleep-onset times that are delayed several hours relative to conventional

Table 1
Cognitive–Behavioral Treatment Approaches for Insomina

Treatment	Description	Considerations
Cognitive therapy	Identifies a person's sleep misconceptions and maladaptive beliefs and attitudes	Typically used in conjuction with sleep-restriction and stimulus-control therapies
	Replaces misconceptions with more adaptive beliefs and facts	Eliminates anxiety previously surrounding sleep
Relaxation training	Practice of deep relaxation for 20–30 minutes on a daily basis before bedtime	A general feeling of relaxation and well-being results
	Commonly includes variations of yoga, meditation, or progressive muscle relaxation	Helps reduce anxiety regarding falling asleep and maintaining sleep
Sleep hygiene	Quiet, dark, relaxing environment conducive to sleep	Important to educate both parents and adolescents regarding sleep hygiene
	Consistent evening routine, bedtime, and rise time	
	Arousing activities should be avoided about 1 hour before bedtime	
	Avoid excessive hunger, but do not eat or drink to excess	
	Try to avoid long, unscheduled and late afternoon/evening naps	
	Avoid caffeine intake during the day, particulary 4–6 hours before sleep	
	Stay away from alcohol and nicotine, as they disturb sleep	
Sleep-restriction therapy	Reduces amount of nonsleeping time in bed by restricting hours the person is in bed to only when sleeping	Approach takes 3–4 weeks to be effective; similar to stimulus-control therapy; some individuals may be sleepy during the day
	Time in bed gradually increases when sleep efficiency is greater than 85% for the current number of hours in bed	
Stimulus-control therapy	Reassociates bedtime and bed with successful sleep	Use your bed/bedroom only for sleep
	Restricts activities that are incompatible with sleep in the bedroom/bed and at bedtime	Go to bed and lie down only when sleepy
	Establishes a consistent sleep–wake cycle	Establish a regular presleep routine; keep sleep environment quiet, dark, and comfortable in temperature
		If you can't fall asleep after about 10–15 minutes, get up, go to another room; choose quiet activity until drowsy, then return to the bedroom to sleep
		Avoid naps and go to bed and wake up at the same time each day, regardless of how much sleep is obtained at night

Adapted form ref. *37.*

bedtimes (3 AM rather than 11 PM). Conversely, the normal time to wake up drifts to correspondingly later in the morning (11 rather than 7 AM). Adolescents with DSPS typically complain of sleep-onset insomnia when attempting to go to bed at a "normal" time and experience extreme difficulty arising at a desired "normal" wake time. However, when on vacation or in a situation where sleep schedule is unimportant, these teenagers have no difficulty with sleep initiation, sleep maintenance, or functioning the next day, as they are able to self-select their sleep and wake times in accordance with their biologically mandated schedule. Because school must be attended, adolescents with DSPS often come home from school and crash for a nap or fall asleep in a friend's parked car, only to then later stay up until all hours of the night in a repetitive cycle. A more detailed discussion of the etiology and factors contributing to the development of DSPS is given in Chapter 6.

There seems to be a strong relationship between depression and DSPS. One study of adolescents with DSPS found that 36% had features of depression. In a more recent study of older adolescents (first-year college students), the researchers concluded that the sleep–wake patterns associated with DSPS and chronic insufficient sleep tend to result in lowered academic performance, depressed mood, and other daytime difficulties *(67)*. The relationship between DSPS and mood difficulties is poorly understood in that the inadequate sleep associated with DSPS may give rise to depression, or there may be a primary mood disorder that evokes the symptoms of DSPS. Students may feel depressed because they failed to attend class; this should be differentiated from school refusals that show a DSPS-like sleep schedule as a means of avoiding school, often failing to advance to the next grade *(67)*.

Assessment and Treatment

The International Classification of Sleep Disorders–Revised (ICSD-R) requires certain minimal criteria for diagnosing DSPS *(68)*. These criteria are as follows:

1. Inability to initiate sleep at the desired time and difficulty awakening.
2. Delayed timing of the habitual sleep episode.
3. Presence of symptoms for 1 month or more.
4. When constraints permit (e.g., when not working or attending classes), the patient opts for delayed timing of the major sleep episode, which is felt to be of good quality and quantity, and can awaken from this sleep episode without difficulty, and remains on this delayed sleep–wake schedule without difficulty.
5. Two weeks or more of subjective sleep data (e.g., sleep–wake diary) verify the presence of the delayed, habitual sleep–wake schedule *(68)*.

Similar to insomnia, assessment of DSPS requires an intake evaluation (e.g., interview with the adolescent and his or her parent/guardian), a 2-week sleep–wake diary, and possibly wrist actigraphy to gain more objective data on patterns of sleep–wake behaviors *(66,69)*. Actigraphy has been established as a valid and reliable method of assessing current sleep–wake patterns in children, adolescents, and adults *(69–71)*.

There are several treatment approaches for DSPS. Individual teenagers may respond to treatments differently, and, therefore, matching the specific treatment with the individual adolescent is crucial. A combination of treatment strategies is often the best approach *(65–67)*. For a complete description of DSPS, *see* Chapter 6.

CONCLUSION

Recognition and efficacious treatment of insomnia and DSPS among adolescents is clearly needed. There are no outcome studies that track the long-term consequences of adolescent and pediatric sleep disorders or their contribution to adult sleep problems, but this is an area of increasing research attention *(72)*. Furthermore, there is growing evidence suggesting that adolescent girls report more insomnia-like difficulties than their male peers and that the risk of insomnia may be tied to the onset of puberty and menstruation for females. Longitudinal, multifaceted research, however, is needed to better understand these trends. Parents, teachers, health care providers, adolescents, and friends should be educated regarding insomnia, DSPS, and related sleep problems so that teenagers are diagnosed and not misdiagnosed, treated appropriately, and are able to obtain the all too important social support.

REFERENCES

1. Carskadon, M.A., C. Acebo, and O.G. Jenni, Regulation of adolescent sleep: implications for behavior. *Ann NY Acad Sci*, 2004;**1021**:276–291
2. Carskadon, M.A., K. Harvey, P. Duke, T.F. Anders, and W.C. Dement, Pubertal changes in daytime sleepiness. *Sleep*, 1980;**2**:453–460.
3. Carskadon, M.A., C. Vieira, and C. Acebo, Association between puberty and delayed phase preference. *Sleep*, 1993;**16**(3):258–262.
4. Carskadon, M., A. Wolfson, C. Acebo, O. Tzischinsky, and R. Seifer, Adolescent sleep patterns, circadian timing, and sleepiness at a transition to early school days. *Sleep*, 1998;**21**(8):871–881.
5. Carskadon, M.A. and C. Acebo, Regulation of sleepiness in adolescents: update, insights, and speculation. *Sleep*, 2002;**25**(6):606–614.
6. Sadeh, A., R. Raviv, and R. Gruber, Sleep patterns and sleep disruptions in school-age children. *Dev Psychol*, 2000;**36**(3):291–301.
7. Wolfson, A.R. and M.A.Carskadon, Sleep schedules and daytime functioning in adolescents. *Child Dev*, 1998;**69**:875–887.
8. Wolfson, A.R., C. Acebo, G. Fallone, and M.A. Carskadon, Actigraphically-estimated sleep patterns of middle school students. *Sleep* (Suppl), 2003;**26**:313.
9. Wolfson, A. Bridging the gap between research and practice: What will adolescents' sleep/wake patterns look like in the 21st century? In: *Adolescent Sleep Patterns: Biological, Social, and Psychological Influences* (M.A. Carskadon, ed.). New York: Cambridge University Press, 2002, pp. 198–219.
10. Carskadon, M.A. Patterns of sleep and sleepiness in adolescents. *Pediatrician*, 1990;**7**:5–12.
11. Comstock, G. *Televison and the American Child*. San Diego, CA: Academic Press, 1991.
12. Wahlstrom, K. Changing times: findings from the first longitudinal study of later high school start times. *NASSP Bull*, 2002;**86**(633):3–21.
13. Wolfson, A.R. and M.A.Carskadon, Understanding adolescents'sleep patterns and school performance: a critical appraisal. *Sleep Med Rev*, 2003;**7**(6):491–506.
14. *Working Group Report on Problem Sleepiness*. Bethesda, MO: National Institutes of Health, National Center on Sleep Disorders Research and Office Prevention, Education, and Control, 1997.
15. Carskadon, M.A. The second decade. In: *Sleeping and Waking Disorders: Indications and Techniques* (C. Guilleminault, ed.). Menlo Park: Addison-Wesley, 1982, pp. 99–125.
16. Strauch, I. and B. Meier, Sleep need in adolescents: a longitudinal approach. *Sleep*, 1988;**11**(4):378–386.
17. Thorleifsdottir, B., J.K. Bjornsson, B. Benediktsdottir, T. Gislason, and H. Kristbjarnarson, Sleep and sleep habits from childhood to young adulthood over a 10-year period. *J Psychosom Res*, 2002;**53**:529–537.

18. Price, V.A., T.J. Coates, C.E. Thoresen, and O.A. Grinstead, Prevalence and correlates of poor sleep among adolescents. *Am J Dis Child*, 1978;**132**:583–586.

19. Carskadon, M.A., J. Orav, and W.C. Dement, Evolution of sleep and daytime sleepiness in adolescents. In: *Sleep/Wake Disorders: Natural History, Epidemiology, and Long-Term Evolution* (C. Guilleminault and E. Lugaresi, eds.). New York: Raven Press, 1983:201–216.

20. Andrade, M.M., A.A. Silva-Benedito, E.E.S. Domenice, I.J.P. Arnhold, and L.M. Menna-Barreto, Sleep characteristics of adolescents: a longitudinal study. *J Adolesc Health*, 1993;**14**:401–406.

21. Ishihara, K., Y. Honma, and S. Miyake, Investigation of the children's version of the morningness-eveningness questionnaire with primary and junior high school pupils in Japan. *Percept Motor Skills*, 1990;**71**:1353–1354.

22. Manber, R., R.E. Pardee, R.R. Bootzin, et al. Changing sleep patterns in adolescence. *Sleep Res*, 1995;**24**:106.

23. Gau, S.F. and W.T. Soong, Pediatric sleep disorders: sleep problems of junior high school students in Taipei. *Sleep*, 1995;**18**:667–673.

24. Laberge, L., D. Petit, C. Simard, F.Vitaro, R.E. Tremblay, and J. Montplaisir, Development of sleep patterns in early adolescents. *J Sleep Res*, 2001;**10**:59–67.

25. Stores, G. Practicioner review: assessment and treatment of sleep disorders in children and adolescents. *J Child Psychol Psychiatry*, 1996;**7**(8):907–925.

26. Mindell, J.A. Insomnia in children and adolescents. In: *Insomnia Principles and Management* (M.P. Szuba, J.D. Kloss, and D.F, Dinges, eds.). New York: Cambridge University Press, 2003:125–135.

27. American Psychiatric Association. *Diagnostic and Statistical Manual of Mental Disorders*, 4th ed., revised. Washington, DC: American Psychiatric Association, 1994.

28. Sack, R.L., R.J. Hughes, M.L.N. Pires, and A.J. Lewy, The sleep-promoting effects of melatonin. In *Insomnia Principles and Management*, ed MP Szuba, JD Kloss, and DF Dinges. New York: Cambridge University Press, 2003:96–114.

29. Boivin, D.B. and F.O. James, Insomnia due to circadian rhythm disturbances. In: *Insomnia Principles and Management* (M.P. Szuba, J.D. Kloss, and D.F. Dinges, eds.). New York: Cambridge University Press, 2003:155–191.

30. Regestein, Q.R. and T.H. Monk, Delayed sleep phase syndrome: a review of its clinical aspects. *Am J Psychiatry*, 1995;**152**:602–608.

31. National Sleep Foundation. *Treating Insomnia in the Primary Care Setting*. Washington, DC: National Sleep Foundation, 2000.

32. Ohayon, M.M. and R.E. Roberts, Comparability of sleep disorders diagnoses using DSM-IV and ICSD classifications with adolescents. *Sleep*, 2001;**24**(8):920–925.

33. Morrison, D.N., R. McGee, and W.R. Stanton, Sleep problems in adolescence. *J Am Acad Child Adolesc Psychiatry*, 1992;**31**(1):94–99.

34. Roberts, R., C. Roberts, and I.G. Chen, Impact of insomnia on future functioning of adolescents. *J Psychosom Res*, 2002;**53**:561–569.

35. Roberts, R.E., E.S. Lee, M. Hernandez, and A.C. Solari, Symptoms of insomnia among adolescents in the Lower Rio Grand Valley of Texas. *Sleep*, 2004;**27**(4):751–759.

36. Roberts, R.E., C.E. Roberts, and I.G. Chen, Ethnocultural differences in sleep complaints among adolescents. *J Nerv Ment Dis*, 2002;**188**(4):222–229.

37. Wolfson, A.R. *The Women's Book of Sleep: A Complete Resource Guide*. Oakland, CA: New Harbinger Publications, Inc., 2001.

38. Bailly, D., I. Bailly-Lambin, D. Querleu, R. Beuscart, and C. Collinet, Sleep in adolescents and its disorders. A survey in schools. *Encephale*, 2004;**30**(4):352–359.

39. Johnson, E.O., T. Roth, and N. Breslau, Epidemiology of DSM-IV insomnia among a community based cohort of adolescents. *Sleep* (Suppl), 2004;**27**:A112.

40. Yang, L., C. Zuo, and L.F. Eaton, Research note: sleep problems of normal Chinese adolescents. *J Child Psychol Psychiatry*, 1987;**28**:162–172.

41. Camhi, S.L., W.J. Morgan, N. Pernisco, and S.F. Quan, Factors affecting sleep disturbances in children and adolescents. *Sleep Med*, 2000;**1**:117–123.

42. Driver, H.S. and F.C. Baker, Menstrual factors in sleep. *Sleep Med Rev*, 1998;**2**(4):213–229.
43. Baker, F.C. and H.S. Driver, Self reported sleep across the menstrual cycle in young, healthy women. *J Psychosom Res*, 2004;**56**:239–243.
44. Dickerson, L.M., P.J. Mazyck, and M.H. Hunter, Premenstrual syndrome. *Am Fam Physician*, 2003;**67**(8):1–15.
45. Derman, O., N.O. Kanbur, N.E. Tokur, and T. Kutluk, Premenstrual syndrome and associated symptoms in adolescent girls. *Eur J Obstet Gynecol Reprod Biol*, 2004;**116**(2):201–206.
46. Krystal, A.D. Insomnia in women. *Chron Insomnia*, 2003;**5**(3):41–50.
47. Spielman, A.J. and P.B.Glovinsky, The diagnostic interview and differential diagnosis for complaints of insomnia. In: *Understanding Sleep: The Evaluation and Treatment of Sleep Disorders* (M.R. Pressman and W.C. Orr, eds.). Washington, DC: American Psychological Association, 1997, pp. 125–160.
48. Dahl, R.E., N.D. Ryan, M.K. Matty, B. et al. Sleep onset abnormalities in depressed adolescents. *Biol Psychiatry*, 1996;**39**(6):400–410.
49. Choquet, M., V. Kovess, and N. Poutignat, Suicidal thoughts among adolescents: an intercultural approach. *Adolescence*, 1993;**28**:649–659.
50. Patten, C.A., W.S. Choi, J.C. Gillin, and J.P. Pierce, Depressive symptoms and cigarette smoking predict development and persistence of sleep problems in U.S. adolescents. *Pediatrics*, 2000;**106**(2):1–17.
51. Van den Bulck, J. Text messaging as a cause of sleep interruption in adolescents, evidence from a cross sectional study. *J Sleep Res*, 2003;**12**(3):263.
52. Van den Bulck, J. Television viewing, computer game playing, and internet use and self-reported time out of bed in secondary school children. *Sleep*, 2004;**27**(1):101–104.
53. Johnson, J.G., P. Cohen, S. Kasen, M.B. First, and J.S. Brook, Association between television viewing and sleep problems during adolescence and early adulthood. *Arch Pediatr Adolesc Med*, 2004;**158**(6):652–568.
54. Carskadon, M.A. and C.Acebo, A self-administered rating scale for pubertal development. *J Adolesc Health*, 1993;**14**:190–195.
55. Morin, C.M. Cognitive-behavioral approaches to the treatment of insomnia. *J Clin Psychiatry*, 2004;**65**(16):33–40.
56. Jacobs, G.D., E.F. Pace-Schott, R. Stickgold, and M.W. Otto, Cognitive behavior therapy and pharmacotherapy for insomnia: a randomized controlled trial and direct comparison. *Arch Intern Med*, 2004;**164**(17):1888–1896.
57. Bastien, C.H., A. Vallieeres, and C.M. Morin, Precipitating factors of insomnia. *Behav Sleep Med*, 2004;**2**(1):50–62.
58. Weil, G. and M.R. Goldfried, Treatment of insomnia in an eleven-year-old child through self-relaxation. *Behav Ther*, 1973;**4**:282–294.
59. Anderson, D.R. Treatment of insomnia in a 13-year-old boy by relaxation training and reduction of parental attention. *J Behav Ther Exp Psychiatry*, 1979;**10**:263–265.
60. Barowsky, E.I., J. Moskowitz, and J.B. Zweig, Biofeedback for disorders of initiating and maintaining sleep. *Ann NY Acad Sci*, 1990;**602**:97–103.
61. LeBourgeois, M.K., F. Giannotti, F. Cortesi, A.R. Wolfson, and J. Harsh, The relationship between reported sleep quality and sleep hygiene in Italian and American adolescents. *Pediatrics*, 2005;**115**:257–265.
62. Spielman, A.J., P. Saskin, and M.J. Thorpy, Treatment of chronic insomnia by restriction of time in bed. *Sleep*, 1987;**10**(1):45–56.
63. Kallepalli, B.R., V.S. Bhatara, B.S. Fogas, R.C. Tervo, and L.K. Misra, Trazadone is only slightly faster than fluoxetine in relieving insomnia in adolescents with depressive disorders. *J Child Adolesc Psychopharmacol*, 1997;**7**:97–107.
64. Labyak, S. Sleep and circadian schedule disorders. *Nurs Clin North Am*, 2002;**37**:599–610.
65. Garcia, J., G. Rosen, and M. Mahowald, Circadian rhythms and circadian rhythm disorders in children and adolescents. *Semin Pediatr Neurol*, 2001;**8**:229–240.
66. Wyatt, J.K. Delayed sleep phase syndrome: pathophysiology and treatment options. *Sleep*, 2004;**27**(6):1195–1203.

67. Okawa, M., U. Michiyama, S. Ozaki, K. Shibui, and H. Ichikawa, Circadian rhythm disorders in adolescents: Clinical trials of combined treatments based on chronobiology. *Psychiatry Clin Neurosci*, 1998;52:483–490.

68. *The International Classification of Sleep Disorders-Revised: Diagnostic and Coding Manual.* Rochester, MN: American Sleep Disorders Association, 1997.

69. Wolfson, A.R., M.A. Carskadon, C. Acebo, R. Seifer, G. Fallone, S.E. Labyak, and J.L. Martin, Evidence for the validity of a sleep habits survey for adolescents. *Sleep*, 2003;26(2):213–216.

70. Sadeh, A., P.J. Hauri, D.F. Kripke, and P. Lavie, The role of actigraphy in the evaluation of sleep disorders. *Sleep*, 1995;**18**:288–302.

71. Acebo, C., A. Sadeh, R. Seifer, et al., Estimating sleep patterns with activity monitoring in children and adolescents: How many nights are necessary for reliable measures? *Sleep*, 1999;**22**(1):95–103.

72. Halbower, A.C. and C.L. Marcus, Sleep disorders in children. *Curr Opin Pulm Med*, 2003;**9**(6):471–476.

III Premenopausal Women

8

Restless Legs Syndrome

An Overview With an Emphasis on Women

David M. Hiestand and Barbara Phillips

INTRODUCTION

Restless legs syndrome (RLS) is a sensorimotor disorder that affects sleep in up to 15% of the population. Individuals experience uncomfortable sensations of the extremities, which occur with inactivity and are relieved with activity. Because of the circadian rhythmicity of these symptoms, RLS symptoms can interfere with sleep onset. Symptom descriptors are varied; some commonly used terms are "creepy-crawly," "uncomfortable," "pins and needles," and "internal itch." Regardless of the descriptor, symptoms of RLS include a compelling urge to move, as they are usually improved with movement, and patients frequently resort to flexing, stretching, and vigorous movement. The end result is typically poor quality of sleep, leading to excessive daytime somnolence and feelings of fatigue. Although the disorder affects both genders, it is more common in women (in most populations studied) and is associated with several medical conditions including uremia, anemia, diabetes, pregnancy, and menopause.

The disorder was described by Karl Ekbom in 1945 *(1)* after an initial description by Sir Thomas Willis in 1865. It was not until 1995, however, that the International Restless Legs Syndrome Study Group standardized criteria for the definition and diagnosis of RLS *(2)*. These criteria were further updated in 2002, and currently the following four diagnostic criteria must be met:

1. The patient must have an urge to move the legs, usually accompanied by an unpleasant sensation in the legs.
2. RLS symptoms must be aggravated by rest.
3. RLS symptoms must be alleviated by movement, in particular, walking.
4. RLS symptoms must be worse in the evening or night either currently or in the past when the condition first started.

Secondary supporting symptoms include having a first-degree relative with RLS, periodic limb movements (PLMs), and relief with dopaminergic agents.

From: *Current Clinical Neurology: Sleep Disorders in Women: A Guide to Practical Management*
Edited by: H. P. Attarian © Humana Press Inc., Totowa, NJ

Diagnosis is based purely on clinical grounds, with history making up the key component of the evaluation. In light of the impact on women, particularly in pregnancy and menopause, and the necessity of clinical diagnosis, the practitioner caring for women must be able to recognize the symptoms of RLS, complete necessary diagnostic studies, and initiate therapy.

Another disorder that can co-exist and is often confused with RLS is periodic limb movement disorder (PLMD). PLMs are defined according to the International Classification of Sleep Disorders criteria based on five elements. First, the patient has a complaint of insomnia or excessive sleepiness, although he or she may be asymptomatic, with movements witnessed by an observer. Second, repetitive highly stereotyped limb movements are present, usually in the leg, with the characteristic movement of extension of the big toe in combination in the partial flexion of the ankle, knee, and sometimes hip. Third, polysomnograpy (PSG) monitoring demonstrates repetitive episodes of muscle contraction (0.5–5 seconds) separated by 20- to 40- second intervals; arousals or awakenings may be associated with these movements. Fourth, the patient should have no evidence of a medical or mental disorder that can account for the primary complaint. Finally, other sleep disorders may be present, but do not account for the symptoms. The subjective complaints in this disorder are typically limited to poor sleep and insomnia, while a heavy emphasis is placed on PSG evidence of events.

Although periodic limb movements may be noted in patients undergoing PSG for other indications, one must remember that PLMs in the absence of symptoms does not establish the syndrome of RLS. Furthermore, a PLM index of more than 5, generally considered pathological, is commonly found both in normal subjects and in patients with other sleep disorders. In a study of 100 patients including controls, insomniacs, hypersomniacs, narcoleptics, and RLS patients, the prevalence of a PLM index greater than 5 was 55% in controls, 40% in insomniacs, 30% in hypersomniacs, 80% in narcoleptics, and 85% in RLS patients *(3)*.

PLMs are also seen in association with commonly prescribed medications. In a study of nine depressed patients on fluoxetine compared with six depressed patients on no medication, PLMs were observed in 44% of the medicated patients *(4)*. This finding has been demonstrated with other antidepressants. Buporopion, in contrast, has been shown to decrease the number of PLMs in depressed patients with this disorder *(5)*.

In addition to the association with medications, PLMs are also associated with other sleep conditions, such as narcolepsy, rapid eye-movement (REM) behavior disorder, and sleep-disordered breathing, including upper airways resistance syndrome *(6,7)*. In the case of obstructive sleep apnea, however, it is unclear whether PLMs are caused by the associated disorder or are merely associated with the arousals that result from that disorder *(8)*.

PLMD can, under appropriate circumstances, be treated with the same medications used to treat RLS. In the absence of subjective symptoms, however, the benefits of therapy must be carefully evaluated. Furthermore, identification and treatment of associated conditions may be a more prudent initial therapy.

EPIDEMIOLOGY

The prevalence of RLS in the population was originally estimated by Ekbom *(1)* to be 5%, based on his clinical population. More recent estimates place the prevalence somewhere between 6 and 15%. These estimates vary in part as a function of the means used to collect the information, the population surveyed, and the definition of RLS utilized. A population-based telephone survey from Kentucky found that 10% of respondents experienced symptoms at least "often." In this study there was an age-related increase in prevalence, with 3% of those affected being 18–29 years of age and 19% aged 80 or older *(9)*. This study demonstrated no difference between prevalence in men and women. More recent studies have validated the correlation between increasing prevalence of symptoms with increasing age and have also identified a clear gender difference in symptom occurrence and prevalence.

A recent and relatively large survey of 2099 rural primary care patients, designed for the purpose of identifying the prevalence of RLS in a general population, revealed that 24% of patients were positive for all four of the cardinal symptoms used to make the diagnosis of RLS. Furthermore, 15.3% of these patients reported symptoms at least weekly *(10)*. In this study RLS was more common in women (59%), and patients reporting symptoms were significantly older than patients without symptoms.

The demonstration of higher prevalence of RLS symptoms in women is most striking in a study conducted in Germany of more than 4300 individuals. This was a cross-sectional survey with face-to-face interviews and physical examinations. In this study, the overall prevalence of RLS was 10.6%, and women were twice as likely to have the disorder as men *(11)*. Furthermore, parity was associated with the prevalence of symptoms. Nulliparous women had equal prevalence to men up to age 64, but those with one child were twice as likely and those with three or more children were 3.5 times more likely to have the disorder. This study was the first to demonstrate an association with parity, which, along with the association with pregnancy and menopause, provides strong support for the role of sex hormones in the etiology and pathophysiology of the disorder.

Although age and gender now appear to have clear roles in the prevalence of RLS, there also appear to be racial and ethnic differences. In a study of African American and Caucasian Americans undergoing hemodialysis, RLS symptoms were less common in the African Americans *(12)* than in the other ethnic groups. To date, there are no specific studies addressing racial differences in a general population, and this remains an area of active investigation.

Similarly, there are few and relatively small studies of RLS prevalence in nonWestern populations. In a study conducted in Singapore, less than 1% of individuals reported symptoms of RLS *(13)*. In a Japanese study, only 5% reported symptoms of RLS, and symptoms were more common in men *(14)*. In a small study conducted in India, only 6.6% of patients undergoing hemodialysis had symptoms, and 0% of a control group of normal individuals had symptoms *(15)*. These studies appear to measure overall prevalence in Eastern populations as somewhat less than the prevalence in Western populations and implicate a complex pathophysiology with multiple potential etiologies.

Although more prevalent with advancing age, RLS has been well described even in children *(16,17)*, in whom the disorder may be misdiagnosed as growing pains or attention deficit hyperactivity disorder. There are no specific data on gender difference among children.

ETIOLOGY AND PATHOPHYSIOLOGY

As a result of the findings in epidemiological studies, the etiology and pathophysiology of RLS remains an area of intense research. The disorder is commonly encountered as an idiopathic disorder, although it has been associated with a number of medical conditions. These associated medical conditions include pregnancy, fibromyalgia, rheumatic disease, diabetes, renal insufficiency, vascular insufficiency, iron-deficiency anemia, thyroid disease, and others. When associated with a chronic medical condition, the disorder is sometimes referred to as secondary. Although symptoms seem to improve in both idiopathic and secondary RLS with standard therapies, as outlined here, it is unclear if primary and secondary forms result from the same mechanism.

An understanding of the etiology of this disorder has been derived from evaluation of anatomical studies, neurotransmitter systems, and iron metabolism. Further postulated mechanisms are derived from associations with pregnancy and menopause, implicating sex hormones in this disorder.

From detailed studies of the peripheral, spinal, subcortical, and cortical components, RLS appears to result from dopaminergic deficits in the central nervous system. This finding has been most convincingly demonstrated from studies of centrally acting dopaminergic agents, which attenuate symptoms, whereas peripherally acting dopaminergic agents do not *(18)*. The specific mechanism of this phenomenon has not been elucidated.

Similarly, the relationship to iron deficiency has been recognized since the studies of Ekbom *(19)*. Further studies have consistently validated this finding. In a study of 18 elderly patients with RLS and 18 age-matched controls, serum ferritin was significantly lower in RLS patients and correlated with severity of symptoms *(20)*. In another study of 27 patients aged 29–81 years, a ferritin level of less than 50 μg/dL was found in all but one patient and correlated with severity of symptoms *(21)*. In a study examining magnetic resonance imaging estimates of brain iron, individuals with RLS had significantly reduced ferritin levels in the substantia niagra *(22)*.

Because the symptoms of RLS typically occur at night, a circadian-related mechanism has been actively investigated. Serum iron levels have been shown to be decreased by 50% at night *(23)*. Iron is an essential element for the synthesis of dopamine, and dopamine production is increased at night. A prevalent hypothesis is that RLS results from low levels of iron in the brain, which interferes with dopamine synthesis.

The specific localization of dopaminergic dysfunction has been more difficult to elucidate. Functional imaging with single photon emission tomography and positron emission tomography have demonstrated conflicting results related to reduced basal ganglia dopamine receptor binding *(24–26)*. Therefore, despite strong support for the role of central iron and dopamine metabolism in the etiology and pathophysiology of RLS, further investigation is still needed.

In light of the circadian cycling of symptoms and the known circadian cycling of hormones, a causative mechanism involving melatonin has been postulated. Michaud and colleagues have shown that PLMs are associated with salivary melatonin secretion *(27)*. Perhaps paradoxically, however, exogenous melatonin improved PLMs in most patients *(28)*. Further complicating this analysis was the finding that urinary excretion of 6-hydroxy melatonin does not vary in patients with RLS compared with controls *(29)*, and therefore the relationship between RLS and melatonin requires further investigation.

Further support for hormonal regulation of RLS in women comes from the increased prevalence of symptoms in pregnancy. Pregnant women have a two- to threefold higher risk of symptoms than does the general population. The severity of these symptoms is generally highest during the third trimester, and they tend to disappear around the time of delivery. Therefore, in addition to possible etiologies, including iron and folate metabolism, several hormonal changes are prevalent in the third trimester. Prolactin, progesterone, and estrogens are elevated, thus lending support to reports of their role in this disorder. Further research is needed in this area, however, because there is currently no definite evidence of a role for these hormones in the pathogenesis of this disorder.

RLS has been identified as a genetically inherited disorder in some individuals. A family history is present in 40–60% of individuals *(30–32)*. In individuals with a family history of RLS, symptoms tend to begin earlier in life *(33)*. In a large study of mono- and dizygotic twins evaluated for RLS symptoms, heritability was estimated at 54% *(34)*. In a study of 12 monozygotic twins, RLS was concordant in 10 pairs *(35)*. Two genetic linkage studies have been conducted, with one family having a linkage mapped to chromosomes 12q *(36)*, and another to 14q *(37)*. Thus far, however, no specific gene has been identified, and the disorder is likely to result from a complex interplay of multiple genetic factors.

DIAGNOSIS

The diagnostic criteria of RLS, as identified by the International Restless Legs Syndrome Association, are listed in Table 1. Emphasis is placed primarily on the history obtained from the patient and, if available, the information from the patient's bed partner. It is important to differentiate between alternative explanations for extremity discomfort. Such alternative diagnoses include diabetic polyneuropathy, leg cramps, and arthritic pains. Upon excluding these diagnoses, a compatible history is all that is needed—and often all that is available—to make a diagnosis. Patients are generally asymptomatic during daytime visits, and physical examination findings are typically normal. Finally, there are no available laboratory markers that can confirm the diagnosis.

In evaluating for alternative diagnoses, a clinical history is generally sufficient. Pain associated with diabetic neuropathy is present during the day and may simply be exacerbated at night. Pain from arthritis also occurs during the daytime, but it

Table 1
Diagnostic Criteria for RLS

Essential criteria:

1. An urge to move the legs, usually accompanied or caused by uncomfortable or unpleasant sensations in the legs. (Sometimes the urge to move is present without the uncomfortable sensations and sometimes the arms or other body parts are involved in addition to the legs.)
2. The urge to move or unpleasant sensations begin or worsen during periods of rest or inactivity such as lying or sitting.
3. The urge to move or unpleasant sensations are partially or totally relieved by movement, such as walking or stretching, at least as long as the activity continues.
4. The urge to move or unpleasant sensations are worse in the evening or night than during the day or only occur in the evening or night. (When the symptoms are very severe, the worsening at night may not be noticeable, but must have been previously present.)

Supportive features:

1. Family history
2. Response to dopaminergic therapy
3. Periodic limb movements (during wakefulness or sleep)

Associated features:

1. Natural clinical course following certain identifiable patterns
2. Sleep disturbance

also affects the joint(s) more than the distal extremities, is associated with some stiffness, and is generally exacerbated by activity. Leg cramps are typically described as a continual, aching pain in the calves, which is worse at night, worse with walking, and associated with palpable knots in the calf muscles.

In patients with a history compatible with RLS, evaluation for potential secondary causes is also warranted. This evaluation should include a history related to possible anemia, including gastrointestinal blood loss, menstruation, and the like. Determination of serum ferritin level is warranted with treatment, as outlined below. Controversy exists regarding the indication for thyroid evaluation. A higher prevalence was found in patients with hyperthyroidism in one study *(11)*, but routine evaluation in the absence of clinical suspicion is likely not warranted. Because of the high prevalence of PLMs in other disorders, PSG is not indicated unless warranted for the evaluation of other sleep disorders.

Diagnosis in children can be difficult, especially in younger children with limited capacity to conceptualize or articulate symptoms. Given the genetic predisposition of the disorder, in individuals with a family history and complaints of poor sleep, insomnia, or growing pains, a high clinic suspicion is warranted. In this scenario, PLMs identified on PSG may be sufficient for diagnosis and treatment.

MANAGEMENT

The goal of therapy is to reduce the severity of symptoms in order to allow the onset and maintenance of sleep. For individuals with infrequent symptoms or symptoms that do not significantly affect quality of life, therapy may be tailored to behavioral and nonpharmacological therapies. Individuals with frequent symptoms or symptoms causing daytime somnolence should be evaluated for secondary etiologies. Once excluded, patients may benefit from the addition of appropriate pharmacotherapeutic agents. Although several agents have been used in RLS, only ropinirole is approved by the US Food and Drug Administration for treatment of RLS.

As previously mentioned, the initial evaluation of patients thought to have RLS should include an evaluation for anemia and iron deficiency. Correction of iron deficiency may be all that is required to alleviate symptoms and is encouraged as a first-line approach to this disorder. In individuals with anemia secondary to iron deficiency, an evaluation for pathological etiologies of blood loss should be initiated and iron supplementation should be instituted. Ferritin levels should be checked at 3-month intervals, with a goal of achieving a serum ferritin level of 50 µg/L orr more *(21)*. Iron can be prescribed in multiple forms. The cheapest preparation, iron sulfate, can be administered in a 325-mg dose three times a day. Most clinicians recommend taking iron sulfate with concurrent administration of 200 mg of vitamin C to enhance oral absorption. Oral iron can cause constipation and abdominal discomfort. It should be taken on an empty stomach to enhance absorption, but if gastrointestinal discomfort occurs, it can be taken with non-dairy-, non-fiber-containing foods.

Upon elimination or treatment of secondary etiologies of RLS, consideration of nonpharmacological treatments should be considered. Such treatments may include nutritional supplementation, exercise, massage, and sleep hygiene *(38)*. The use of nonpharmacological approaches to symptoms is particularly important for pregnant women. The best methods are usually discovered by patients in the course of the illness, often prior to seeking medical advice. Physical activity such as active stretching prior to bedtime may be of benefit. Hot baths, cold baths, or alternating hot and cold baths may provide some relief of symptoms. Massage can be comforting and alleviate symptoms temporarily. Maintenance of appropriate sleep hygiene is encouraged, because sleep deprivation and fragmentation can exacerbate symptoms. An excellent and up-to-date website for support and medically reviewed information is the Restless Legs Syndrome Foundation website (www.rls.org).

For those attempting to utilize nonpharmacological therapies, the avoidance of several medications and dietary substances will also be of benefit. Elimination or restriction of caffeine, nicotine, alcohol, antihistamines, most antidepressants, older antiemetic agents, and antipychotics may alleviate symptoms.

Although alcohol can promote sleep and reduce RLS symptoms, this effect lasts only 30–90 minutes, and rebound (discussed later) may occur. Although some patients show some improvement from tricyclic and selective serotonin reuptake inhibitor antidepressants, these agents often intensify symptoms *(4)*. For patients with depression or nicotine-withdrawal issues, bupropion may be considered. As previously noted, most antidepressants appear to worsen symptoms. Bupropion, a dopamine-active antidepressant, has been shown in one small study to reduce limb movements *(5)*. H1 antihistamines probably exacerbate RLS symptoms owing to their effects on dopamine receptors. Similarly, older antiemetic agents act on the

Table 2
Agents Used to Treat RLS

Agents	Starting dose (mg)	Dose range (mg)	Class side effects
Dopaminergic agents			
Dopamine precursors			
Carbidopa/levodopa	25/100	25/100–100/400	Rebound Augmentation
Dopamine receptor agonists			
Pramipexole	0.125	0.5–2	Nausea/lightheadedness
Ropinirole	0.25	2–4	Nasal stuffiness Constipation Insomnia
Others			
Opioids			Abuse potential
Oxycodone	5	5–15	Constipation/gastro-
Hydrocodone	5	5–15	intestinal upset
Metadone	5	5–10	Daytime somnolence
Tramadol	50	50–100	
Benzodiazepines			REM sleep suppression
Clonazepam	0.5	0.5–4	Daytime somnolence
Temazepam	15	15–30	Abuse potential
Triazolam	0.125	0.125–0.5	
Nonbenzodiazepine sleeping aids			Atazia
Zolpidem	5	5–10	Hallucinations
Zaleplon	10	10–20	Daytime somnolence
Anticonvulsants			
Gabapentin	200 tid	up to 2700 in divided doses	Daytime somnolence Ataxia

REM, rapid eye movement.

dopaminergic system, thus potentiating symptoms. Newer antiemetic agents, which are selective 5-HT3 receptor antagonists, will likely have little effect on RLS symptoms.

For patients who fail to demonstrate improvement with conservative, nonpharmacological methods, the choice of medication initiated should be focused on providing the most effective symptom relief with the least number of side effects. Table 2 shows the general categories of agents used to treat this disorder.

Although the primary pharmacological agents used have traditionally been dopamine precursors, benzodiazepines, and opioids, newer dopamine receptor agonists are increasingly being used as first-line agents (18), particularly for individuals with frequent, chronic symptoms. Dopamine precursors such as carbidopa/levodopa are still used, but patients frequently experience rebound or augmentation.

Rebound is defined as the tendency for symptoms to worsen at the end of the dosing period. This leads to recurrence of symptoms in the late night or early morning. This phenomenon is most common with short-acting, regular-release preparations of carbidopa/levodopa. Augmentation is defined as the tendency for symptoms to develop earlier in the day and to be more severe than the symptoms that occurred before treatment began. Augmentation is the most common complication of carbidopa/levodopa therapy. It is treated by withdrawal of the agent over a few days, followed by initiation of a dopamine agonist.

The nonergot agonists pramipexole and ropinirole are currently preferred to ergot agonists because of their more favorable side-effect profiles. Ropinirole has been demonstrated in several studies to improve symptoms of RLS *(39,40)*. The typical starting dose is 0.25 mg taken 2 hours prior to major RLS symptom onset. The dose is increased by 0.25 mg every 2–3 days to eliminate symptoms. Most patients typically require 2 mg or less, but some patients may require 4 mg or more. Pramipexole has also been shown to have efficacy in RLS *(41–43)*. Pramipexole is usually initiated at 0.125 mg, taken 2 hours prior to major symptom onset. The dose is increased by 0.125 mg every 2–3 days until symptom relief is achieved. Common daily dosage is usually between 0.375 and 0.75 mg. Augmenation is less common with dopamine agonists than with precursors, but it has been demonstrated in patients taking pramipexole for 2 years *(44)*.

Because of the effectiveness of these dopamine agonists, individuals rarely require treatment with other agents. The use of opioids was described by Willis in the 17th century. Their use has been largely abandoned as a result of the possibility of overuse and dependence. They are, however, generally well tolerated and offer good long-term efficacy *(45)*.

Benzodiazepines also produce an improvement in symptoms and have been used for decades in the treatment of RLS. Similarly, their use has been avoided recently because of the risk of abuse, side effects, and intolerance. Furthermore, benzodiazepines have a detrimental effect on sleep architecture, suppressing REM sleep.

The final class of medications used includes anticonvulsant agents, with gabapentin currently being the most promising. In one small double-blind, placebo-controlled, crossover study, gabapentin significantly improved RLS symptoms and PLMs *(46)*. Dosage requirements may be as high as 2700 mg a day in three divided doses. Patients complaining of pain had the greatest benefit in this study.

For women who are pregnant or who are considering pregnancy, few data on pharmacotherapy for RLS are available. Iron and folate supplementation should be strongly encouraged, not only as part of routine pregnancy counseling, but also because of the beneficial effects on RLS symptoms in pregnancy *(47)*. In individuals having symptoms despite appropriate iron and folate supplementation, the choice of therapeutic agent is somewhat limited.

Dopaminergic agonists and precursors are category C agents; therefore, few data are available on which to base recommendations for or against their use. Benzodiazepines are listed as category D agents, and therefore should be avoided in pregnancy. Among opiates, only oxycodone is a category B agent, with all other commonly utilized opiates being either class C or D. The antiepileptic drugs most commonly used, carbamazepine and gabapentin, belong to categories D and C, respectively. The decision to treat women with RLS during pregnancy, therefore, requires thoughtful discussion about possible risks to the fetus. In women who are not pregnant and who are not attempting to become pregnant, all therapeutic choices are available. Women are encouraged to take precaution in utilizing these medications without proper birth control methods. Fortunately, there are no specific drug interactions with dopaminergic agonists, dopamine precursors, opioids, benzodiazepines, or antiepileptic agents.

CONCLUSION

RLS commonly affects women and can significantly affect sleep and quality of life. The etiology of the disorder is multifactorial, but in women it may be influenced by higher rates of anemia and sex hormone levels. Treatment includes correction of iron deficiency, if present, and both nonpharmacological and pharmacological treatments. Current first-line agents include the nonergotamine dopamine agonists ropinirole and pramipexole. The use of these agents in women who are pregnant or considering pregnancy should be carefully considered due to potential risks to the fetus. Alternative agents are available and may need to be considered if rebound or augmentation occurs.

REFERENCES

1. Ekbom, K., Restless legs: a clinical study. *Acta Med Scand Suppl*, 1945;**158**:1–123.
2. Walters, A.S., Toward a better definition of the restless legs syndrome. The International Restless Legs Syndrome Study Group. *Mov Disord*, 1995;**10**(5):634–642.
3. Montplaisir, J., M. Michaud, R. Denesle, and A.Gosselin, Periodic leg movements are not more prevalent in insomnia or hypersomnia but are specifically associated with sleep disorders involving a dopaminergic impairment. *Sleep Med*, 2000;**1**(2):163–167.
4. Dorsey, C.M., S.E. Lukas, and S.L. Cunningham, Fluoxetine-induced sleep disturbance in depressed patients. *Neuropsychopharmacology*, 1996;**14**(6):437–442.
5. Nofzinger, E.A., A. Fasiczka, S. Berman, and M.E. Thase, Bupropion SR reduces periodic limb movements associated with arousals from sleep in depressed patients with periodic limb movement disorder. *J Clin Psychiatry*, 2000;**61**(11):858–862.
6. Fantini, M.L., M. Michaud, N. Gosselin, G. Lavigne, and J. Montplaisir, Periodic leg movements in REM sleep behavior disorder and related autonomic and EEG activation. *Neurology*, 2002;**59**(12):1889–1894.
7. Exar, E.N. and N.A. Collop, The association of upper airway resistance with periodic limb movements. *Sleep*, 2001;**24**(2):188–192.
8. Baran, A.S., A.C. Richert, A.B. Douglass, W. May, and K. Ansarin, Change in periodic limb movement index during treatment of obstructive sleep apnea with continuous positive airway pressure. *Sleep*, 2003;**26**(6):717–720.
9. Phillips, B., T.Young, L. Finn, K. Asher, W.A. Hening, and C. Purvis, Epidemiology of restless legs symptoms in adults. *Arch Intern Med*, 2000;**60**(14):2137–2141.
10. Nichols, D.A., R.P. Allen, J.H. Grauke, et al., Restless legs syndrome symptoms in primary care: a prevalence study. *Arch Intern Med*, 2003;**63**(19):2323–2329.
11. Berger, K, J. Luedemann, C. Trenkwalder, U. John, and C. Kessler, Sex and the risk of restless legs syndrome in the general population. *Arch Intern Med*, 2004;**164**(2):196–202.
12. Kutner, N.G. and D.L. Bliwise, Restless legs complaint in African-American and Caucasian hemodialysis patients. *Sleep Med*, 2002;**3**(6):497–500.

13. Tan, E.K., A. Seah, S.J. See, E. Lim, M.C. Wong, and K.K. Koh, Restless legs syndrome in an Asian population: a study in Singapore. *Mov Disord*, 2001;**16**(3):577–579.

14. Kageyama, T, M. Kabuto, H. Nitta, et al., Prevalences of periodic limb movement-like and restless legs-like symptoms among Japanese adults. *Psychiatry Clin Neurosci*, 2000;**4**(3):296–298.

15. Bhowmik, D., M. Bhatia, S. Gupta, S.K. Agarwal, S.C. Tiwari, and S.C. Dash, Restless legs syndrome in hemodialysis patients in India: a case controlled study. *Sleep Med*, 2003;**4**(2):143–146.

16. Rajaram, S.S., A.S. Walters, S.J. England, D. Mehta, and F. Nizam, Some children with growing pains may actually have restless legs syndrome. *Sleep*, 2004;**27**(4):767–773.

17. Walters, A.S., D.L. Picchietti, B.L. Ehrenberg, and M.L. Wagner, Restless legs syndrome in childhood and adolescence. *Pediatr Neurol*, 1994;**11**(3):241–245.

18. Hening, W., R. Allen, C. Earley, C. Kushida, D. Icchietti, and M. Silber, The treatment of restless legs syndrome and periodic limb movement disorder. An American Academy of Sleep Medicine Review. *Sleep*, 1999;**22**(7):970–999.

19. Ekbom, K.A., Restless legs syndrome. *Neurology*, 1960;**10**:868–873.

20. O'Keeffe, S.T., K.Gavin, and J.N. Lavan, Iron status and restless legs syndrome in the elderly. *Age Ageing*, 1994;**23**(3):200–203.

21. Sun, E.R., C.A. Chen, G. Ho, C.J. Earley, and R.P. Allen, Iron and the restless legs syndrome. *Sleep*, 1998;**21**(4):371–377.

22. Allen, R.P., P.B. Barker, F. Wehrl, H.K. Song, and C.J. Earley, MRI measurement of brain iron in patients with restless legs syndrome. *Neurology*, 2001;**56**(2):263–265.

23. Tarquini, B., Iron metabolism: clinical chroniological aspects. *Chronobiologia*, 1978;**5**:315–336.

24. Ruottinen, H.M., M. Partinen, C. Hublin, et al., An FDOPA PET study in patients with periodic limb movement disorder and restless legs syndrome. *Neurology*, 2000;**54**(2):502–504.

25. Turjanski, N., A.J. Lees, and D.J. Brooks, Striatal dopaminergic function in restless legs syndrome: 18F-dopa and 11C-raclopride PET studies. *Neurology*, 1999;**52**(5):932–937.

26. Eisensehr, I., T.C. Wetter, R. Linke, et al., Normal IPT and IBZM SPECT in drug-naive and levodopa-treated idiopathic restless legs syndrome. *Neurology*, 2001;**57**(7):1307–1309.

27. Michaud, M., M. Dumont, B. Selmaoui, J. Paquet, M.L. Fantini, and J. Montplaisir, Circadian rhythm of restless legs syndrome: relationship with biological markers. *Ann Neurol*, 2004;**55**(3):372–380.

28. Kunz, D., and F. Bes, Exogenous melatonin in periodic limb movement disorder: an open clinical trial and a hypothesis. *Sleep*, 2001;**24**(2):183–187.

29. Tribl, G.G., F. Waldhauser, T. Sycha, E. Auff, and J. Zeitlhofer, Urinary 6-hydroxy-melatonin-sulfate excretion and circadian rhythm in patients with restless legs syndrome. *J Pineal Res*, 2003;**35**(4):295–296.

30. Ondo, W. and J. Jankovic, Restless legs syndrome: clinicoetiologic correlates. *Neurology*, 1996;**47**(6):1435–1441.

31. Walters, A.S., K. Hickey, J. Maltzman, et al., A questionnaire study of 138 patients with restless legs syndrome: the 'Night-Walkers' survey. *Neurology*, 1996;**46**(1):92–95.

32. Winkelmann, J., T.C. Wetter, V. Collado-Seidel, et al., Clinical characteristics and frequency of the hereditary restless legs syndrome in a population of 300 patients. *Sleep*, 2000;**23**(5):597–602.

33. Bassetti, C.L., D. M auerhofer, M. Gugger, J. Mathis, and C.W. Hess, Restless legs syndrome: a clinical study of 55 patients. *Eur Neurol*, 2001;**45**(2):67–74.

34. Desai, A.V., L.F.Cherkas, T.D. Spector, and A.J. Williams, Genetic influences in self-reported symptoms of obstructive sleep apnoea and restless legs: a twin study. *Twin Res*, 2004;**7**(6):589–595.

35. Ondo, W.G., K.D. Vuong, and Q. Wang, Restless legs syndrome in monozygotic twins: clinical correlates. *Neurology*, 2000;**55**(9):1404–1406.

36. Desautels, A., G. Turecki, J. Montplaisir, A. Sequeira, A. Verner, and G.A. Rouleau, Identification of a major susceptibility locus for restless legs syndrome on chromosome 12q. *Am J Hum Genet*, 2001;**69**(6):1266–1270.

37. Bonati, M.T., L. Ferini-Strambi, P. Aridon, A .Oldani, M. Zucconi, and G. Casari, Autosomal dominant restless legs syndrome maps on chromosome 14q. *Brain*, 2003;**126**(Pt 6):1485–1492.

38. Paulson, G.W. Restless legs syndrome. How to provide symptom relief with drug and nondrug therapies. *Geriatrics*, 2000;**55**(4):35–47.
39. Trenkwalder, C., D. Garcia-Borreguero, P. Montagna, et al., Ropinirole in the treatment of restless legs syndrome: results from the TREAT RLS 1 study, a 12 week, randomised, placebo controlled study in 10 European countries. *J Neurol Neurosurg Psychiatry*, 2004;**75**(1):92–97.
40. Adler, C.H., R.A. Hauser, K. Seth, et al., Ropinirole for restless legs syndrome: a placebo-controlled crossover trial. *Neurology,* 2004;**62**(8):1405–1407.
41. Lin, S.C., J. Kaplan, C.D. Burger, and P.A. Fredrickson, Effect of pramipexole in treatment of resistant restless legs syndrome. *Mayo Clin Proc*, 1998;**73**(6):497–500.
42. Becker, P.M., W. Ondo, and D. Sharon, Encouraging initial response of restless legs syndrome to pramipexole. *Neurology*, 1998;**51**(4):1221–1223.
43. Montplaisir, J., R. Denesle, and D. Petit, Pramipexole in the treatment of restless legs syndrome: a follow-up study. *Eur J Neurol*, 2000;**7** (Suppl 1):27–31.
44. Winkelman, J.W. and L. Johnston, Augmentation and tolerance with long-term pramipexole treatment of restless legs syndrome (RLS). *Sleep Med*, 2004;**5**(1):9–14.
45. Walters, A.S., J. Winkelmann, C. Trenkwalder, et al., Long-term follow-up on restless legs syndrome patients treated with opioids. *Mov Disord*, 2001;**16**(6):1105–1109.
46. Garcia-Borreguero, D., O. Larrosa, de la LY, K. Verger, X. Masramon, and G. Hernandez, Treatment of restless legs syndrome with gabapentin: a double-blind, cross-over study. *Neurology*, 2002;**59**(10):1573–1579.
47. Lee, K.A., M.E. Zaffke, and K. Baratte-Beebe, Restless legs syndrome and sleep disturbance during pregnancy: the role of folate and iron. *J Womens Health Gend Based Med*, 2001;**10**(4):335–341.

9

Nonhormonal Treatments for Insomnia

Catherine C. Schuman

INTRODUCTION

Insomnia is a common and growing complaint; 54% of adults report experiencing at least one symptom of insomnia a few nights a week, and 33% of adults report experiencing at least one symptom every night, according to the National Sleep Foundation's 2005 Sleep in America poll *(1)*. Of those adults experiencing at least one symptom of insomnia a few nights a week, women comprise 57%, whereas men comprise 51% *(1)*, although women are 1.5 times more likely than men to experience insomnia when using full diagnostic criteria *(2)*.

Insomnia is a disruption in sleep that is defined as difficulty initiating and/or maintaining sleep or the complaint of nonrestorative sleep that causes clinically significant distress or impairment in functioning *(3)*. Sleep disruption may present as difficulty falling asleep, awakenings during the night with delays in returning to sleep, early morning awakening, decreased total sleep time, and increased ratio of time in bed to sleep time, and/or a decrease in the restorative nature of sleep. The disruption can be caused by psychiatric, medical, or developmental disorders, environmental factors, and medication reactions.

There are three major classification systems for insomnia that have led to some confusion when comparing research findings because the results are affected by the definitions of insomnia and the populations examined. For the purposes of this chapter, we use the criteria laid out in the fourth edition of the *Diagnostic and Statistical Manual of Mental Disorders* (DSM-IV-TR) *(3)*, which defines primary insomnia as a predominant complaint of difficulty initiating or maintaining sleep, or nonrestorative sleep for at least 1 month. The sleep disturbance must cause clinically significant distress or impairment in important daily functions and not occur exclusively during an additional sleep, mental, or medical disorder and not be the physiological result of a substance. The other major classification systems used by professionals include the second edition of *The International Classification of Sleep Disorders (3a)*, and 10th revision of the *International Statistical Classifications of Diseases and Related Health Problems (3b)*.

From: *Current Clinical Neurology: Sleep Disorders in Women: A Guide to Practical Management*
Edited by: H. P. Attarian © Humana Press Inc., Totowa, NJ

TREATMENTS

Pharmacological treatments are often the first line of treatment used when patients present with insomnia. However, cognitive–behavioral therapies (CBTs) have been shown to have effects comparable to medical interventions in the short term and substantially better effects over time *(4–6)*.

Cognitive–Behavioral Therapies

CBT uses a myriad of techniques to improve sleep, including sleep restriction, stimulus control, sleep hygiene, diaphragmatic breathing and relaxation training, and cognitive therapy. In individualized combinations, CBTs are effective in addressing the complex factors of the "3 Ps" model: the predispose, precipitate, and perpetuate factors of insomnia *(7)*. Treatment is usually started with an initial evaluation that lasts 60–90 minutes, followed by 5–12 sessions lasting 50 minutes each. Treatment tends to last longer when there are simultaneous sleep, mental, or medical disorders.

Insomnia usually starts with a psychological, social, or medical stressor and is then perpetuated, sometimes for long periods of time, by heightened arousal and conditioning. To start the process of treatment, it is beneficial to begin with a baseline measurement of the individual's sleep using a sleep log; a sample sleep log that we use at the University of Vermont and the Vermont Regional Sleep Center, a division of Fletcher Allen Health Care, is shown in Fig. 1. The sleep log monitors bedtime, sleep-onset latency, number and length of awakenings, wake time, time to get out of bed, substance intake, exercise, and medication use. Generally speaking, it is important to start with improving the complaint of difficulty initiating or maintaining sleep by first focusing on changing sleep behaviors, with less of an emphasis on changing cognitive factors, but, as sleep improves, shifting the focus to cognitive changes with less of an emphasis on sleep behaviors. For most patients, it is good to start with sleep restrictions, stimulus control, and good sleep hygiene behaviors, which may be combined with medication. Once patients start to experience even the slightest improvement in their sleep, they are more open to work on cognitive treatment.

Sleep restriction, stimulus control, and relaxation techniques can easily be taught to a variety of health care providers, but it is often helpful to seek the care of a clinical psychologist who is part of a multidisciplinary team in a sleep clinic or a clinical psychologist who specializes in sleep. The specialized training of a psychologist with a behavioral medicine background is uniquely beneficial in addressing the psychological, medical, and behavioral issues involved in insomnia. It may seem fairly easy to describe these treatments to a patient, but the patient must be motivated and the therapist must have the skill and ability to educate the patient in a way that allows the patient to persevere through the uncomfortable periods of treatment. If you do not have the luxury of a multidisciplinary team, it is recommended that a psychologist or psychiatrist be available for easy referral in the event that a mental disorder is either exacerbated or impeding treatment.

Sleep Restriction

Sleep restriction is useful in consolidating sleep because it works on both initiation and maintenance issues. It focuses on the amount of time in bed vs the amount of time sleeping and reconditioning the bed and bedroom as being a place for sleep.

It is essential to have at least a 1-week sleep diary, and preferably a 2-week diary, to accurately calculate the average actual time sleeping vs time in bed. Once the sleep log is completed, the average time sleeping is calculated by adding hours slept and dividing by days recorded. The average time sleeping becomes the window of time that the patient is allowed to sleep. One should not recommend a less than a 5-hour window of time in bed except under extraordinary conditions. If the actual average time sleeping is less than 5 hours, the window of time in bed becomes 5 hours. This process leads to an initial decrease in the time sleeping caused by the decrease in time in bed, which results in increased sleepiness and daytime fatigue. The increase in sleepiness then translates into more time sleeping during the window of time in bed. The changes in time can be measured using the process initially described by Spielman et al. *(7)*, in which a sleep efficiency ratio is calculated by dividing the total sleep time by the total time in bed and multiplying by 100. Spielman et al. *(7)* recommend that as the sleep efficiency ratio reaches 90%, 15 minutes of sleep be added per week;when the ratio falls below 85% sleep time should be decreased by 15 minutes. When calculating the ratio on a weekly basis, the additional time can be changed to 30-minute increments until the patient indicates a feeling of being rested.

Stimulus Control

Stimulus control is useful in increasing a restorative sleep pattern by addressing both initiation and maintenance issues. This treatment, developed by Bootzin and Nicassio *(8)*, focuses on stimuli that affect patients' sleeping patterns, including many items that patients have introduced to help initiate and gain more sleep. In an effort to improve their sleep, many patients end up conditioning themselves not to sleep by engaging in a plethora of activities, including spending increasing amounts of time in bed, taking naps during the day, and engaging in stimulating activities in bed such as reading and watching television.

The main idea behind this treatment is to recondition the patient to sleep in his or her bedroom by focusing on the patient's environment and behaviors. This treatment is based on learning theory. Stimulus control is often used in conjunction with sleep restriction to achieve synergistic results. When using stimulus control, the patient is instructed to (1) get into bed only when sleepy, (2) only use the bed for sleep and sexual activity and avoid activities such as reading and watching television, (3) if not asleep within 10 minutes of going to bed or after an awakening, get out of bed and only return to the bedroom when feeling sleepy, (4) get out of bed consistently when awake for more than 10 minutes and get out of bed at the same time every day, and (5) take no naps during the day.

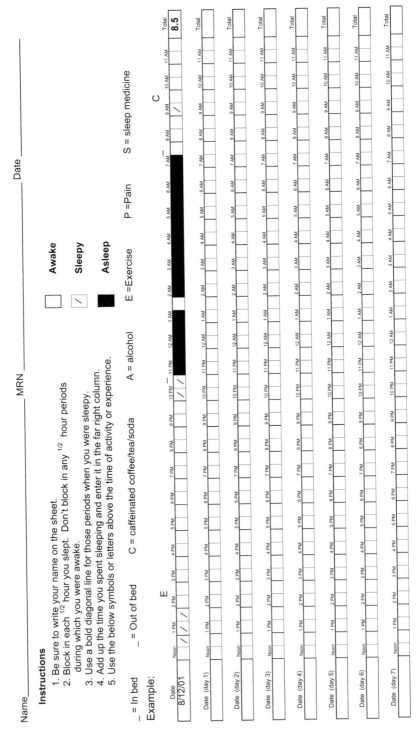

Name _____ MRN _____ Date _____

Instructions

1. Be sure to write your name on the sheet.
2. Block in each $^{1/2}$ hour you slept. Don't block in any $^{1/2}$ hour periods during which you were awake.
3. Use a bold diagonal line for those periods when you were sleepy.
4. Add up the time you spent sleeping and enter it in the far right column.
5. Use the below symbols or letters above the time of activity or experience.

☐ Awake | ╱ Sleepy | ■ Asleep

_ = In bed   _ = Out of bed   C = caffeinated coffee/tea/soda   A = alcohol   E =Exercise   P =Pain   S = sleep medicine

Example:

Date	Noon	1 PM	2 PM	3 PM	4 PM	5 PM	6 PM	7 PM	8 PM	9 PM	10 PM	11 PM	12 AM	1 AM	2 AM	3 AM	4 AM	5 AM	6 AM	7 AM	8 AM	9 AM	10 AM	11 AM	Total
Date (day 8)																									
Date (day 9)																									
Date (day 10)																									
Date (day 11)																									
Date (day 12)																									
Date (day 13)																									
Date (day 14)																									

Fig. 1. Sleep log.

Sleep Hygiene

Every clinic and provider has its own list of lifestyle and environmental factors that, if followed, will aid in providing a condition where sleep is more likely, but all sleep hygiene lists include a core group of behaviors that have been shown to improve the likeliness of sleep. At the University of Vermont and the Vermont Regional Sleep Center, we encourage individuals experiencing primary insomnia to follow certain behaviors (*see* below). An important caveat to building a therapeutic alliance and willingness to change ingrained behaviors is to use a framework of 2–4 weeks during which the patient will change their behaviors. It is important for individuals to know that there is an end in sight and that they have control. Also, it is helpful to stress that the changes are not necessarily permanent and that once a good sleeping pattern is restored, the patient may be able to engage in many of his or her original behaviors. If patients make a hierarchical list of all the behaviors they do not want to change and attempt to step them back into their routine one behavior per week to determine what they can and cannot do and maintain good restorative sleep, they are much more willing to engage in change. Sometimes flexibility is very important to patients, and they would rather take an extra week or two to incorporate the new behaviors, acknowledging the consequence of an extended period to achieve consolidated and restorative sleep.

Good Sleep Hygiene Behaviors
1. Only go to bed when you are tired, and set a consistent wake time every day of the week.
2. Only use your bed and bedroom for sleep or sexual activity and sleep nowhere but your bed. Move televisions, computers, and stereos out of the bedroom. No eating, reading, or relaxing in the bedroom.
3. Leave the bedroom for awakenings longer than 20 minutes and engage only in nonstimulating tasks. Remember, your only job during awakenings is to get yourself back to sleep.
4. During awakenings, keep lights low or off.
5. Avoid naps at any time unless safety or health is an issue.
6. Prepare your bedroom to be a relaxing, quiet, calming, and sleep-conducive place. Be aware of light, noise, and temperature in the bedroom.
7. Avoid all alcohol.
8. Avoid smoking tobacco products.
9. Avoid all caffeinated products, including coffee, tea, soda, chocolate, and over-the-counter (OTC) medications.
10. Avoid excessive consumption of liquids within 2 hours of bedtime.
11. Engage in regular exercise (with that occurring 5–6 hours prior to bedtime being the most beneficial).
12. Eat a balanced diet at regular intervals. Do not go to bed hungry.
13. If you find yourself watching the clock, turn it away or put it on the floor.
14. Take time prior to going to bed to review and let go of negative thoughts and worries. If you are worried about falling asleep, it will interfere with the sleep process.
15. Set up a pre-bedtime routine that signals to your body that it is time to sleep.

Cognitive Therapy

Individuals who experience insomnia tend to experience high arousals associated with stressors in their life. During these periods of high arousal, they tend to experience difficulty initiating and maintaining sleep. During these episodes of disrupted sleep, they tend to focus on their inability to sleep for long enough periods to feel rested. The anxiety and negative ruminations concerning sleep eventually become the focus of an insomniac's description of sleep. Insomnia has been thought of as merely a symptom of a psychological disorder such as anxiety and depression, but we now know that insomnia is also a predisposing factor to psychological disorders. Cognitive therapy and CBT have become the gold standard in treating depression, anxiety, and disorders involving autonomic arousal. It is helpful to educate and introduce relaxation with imagery and diaphragmatic breathing as a way to experience immediate change in symptoms of arousal by addressing the activated sympathetic nervous system and teaching patients to activate the parasympathetic nervous system, which in turn deactivates the sympathetic nervous system. Once they have experienced the relatively immediate decrease in arousal, it is important to educate them as to how their thoughts affect the nervous system and eventually their endocrine system.

The focus of this treatment is to educate the patient about the process of how negative thoughts affect emotions and how negative emotions affect behavior. With some practice, patients become very good at identifying negative thoughts that they may have initially denied having because they were unaware of their automatic thoughts. One way to aid patients in identifying negative thoughts is to have them keep a log for a week or two in which they identify how they responded cognitively, emotionally, and behaviorally to events. Once patients are able to identify their negative thoughts, it is important to teach them how to shift their negative thoughts to more positive ones. This process is facilitated by having them respond to every negative thought with four positive ones that specifically refute the negative thought. It is most useful when the patient keeps this in a small notebook that they can easily carry with them. Patients are initially instructed to fill out the easier parts of the log, and the rest is completed in session. Eventually, patients are able to shift their automatic negative thoughts to more positive ones, and their negative thoughts start to stand out more as being different.

Diaphragmatic Breathing and Relaxation Therapy

The physiological arousal that goes along with insomnia can be addressed using diaphragmatic breathing, progressive muscle relaxation, and self-hypnosis. As explained in the section on CBT, it is important to explain how the use of therapies can decrease the arousal that can affect and be affected by insomnia. Patients are instructed in the process of initiating diaphragmatic breathing or belly breathing vs short, shallow chest breaths. Patients are also instructed in the method of using progressive muscle relaxation to decrease their arousal, which is simply a process of starting at one end of the body and focusing on each muscle group by tensing and releasing to give patients a sense of how much they are tensing their bodies and what tension feels like in their muscles. Clinical experience with patients who have experienced chronic pain and medical disorders has led to a slight modification in this process. It can be useful to just have the patient focus on the body part and then release any tension from that area without tensing, because when patients have been tensing their muscles chronically, the traditional progressive muscle relaxation can lead to muscle spasms. If patients have a negative experience, such as a spasms, while relaxing, it is important to depict this as a signal of how much tension they have been carrying in their bodies and suggest that as they practice they will have more positive experiences. Self-hypnosis is another useful tool that can be used to teach patients to become more aware of their bodies and turn down the arousal using imagery. As with all treatment, it is important to have an experienced provider who is able to provide a safe environment in which patients can allow themselves to let their guard down. Knowing how to teach relaxation and being able to provide a safe experience once relaxation has occurred are two different processes. Individuals with chronic psychological histories are at risk of emotional degeneration when their shields have been disarmed hastily or should treatments be perceived as ineffective.

Pharmacological Treatments

It bears repeating that CBTs have been shown to have effects comparable to medical interventions in the short term and substantially better effects over time for insomnia *(4–6)*. Despite this information, pharmacological modalities have often been the first line of treatment. Ideally, pharmacological treatments are used to elicit a more rapid decrease in sleep deficits while at the same time pursuing longer lasting effects using CBTs.

When treating patients who are experiencing insomnia, it is important to keep in mind that 25–30% self-medicate with either alcohol, OTC hypnotics, or a combination of the two *(9)*. Alcohol is the most common substance used when self-medicating for insomnia. With this information in mind, it is important to educate even the most unsuspecting and denying patient of its deleterious effects on sleep.

Even though there are no reliable studies showing the efficacy of antihistamines or other OTC hypnotics in treating insomnia, they are the most used and most recommended hypnotics. Diphenhydramine is the active ingredient in most OTC hypnotics, but unfortunately it has significant adverse effects and impairs driving performance more than alcohol *(10)*.

Pharmacological treatments of insomnia consist of hypnotic medications, including benzodiazepines and benzodiazepine receptor agonists, as well as antidepressants, herbals, and a new class of medication—an MT1/MT2 receptor agonist—which are usually categorized as short-acting, intermediate-acting, and long-acting (*see* Table 1). Each medication has properties that, when used correctly or in combination with other treatments, can give an optimal outcome. However, each medication has side effects that need to be taken into consideration when prescribing.

Benzodiazepines include, in order of increasing half-life: Halcion® (triazolam), Restoril® (temazepam), Prosom® (estazolam), Doral® (quazepam), and Dalmane® (flurazepam). Until the advent of the benzodiazepine receptor agonist, benzodiazepines were the only hypnotics of choice for insomnia. Benzodiazepine receptor agonist medications include, in order of increasing half-life: Sonata® (zaleplon),

Table 1
Benzodiazepines Approved in the United Sates for the Treatment of Insomina

Drug	Elimination half-life (h)	Peak plasma level	Active metabolites
Short-acting			
Sonata® (zaleplon)	1	60 min	No
Ambien® (zolpidem)	2.2	1.5 h	No
Dalmane® (flurazepam)	2.3	20 min	Yes
Intermediate-acting			
Halcion® (triazolam)	1.5–5.5	15–30 min	No
Lunesta® (eszopiclone)	6	60 min	No
Long-acting			
Restoril® (temazepam)	8–15	30–60 min	No
Prosom® (estazolam)	10–15	0.5–2 h	No
Doral® (quazepam)	39	2 h	Yes

Ambien® (zolpidem), and Lunesta® (eszopiclone). Benzodiazepines and benzodiazepine receptor agonist medications differ from each other mainly in their speed of absorption and elimination half-life (*see* Table 1). All of the benzodiazepine receptor agonists have been shown to be effective and safe hypnotics with minimal adverse effects and with no dependence, withdrawal, tolerance, or rebound insomnia over long-term use *(11–15)*.

Sedating antidepressants are frequently used as off-label prescriptions to treat primary insomnia, usually because of concerns of tolerance, addiction, and dependence associated with benzodiazepines. They can be very helpful when treating secondary insomnia as it relates to psychological disorders such as depression and anxiety. Elavil® (amitriptyline) and Desyrel® (trazodone) are the primary antidepressants used for this purpose. However, Desyrel (trazodone) is currently the only available antidepressant that has literature to supports its use for insomnia, and its half-life is biphasic and lasts 3–6 hours and 5–9 hours *(16,17)*. Unfortunately, Desyrel (trazodone) has a side effect of increased slow-wave sleep, delaying rapid eye-movement sleep and increasing daytime sedation as the result of a long half-life that does not change the objective duration of sleep but does decrease the quality of sleep *(18)*. Desyrel (trazodone) often causes residual daytime sedation and can cause rebound insomnia, but does not tend to worsen other sleep disorders, such as restless legs syndrome (RLS) and periodic limb movement disorder. There is also no evidence that Desyrel (trazodone) improves sleep in patients with primary insomnia without co-morbid depression *(14)*. Tricyclics as a category tend to result in lingering daytime sedation after nighttime administration and also tend to worsen other sleep disorders, such as RLS, which ultimately makes them a poor treatment choice for primary insomnia. Table 2 more fully addresses the differences between benzodiazepines, benzodiazepine receptor agonists, and other treatment options, indicating their speed of absorption and elimination half-life.

Table 2
Antidepressants and Herbals Used for the Treatment of Insomnia

Drug	Elimination half-life (h)	Peak plasma level	Active metabolites
Antidepressants			
Desyrel® (Trazodone)	3–6, 5–9		No
Elavil® (Amitriptyline)	10–26	4–5 h	Yes
Herbals			
Melatonin	1	60 min	No
Valerian root	Pending	Pending	Pending
New melatonin receptor agonist			
Rozerem® (Ramelteon)	1–2.6	45 min	Yes

Melatonin is a treatment that has some supporting evidence, indicating that it may be helpful in the treatment of age-related insomnia *(19)* and for chronic sleep-onset insomnia in children *(20)*. However, there are no data to support its use as a wide-spectrum hypnotic for primary insomnia *(21–24)*. Valerian root is another OTC treatment often used by insomniacs that has received mixed results from the literature. A few studies have found it to show clinically significant polygraphic and subjective improvement in sleep *(25–29)*. Valerian root has also been shown to improve sleep after benzodiazepine withdrawal *(30)*.

Ramelteon, a new medication, is a melatonin receptor agonist statistically found to significantly reduce latency to persistent sleep. It has shown no evidence of next-day residual psychomotor, memory, or cognitive side effects *(31)*.

CONCLUSION

Although women are more likely than men to experience insomnia, it is important to understand that nonhormonal treatments do not vary according to gender. There are many effective and widely available treatments for insomnia, and it is important that we adequately assess and offer those treatments, including both pharmacological and CBTs.

REFERENCES

1. National Sleep Foundation. *Sleep in America Poll.* www.sleepfoundation.org/content/hottopics/2005summaryoffindings.pdf, 2005.
2. Doghramji, P.P., Detection of insomnia in primary care. *J Clin Psychiatry*, 2001;**62** (Suppl 10):18–26.
3. Anonymous, Sleep disorders. In: *Diagnostic and Statistical Manual of Mental Disorders*, Washington DC: American Psychiatric Publishing. 2000:597–662.
3a. American Academy of Sleep Medicine, The International Classification of Sleep Disorders, Revised Diagnostic and Coding Manual. 2nd ed. Chicago, IL: Author; 2005.
3b. World Health Organization, F50-F59: Behavioural syndromes associated with psychological disturbances and physical factors. The International Statistical Classification of Diseases and Related Health Problems, 10th revision. 1992:174–197.

4. McClusky, H.Y., J.B. Milby, P.K. Scoitzer, V. Williams, and V. Wooten, Efficacy of behavioral versus triazolam treatment in persistent sleep-onset insomnia. *Am J Psychiatry*, 1991;**148**(1):121–126.

5. Morin, C.M., C. Colecchi, J. Stone, R. Sood, and D. Brink, Behavioral and pharmacological therapies for late-life insomnia: a randomized controlled trial. *JAMA*, 1999;**281**(11):991–999.

6. Smith, M.T., M.L. Perlis, A. Park, et al., Comparative meta-analysis of pharmacotherapy and behavior therapy for persistent insomnia. *Am J Psychiat*ry, 2002;**159**(1):5–11.

7. Spielman, A.J., L.S. Caruso, and P.B. Glovinsky, A behavioral perspective on insomnia treatment. *Psychiatr Clin North Am*, 1987;**10**(4):541–553.

8. Bootzin, R.R. and Nicassio, P.M., Behavioral treatments for insomnia. In: *Progress in Behavior Modification* (M. Hersen, R. Eissler, P. Miller, eds.). 1978:1–45.

9. Roehrs, T., E. Hollebeek, C. Drake, and T. Roth, Substance use for insomnia in metropolitan Detroit. *J Psychosom Res*, 2002;**53**(1):571–576.

10. Weiler, J.M., J.R. Bloomfield, G.G. Woodworth, et al., Effects of fexofenadine, diphenhydramine, and alcohol on driving performance. A randomized, placebo-controlled trial in the Iowa driving simulator. *Ann Intern Med*, 2000;**132**(5):354–363.

11. Hedner, J., R. Yaeche, G. Emilien, I. Farr, and E. Salinas, Zaleplon shortens subjective sleep latency and improves subjective sleep quality in elderly patients with insomnia. The Zaleplon Clinical Investigator Study Group. *Int J Geriatr Psychiatry*, 2000;**15**(8):704–712.

12. Israel, A.G. and J.A. Kramer, Safety of zaleplon in the treatment of insomnia. *Ann Pharmacother*, 2002;**36**(5):852–859.

13. Krystal, A.D., J.K. Walsh, E. Laska, et al., Sustained efficacy of eszopiclone over 6 months of nightly treatment: results of a randomized, double-blind, placebo-controlled study in adults with chronic insomnia. *Sleep*, 2003;**26**(7):793–799.

14. Mendelson, W.B., T. Roth, S. Cassella, et al., The treatment of chronic insomnia: drug indications, chronic use and abuse liability. Summary of a 2001 New Clinical Drug Evaluation Unit meeting symposium. *Sleep Med Rev*, 2004;**8**(1):7–17.

15. Saletu-Zyhlarz, G., P. Anderer, N. Brandstatter, et al., Placebo-controlled sleep laboratory studies on the acute effects of zolpidem on objective and subjective sleep and awakening quality in nonorganic insomnia related to neurotic and stress-related disorder. *Neuropsychobiology*, 2000;**41**(3):139–148.

16. Saletu-Zyhlarz, G.M., M.H. Abu-Baker, P. Anderer, et al., Insomnia in depression: differences in objective and subjective sleep and awakening quality to normal controls and acute effects of trazodone. *Prog Neuropsychopharmacol Biol Psychiatry*, 2002;**26**(2):249–260.

17. Saletu-Zyhlarz, G.M., M.H. Abu-Baker, P. Anderer, et al., Insomnia related to dysthymia: polysomnographic and psychometric comparison with normal controls and acute therapeutic trials with trazodone. *Neuropsychobiology*, 2001;**44**(3):139–149.

18. Montgomery, I., I. Oswald, K. Morgan, and K. Adam, Trazodone enhances sleep in subjective quality but not in objective duration. *Br J Clin Pharmacol*, 1983;**16**(2):139–144.

19. Zhdanova, I.V., R.J. Wortman, M.M. Regan, J.A. Taylor, J.P. Shi, and O.U. Leclair, Melatonin treatment for age-related insomnia. *J Clin Endocrinol Metab*, 2001;**86**(10):4727–4730.

20. Smits, M.G., E.E. Nagtegaal, J. van der Heijden, A.M. Coenen, and G.A. Kerkhof, Melatonin for chronic sleep onset insomnia in children: a randomized placebo-controlled trial. *J Child Neurol*, 2001;**16**(2):86–92.

21. Almeida Montes, L.G., H.P. Ontiveros Uribe, J. Cortes Sotres, and G. Heinze Martin, Treatment of primary insomnia with melatonin: a double-blind, placebo-controlled, crossover study. *J Psychiatry Neurosci*, 2003;**28**(3):191–196.

22. Arendt, J., Complex effects of melatonin. *Therapie*, 1998;**53**(5):479–488.

23. Sack, R.L., A.J. Lewy, and R.J. Hughes, Use of melatonin for sleep and circadian rhythm disorders. *Ann Med*, 1998;**30**(1):115–121.

24. Stone, B.M., C. Turner, S.L. Mills, and A.N. Nicholson, Hypnotic activity of melatonin. *Sleep*, 2000;**23**(5):663–669.

25. Doghramji, P.P., Treatment of insomnia with zaleplon, a novel sleep medication. *Int J Clin Pract*, 2001;**55**(5):329–334.

26. Donath, F., S. Quispe, K. Diefenbach, A. Maurer, I. Fietze, and I. Roots, Critical evaluation of the effect of valerian extract on sleep structure and sleep quality. *Pharmacopsychiatry*, 2000;**33**(2):47–53.

27. Dorn, M., (Efficacy and tolerability of Baldrian versus oxazepam in non-organic and non-psychiatric insomniacs: a randomised, double-blind, clinical, comparative study). *Forsch Komplementarmed Klass Naturheilkd*, 2000;**7**(2):79–84.

28. Fussel, A., A. Wolf, and A. Brattstrom, Effect of a fixed valerian-Hop extract combination (Ze 91019) on sleep polygraphy in patients with non-organic insomnia: a pilot study. *Eur J Med Res*, 2000;**5**(9):385–390.

29. Ziegler, G., M. Ploch, A. Miettinen-Baumann, and W. Collett, Efficacy and tolerability of valerian extract LI 156 compared with oxazepam in the treatment of non-organic insomnia—a randomized, double-blind, comparative clinical study. *Eur J Med Res*, 2002;**7**(11):480–486.

30. Poyares, D.R., C. Guilleminault, M.M. Ohayon, and S. Tufik, Can valerian improve the sleep of insomniacs after benzodiazepine withdrawal? *Prog Neuropsychopharmacol Biol Psychiatry*, 2002;**26**(3):539–545.

31. Zammit, G., T. Roth, M. Erman, S. Sainati, S. Weigand, and J. Zhang, Polysomnography and outpatient study to determine the efficacy of Ramelten in adults with chronic insomnia. 2005;**227**.

10

Obstructive Sleep Apnea–Hypopnea Syndrome in Premenopausal Women

Kanika Bagai and Beth A. Malow

INTRODUCTION

Obstructive sleep apnea–hypopnea syndrome (OSAHS) is characterized by recurrent sleep-induced collapsibility of the pharyngeal airway. Normal adult women (20–45 years of age) are a cohort of women in whom menstrual cycles, use of oral contraceptives, pregnancy, and lactation are associated with a varied hormonal environment. These differences in hormonal status may, in turn, potentially change the likelihood of development of OSAHS in premenopausal women. The clinical spectrum of sleep-disordered breathing (SDB) includes apnea, hypopnea, and upper airway resistance syndrome (UARS).

PREVALENCE

The prevalence of OSAHS in premenopause is low (0.5%, according to an interview and polysomnography-based survey in a large cohort of women) (1). Interestingly, postmenopausal women on hormone replacement were found to have a similar low prevalence in the same study (0.5%). In these two groups, sleep apnea was exclusively associated with obesity (defined as body mass index [BMI] ≥32.3 kg/m^2). The prevalence of obstructive sleep apnea (OSA) was significantly higher (2.7%) in postmenopausal women not on hormone replacement.

In another study comparing the prevalence and severity of sleep apnea between premenopausal (n = 797) and postmenopausal (n = 518) women, Dancey et al. (2) found that postmenopausal women had a higher prevalence of OSAHS (47 vs 21% in premenopausal women, with OSA defined as apnea–hypopnea index [AHI] >10 per hour). In the same study, BMI and neck circumference were higher in postmenopausal women with sleep apnea than in premenopausal women with sleep apnea. Whereas AHI increased with BMI and neck circumference in both groups, in premenopausal women the relationship between BMI and AHI was less linear, with a steep slope in the most obese range. The relationship between neck cir-

From: *Current Clinical Neurology: Sleep Disorders in Women: A Guide to Practical Management*
Edited by: H. P. Attarian © Humana Press Inc., Totowa, NJ

cumference and AHI was similar in both groups. Furthermore, sleep apnea severity was noted to be higher in the postmenopausal group, even after adjusting for neck circumference and BMI, suggesting functional differences in the upper airway between the two groups.

In the Wisconsin Sleep Cohort Study *(3)* *(N* = 589), the prevalence of SDB, indicated by AHI cut points of 5–15 events per hour, increased across menopausal categories: 10.8% in premenopausal, 18.4% in perimenopausal, 27% in perimenopausal/postmenopausal, and 29.1% in postmenopausal women, respectively. Therefore, menopause seems to increase and premenopausal status and hormone replacement to decrease the risk for sleep apnea, suggesting an important role of hormones in the pathogenesis of OSA.

EFFECT OF HORMONES ON SLEEP AND BREATHING AND ROLE OF HORMONES IN PATHOGENESIS OF OSAHS

Progesterone

The effect of progesterone on sleep in experimental models resembles that of benzo-diazepines. Non-rapid eye-movement (NREM) sleep latency is shortened, low-frequency (τ and δ) electroencephalogram activity is reduced, and high-frequency (>10 Hz) activity is increased. High doses of progesterone suppress REM sleep in rats *(4)*.

Progesterone is a respiratory stimulant. Basal minute ventilation and ventilatory responsiveness to hypercarbia were augmented in men receiving medroxyprogesterone acetate, a synthetic progesterone used to stimulate respiration in high-altitude poly-cythemia, chronic obstructive pulmonary disease, and the obesity–hypoventilation syndrome. In nonhypercapnic men with OSA, however, medroxyprogesterone did not reduce apnea frequency, duration, or arterial oxygen desaturation *(5)*.

Women experience an increase in ventilatory drive during the luteal phase of the menstrual cycle and during pregnancy. This is thought to be secondary to the increased levels of progesterone *(6,7)*.

Popovic and White *(8)* determined the level of the awake genioglossus elec-tromyogram and upper airway resistance in 12 premenopausal and 12 postmeno-pausal women under basal conditions and during the application of an inspiratory resistive load. They determined that the waking peak phasic and tonic genioglossus electromyographic (EMG) activity in women tended to be higher in the luteal phase of the menstrual cycle, lower in the follicular phase, and lowest in the postmeno-pausal phase. There was a weak but significant positive correlation between proges-terone levels and both peak phasic and tonic EMG activity. They concluded that female hormones (possibly progesterone) have a substantial impact on upper air-way dilator muscle activity. They did not, however, study the effect of sleep on upper airway tone.

Estrogen

Estrogen may have an indirect influence in the control of breathing. Estradiol, via an upregulation of progesterone receptors, may enhance the respiratory stimu-lant effects of progesterone *(9)*.

Small patient numbers limit almost all of the studies comparing the effect of hormone replacement therapy (HRT) on the severity of sleep apnea, and the results have been varied. In a group of nine healthy, surgically postmenopausal women, Pickett et al. *(10)* found that combined estrogen–progestin treatment was superior to placebo in reducing episodes of SDB and in decreasing the duration of hypopneas. Cistulli et al. *(11)* could not show any benefit with estrogen or with combined estrogen–progestin treatment in 15 postmenopausal women with moderate OSA. A recent pilot study *(12)* evaluated four postmenopausal women and one perimenopausal woman with clinical symptoms and OSAHS, with polysomnography before and after HRT (estradiol and trimegeston). The subjects had a 75% mean reduction of the severity of sleep apnea as measured by AHI. The variable results of HRT in different studies possibly indicate variability in hormone metabolism in different individuals. Further studies comparing the effects of estrogen replacement and combined HRT are needed to clarify the role of estrogens in the control of breathing and sleep apnea syndrome.

Estrogen replacement therapy has been reported to cause a worsening of asthma symptoms in postmenopausal women with mild-to-moderate asthma. In a study by Lange et al. *(13)*, a weak but positive association was reported between HRT and self-reported asthma and asthma-like symptoms.

Estrogen deficiency has been suggested to play a role in menopause-associated changes in body fat distribution. During the menopause transition, estrogen levels decline while the ovary continues to secrete small amounts of androgens. Both overall body fat and upper body adiposity have been associated with increased testosterone levels. In some studies, HRT attenuated the menopause-related acceleration of adipose tissue deposits, which has been attributed to decreased lipoprotein lipase activity *(14)*. Hormone treatment with either unopposed estrogen or with estrogen in combination with progesterone stimulated liprotein lipase activity, minimizing adipose tissue deposits. Changes in body fat distribution, especially in the neck region, influence upper airway muscle tone and may facilitate OSA.

GENDER DIFFERENCES IN UPPER AIRWAY RESISTANCE

Gender plays a role in determining the incidence of OSA in men and women. This has been attributed to the differences in upper airway function during sleep in patients with OSA.

Trinder et al. *(15)* studied changes in ventilation and upper airway resistance (UAR) both during sleep onset and over a full NREM sleep period from wakefulness to slow-wave sleep (SWS) in a group of 14 men and 14 women. Airflow was measured by attaching the mask to a pneumotachograph. UAR was calculated by using simultaneous recordings of airflow, mask pressure, and epiglottal pressure. They found that changes in ventilation and UAR from wakefulness to early stage 2 NREM sleep were similar in male and female subjects. Once NREM sleep became established and developed to SWS, the pattern of change in UAR varied between men and women. In men, there was a progressive increment in UAR over the sleep period, whereas in women UAR during SWS remained at a level similar to, or only slightly above, that observed in subjects who did not obtain SWS. Ventilation was maintained at similar levels despite the marked difference in UAR. This difference in the effect of sleep on upper airway muscle activity in males and females may contribute to a male predisposition to SDB.

In a study of UAR and dimensions in healthy young and old men and women *(16)*, young women (mean age 27 ± 1 [18–34]) had narrower airways at all sites compared with young men and older men and women in both sitting and supine positions. Young women had a greater percentage increase in oropharyngeal resistance at high flows between awake and NREM sleep compared with young men. Total respiratory resistance increased between awake and REM sleep in young women and older men only. However, when overall changes from awake to sleep were considered, there were no significant differences between groups of younger and older men and women, and therefore, the significance of these findings is not known.

Obesity predisposes to OSA. Even though women have greater total body fat and are more likely to be obese than men, the prevalence of OSA is higher in men. In a study *(17)* comparing the upper airway size in 78 male and 52 female patients, both oropharyngeal junction and pharyngeal cross-sectional areas were significantly smaller in females than in male patients with comparable BMI. There was no correlation between BMI and pharyngeal size in either gender. There was a positive correlation between BMI and AHI in both men and women. Obesity may predispose to UAR through mass loading and alteration of tissue characteristics, in addition to fat deposition. Other studies *(18)* have shown that normal men, despite larger pharyngeal areas as compared with normal women, have a higher pharyngeal resistance than women. This may be the result of gender differences in airway compliance and tissue characteristics.

SYMPTOMS

The most common presenting symptoms of OSA are loud snoring, excessive daytime sleepiness, choking arousals, restless sleep, and witnessed apneas. All aspects of quality of life, from physical and emotional health to social functioning, are markedly impaired by OSA *(19)*. Other symptoms in premenopausal women can include mood disturbances, irritability, disrupted social interactions, reduced libido, nocturia with disrupted nocturnal sleep, morning headaches, and dry mouth upon awakening. In one study, 43% of women reported menstrual irregularities *(20)*. As many as 40% of the women with SDB disorder attributed divorce or dissolution of a romantic relationship to their chronic sleepiness and fatigue, and their social isolation to a physical and not a psychiatric problem, such as depression.

SBD in women may be poorly recognized because women are more likely than men to complain of fatigue and morning headache, less likely to report restless sleep, or have been told of witnessed apneas during sleep *(21)*. Despite daytime sleepiness, women are more likely to complain of difficulty falling asleep, and their concerns may be attributed to insomnia.

Before referral to a physician, women tend to have sleepiness or other symptoms related to SDB for 9.7 ± 3.1 years. The problem receives faster attention in elderly or obese women *(20)*. When a population with mild OSA and sleepiness was analyzed, 72% of the men were initially given the diagnosis of hypersomnolence or narcolepsy, and one was diagnosed as chronic fatigue syndrome. In contrast, 53% of the women were initially diagnosed and treated for chronic fatigue syndrome *(20)*. Some groups have found that because women are vastly underdiagnosed, they tend to present with considerably more severe and greater coexisting medical problems. In some series, hypothyroidism was present in almost 20% of the women with OSA *(22)*.

SIGNS

Morbid obesity is the dominant factor for the appearance of OSAHS in premenopausal women. In one study *(23)* with 27 women (one-third of whom were premenopausal) referred to a sleep disorder clinic for clear symptoms of OSA syndrome, the women with OSAHS were found to be much more overweight than the 110 men with OSAHS.

Schellenberg et al. *(24)* studied the physical findings and risk for OSA in 420 patients. They tried to identify the upper airway bony and soft tissue structural abnormalities by physical examination (lateral pharyngeal wall narrowing, tonsillar enlargement, enlargement of the uvula or tongue, low-lying palate, retrognathia, or overjet) associated with an increased risk for OSAHS. After controlling for BMI and neck circumference, narrowing of the airway by the lateral pharyngeal walls and tonsillar enlargement had a significant statistical association (odds ratio 2.0 and 2.6, respectively) with OSA. A subgroup analysis studying differences between men and women showed that no oropharyngeal risk factor achieved significance in women, whereas lateral narrowing was the sole independent risk factor in men. This study, however, did not distinguish the characteristics of pre- and postmenopausal women.

Another study *(25)* compared 10 premenopausal women with 13 postmenopausal women and 32 men with OSAHS. Two premenopausal women had structural abnormalities of the pharynx, and the remaining eight were significantly more obese than the men with OSA. Thus, premenopausal women with OSAHS were more likely than men and postmenopausal women to have structural abnormalities of the upper airway and to be extremely obese.

ADVERSE CONSEQUENCES

OSA has many adverse consequences. Several studies have implicated OSA as a risk factor for the development of hypertension and cardiovascular disease *(26,27)*. A study of a large community-based cohort of 6132 subjects indicated that SDB was associated with systemic hypertension in middle-aged and older individuals of different genders and ethnic backgrounds *(27)*. A prospective study found a dose–response relationship between OSA and the presence of hypertension 4 years later that was independent of confounding variables *(28)*. Muscle sympathetic nerve activity and nocturnal norepinephrine levels are elevated and thought to be a possible cause for OSA-induced hypertension. OSA has been associated with an increased risk for transient ischemic events and strokes *(29)*. Intracranial pressures may rise secondary to apneic events, contributing to morning headaches, cognitive impairment, or vascular complications. Dysmenorrhea and amenorrhea are complaints in some women with OSA and may improve with treatment. Finally, there is a strong association between OSA and the risk for motor vehicle accidents *(30)*.

SLEEP APNEA RELATED TO MENSTRUAL CYCLE

Menstrual cycle fluctuations in progesterone influence ventilation. During the luteal phase of the menstrual cycle, women have a greater central chemoreceptor drive. Both minute ventilation and ventilatory responsiveness to hypercapnia increase during this phase, presumably because of the physiological rise in progesterone *(31)*. However, these ventilatory effects do not ameliorate OSAHS. In studies of premenopausal women with OSAHS, there were no changes in the rate or length of apneas or hypopneas or in oxygen desaturation throughout the menstrual cycle during NREM sleep *(31)*. Only marginal improvements in these parameters occurred during REM sleep in the luteal phase of the cycle. However, mean arterial pressure responses to apneic events increased significantly in the luteal phase as compared with the follicular phase for both NREM and REM sleep. In women with obesity or anatomically narrow airways, progesterone protects the airways from obstruction by acting as a respiratory stimulant, although this protective effect is counterbalanced by factors that exacerbates upper airway obstruction *(32)*.

SLEEP APNEA RELATED TO PREGNANCY AND PRE-ECLAMPSIA

Pregnancy affects sleep-related respiration independent of changes in sleep *(33)*. Some variables are detrimental, whereas others are protective. Detrimental variables include weight gain, uterine enlargement, and nasal obstruction. Weight gain during pregnancy has been correlated with increased upper airway obstruction during laryngoscopy and with increased difficulty with obstetrical intubation *(34)*. Apart from weight gain, the most obvious mechanical abnormality causing respiratory changes during pregnancy is the enlarging uterus, which elevates the diaphragm. The effect is a decrease in expiratory reserve volume and residual volume, which cause a decrease in the functional residual capacity. This decrease can potentially produce shunting and hypoxemia, as well as reduced lung oxygen stores, contributing to hypoxemia during hypoventilation *(33)*. During the second and third trimester, nasal obstruction is very common. Increased estrogen levels cause hyperemia and edema of the nasal mucosa with increased secretions. The increased resistance to airflow in the nasopharynx contributes to OSAHS and UARS by creating excessive negative pressure in the collapsible pharyngeal airway.

Protective variables include an increased ventilatory drive from circulating progesterone (reviewed previously), avoidance of the supine position later in pregnancy owing to discomfort, decreased REM sleep (a state during which sleep apnea may occur preferentially because of upper airway hypotonia) as a result of the effects of high levels of estrogen and progesterone, and the rightward shift of the oxyhemoglobin dissociation curve, which enhances oxygenation to the fetal circulation.

The precise incidence and consequences of SDB during pregnancy are unknown. Polysomnographic studies performed on six pregnant women at 36 weeks gestation and at postpartum showed that oxygenation was well maintained and that the frequency of apneas and hypopneas was significantly reduced during pregnancy *(35)*. These findings were observed despite reduced functional residual capacity and residual volume, increased alveolar–arterial differences for oxygen, and reduced cardiac output in the supine position.

Several studies have reported an increase in self-reported snoring in pregnancy. A questionnaire study reported frequent snoring as being common in 350 pregnant women compared with 110 age-matched nonpregnant women, but snoring mothers were not at an increased risk for delivering infants with fetal compromise *(36)*. In a separate investigation of 502 women screened on the day of delivery with a questionnaire, 23% reported snoring nightly, 14% developed hypertension (compared with only 6% of nonsnorers), and 10% developed pre-eclampsia (vs 4% of nonsnorers). Witnessed apneas were observed in 11% of habitual snorers, compared to 2% of nonsnorers. Intrauterine growth retardation occurred in 7.1% of the infants of snoring mothers and 2.6% of the remaining infants. Despite the limitations of the study, it suggests that the consequences of UAR could affect the fetus *(37)*.

Maasilta et al. *(38)* evaluated SBD in obese (mean prepregnancy BMI >30 kg/m^2) and nonobese (mean BMI 20–25 kg/m^2) pregnant women. During early pregnancy, there were significant differences in the AHI: 1.7 events per hour in the obese group vs 0.2 events per hour in the nonobese pregnant group ($p = 0.05$). There were significant differences in the snoring frequency—32% vs 1% ($p < 0.001$)—between obese and nonobese pregnant women.

Izci et al. *(39)* studied upper airway dimensions in 37 women with pre-eclampsia and 50 nonpregnant and 50 pregnant women in their third trimester. Snoring was reported by 75% of the women with pre-eclampsia. Women with pre-eclampsia had upper airway narrowing in both upright and supine postures as compared with nonpregnant and pregnant women. These changes could contribute to the upper airway resistance episodes during sleep in women with pre-eclampsia. These alterations during sleep could further increase the blood pressure of this group of pregnant women.

SLEEP APNEA RELATED TO POLYCYSTIC OVARY SYNDROME

Polycystic ovary syndrome (PCOS) is a common endocrine disorder of premenopausal women, clinically characterized by oligomenorrhea, signs of androgen excess, and insulin resistance. Obesity is seen commonly in these women and is frequently central (increased waist-to-hip ratio).

Vgontzas et al. *(40)* compared the polysomnograms of 53 women with PCOS (age range 16–45 years) and 452 control premenopausal women without PCOS (20–42 years). PCOS patients were 30 times more likely to suffer from SDB than controls, even when corrected for BMI differences between the two groups. In addition, PCOS patients reported more frequent daytime sleepiness than the controls (80.4 vs 27.0%; $p < 0.001$). The subgroup of PCOS patients, who were recommended to seek treatment for SDB, had significantly higher fasting plasma insulin levels and lower glucose-to-insulin ratios compared with patients who did not receive treatment. Plasma-free and total testosterone and fasting blood glucose concentrations were not different between the two subgroups of PCOS women. It was concluded that higher fasting plasma insulin levels and low glucose-to-insulin ratio could be a stronger marker of sleep apnea than testosterone levels in this group of premenopausal women. Other case series *(41)* have confirmed the higher prevalence of sleep apnea symptoms and higher AHI in patients with PCOS compared with women without PCOS.

SLEEP APNEA RELATED TO HYPOTHYROIDISM

Routine testing for hypothyroidism in women with symptoms of SDB is unlikely to be useful *(42)*. However, it is important to recognize that hypothyroidism predisposes to OSAHS. Patients with hypothyroidism should be screened for possible OSAHS with questions regarding snoring and daytime somnolence. If clinically suspected, this should be confirmed with overnight polysomnography.

GENDER DIFFERENCES IN THE POLYSOMNOGRAPHIC FEATURES OF OSA

In several studies, women demonstrate a lower AHI compared with BMI- and age-matched men *(43,44)*. Ware and colleagues *(44)* found that both young and middle-aged women had fewer apneic events compared with men of similar age, but older women (60–88 years) had apnea severity similar to that of age-matched older men. They postulated that menopausal status and upper airway muscle tone might have played a role. Female gender and younger age seem to confer benefit by preventing airway collapse in spite of an increased BMI. In other words, for a given value of AHI, women can be more obese than men.

Along the same lines, Walker et al. *(45)* found a weaker correlation between AHI and BMI in women than in men. They postulated that weight loss in women, therefore, might not be associated with as marked an improvement in apnea severity compared to men.

In a retrospective study of 830 patients, O'Connor and colleagues *(46)* studied the influence of gender on the polysomnographic features of OSA. They found that OSAHS is less severe in women because of milder OSA during NREM sleep and because women had a greater clustering of respiratory events during REM sleep compared with men. They found that REM-related OSA (mild OSA that occurred predominantly during REM sleep with total AHI 5–15 events per hour, AHI REM/AHI NREM greater than 2 and AHI NREM less than 15 events per hour) was disproportionately more common in women that in men. Supine OSA (OSA of any severity that occurred predominantly in the supine position) was disproportionately more common in men than in women. They further compared the REM difference for men and women within different ranges of BMI (<30, 30–40, >40 kg/m^2) and found no significant effect of BMI.

PREMENOPAUSAL VS POSTMENOPAUSAL OSAHS

In the Wisconsin Sleep Cohort Study *(47)*, perimenopausal and postmenopausal women were twice as likely to be dissatisfied with their sleep as compared with premenopausal women, but menopause was not associated with decreased sleep quality as assessed by polysomnography. As the severity of SDB indicated by AHI categories increased, sleep architecture became less favorable in both pre- and post-menopausal women. At any AHI level, postmenopausal women had more favorable objectively measured sleep quality than did premenopausal women. Thus, menopause is not independently associated with objectively measured diminished sleep quality, and abnormal sleep in midlife women should not be treated as a simple menopausal symptom.

Management

The decision to treat patients should be based on the symptoms and signs of OSAHS and the polysomnography results. Methods used to treat sleep apnea include behavioral treatment, including weight loss; treatment of nasal symptoms; continuous positive airway pressure (CPAP); oral appliances; and surgery.

Behavioral Treatment

It is important to identify any coexisting conditions that contribute to or promote upper airway collapsibility. The same lifestyle modifications recommended to patients with OSAHS apply to the treatment of premenopausal women.

Weight Loss

An association has been noted between OSAHS in premenopausal women and a higher BMI and neck circumference. Dancey et al. *(2)* noted a steep increase in AHI with increasing BMI in the most obese women. It has also been noted that pre-eclamptic women were heavier than healthy pregnant and nonpregnant women and had higher BMIs than the healthy pregnant women before pregnancy *(48)*.

Weight loss, using a combination of diet change and exercise, is of prime importance in decreasing the severity of OSAHS. The degree of weight reduction that will result in an improvement of the AHI varies, and even modest weight loss can result in substantial benefits in some patients *(49)*. Bariatric surgery has consistently been shown to cause significant improvement in sleep apnea severity *(50)*.

Positional Treatment

Sleeping on the side is recommended to prevent the tongue from falling back in the supine position and decreasing upper airway dimensions. It is also the preferred body position during sleep in pregnant women to prevent pressure on the inferior vena cava by the gravid uterus. Elevation of the head of the bed can also be useful.

Avoidance of Agents That Promote Upper Airway Collapsibility

Alcohol should be avoided for at least 6 hours before bedtime. Sedatives and heavy meals should also be avoided before bedtime. Sleep deprivation should be avoided as it increases sleep drive on subsequent nights.

Treatment of Nasal Symptoms

It is important to promptly treat allergic symptoms, which cause nasal congestion, as they compound upper airway obstruction. A trial of an inhaled nasal steroid, such as fluticasone with or without a nonsedating antihistamine, should be used for 4–6 weeks. Surgery may be indicated for a deviated nasal septum or turbinate hypertrophy. Smoking cessation should be encouraged to improve upper airway health.

Continuous Positive Airway Pressure

CPAP is considered the gold standard for the treatment of moderate to severe sleep apnea. In 1994, the American Thoracic Society (ATS) published an official statement on the use of CPAP in sleep apnea syndromes and reported that CPAP is effective in the treatment of patients with clinically important OSAHS and that it is a safe, effective form of therapy with rare complications. The ATS did not present specific diagnostic criteria, but noted that patients with more than 20 apneas or hypopneas per hour have been selected for studies examining clinical responses to treatment.

In 1999, Loube and colleagues *(51)* published a consensus statement indicating that CPAP treatment should be indicated for all OSA patients with a respiratory disturbance index score (RDI) of 30 events per hour, regardless of symptoms, based on the increased risk of hypertension evident from the Wisconsin Sleep Cohort data. They further stated that treatment with CPAP is indicated for patients with an RDI of 5–30 events per hour accompanied by symptoms of excessive daytime sleepiness, impaired cognition, mood disorders, insomnia, or documented cardiovascular diseases including hypertension, ischemic heart disease, or stroke.

In a study of 334 women with SBD *(20)*, treatment with CPAP led to improvement in sleepiness in all cases as well as other symptoms, including dysmenorrhea in the premenopausal group.

CPAP has been tried as the first-line therapy for UARS and is often used as a therapeutic trial to demonstrate improvement in symptoms. In a randomized study conducted on postmenopausal women with UARS and chronic insomnia, radiofrequency reduction of nasal turbinates or turbinectomy or a trial of CPAP showed better relief in daytime fatigue than behavioral treatment alone at 6 months *(52)*. Some patients with UARS may benefit from CPAP treatment even with a normal apnea index and absence of snoring *(50)*.

In pregnant women with pre-eclampsia, low-level autosetting nasal continuous positive airway pressure has been safely and effectively used to eliminate inspiratory flow limitation, resulting in a significant lowering of nocturnal blood pressure *(53)*.

Oral Appliances

Oral appliances can be used for the improvement of snoring, OSA, or both. The possible mechanisms include mandibular repositioning, tongue advancement, and alteration of palatal and mandibular position or dynamics. According to the American Sleep Disorders Association practice parameters for the use of oral appliances in the treatment of snoring and OSA *(54)*, oral appliances are indicated for use in patients with primary snoring or mild OSA who do not respond to or are not appropriate candidates for treatment with behavioral measures such as weight loss or sleep-position change. Oral appliances may also be useful during the period of weight loss or adaptation to sleep-position changes. Oral appliances can also achieve satisfactory outcomes in UARS *(55)*. It is recommended that patients with moderate to severe OSA should have an initial trial of nasal CPAP because greater effectiveness has been shown with CPAP than with the use of oral appliances.

Oral appliances are also indicated for patients with moderate to severe OSA who are intolerant of or refuse treatment with nasal CPAP and for patients who refuse or are not candidates for tonsillectomy and adenoidectomy, cranofacial operations, or tracheostomy. Follow-up polysomnography is not indicated for patients with either primary snoring or mild OSA unless symptoms worsen or do not resolve. However, patients with moderate to severe OSA should undergo polysomnography to ensure therapeutic benefit with the oral appliance in place after final adjustments of fit have been performed and should have follow-up office visits to monitor compliance.

Oral appliances may cause a worsening of OSA in some patients, and appropriate follow-up care is therefore essential. Intolerance and improper use of the device are potential problems for patients using oral appliances, which require patient effort to use properly. Oral appliances may aggravate temporomandibular joint disease and may cause dental misalignment and discomforts that are unique to each device.

Surgery

According to the American Sleep Disorders Association practice parameters *(56)*, nasal positive airway pressure is the recommended therapy for patients with moderate to severe OSA. Nasal positive airway pressure may also be the preference of symptomatic patients with mild apnea. Surgery is indicated to treat OSA in patients who have an underlying specific surgically correctable abnormality that is causing the sleep apnea. Surgery may be indicated to treat OSA in patients for whom other noninvasive treatments have been unsuccessful or have been rejected, who desire surgery, and who are medically stable to undergo the procedure.

Uvulopalatopharyngoplasty, whether performed by traditional or laser-assisted method, has been shown to have variable effectiveness. It is not recommended as a sole therapy in patients with severe sleep apnea. Patients need to be carefully selected in order to minimize failure rates, and the procedure should only be performed when nonsurgical treatment options, such as nasal positive airway pressure, have been considered.

Upper-airway surgery, including tonsillectomy and adenoidectomy, craniofacial operations, including sagittal mandibular osteotomy and genioglossal advancement with or without hyoid myotomy and suspension, and tracheotomy may be indicated for patients for whom these operations are predicted to be highly effective in treating sleep apnea. Inadequate data are available on the effectiveness of laser midline glossectomy and lingualplasty.

The patient should be advised about potential surgical success rates and complications, the availability of alternative treatment options, such as nasal positive airway pressure and oral appliances, and the levels of effectiveness and success rates of these alternative treatments.

REFERENCES

1. Bixler, E.O., A.N. Vgontzas, H.M. Lin, et al., Prevalence of sleep-disordered breathing in women: effects of gender. *Am J Respir Crit Care Med*, 2001;**163**(3 Pt 1):608–613.

2. Dancey, D.R., P.J. Hanly, C. Soong, B. Lee, and V. Hoffstein, Impact of menopause on the prevalence and severity of sleep apnea. *Chest*, 2001;**120**(1):151–155.

3. Young, T., L. Finn, D. Austin, and A. Peterson, Menopausal status and sleep-disordered breathing in the Wisconsin Sleep Cohort Study. *Am J Respir Crit Care Med*, 2003;**167**:1181–1185.

4. Lancel, M., J. Faulhaber, F. Josboer, and R. Rupprecht, Progesterone induces changes in sleep comparable to those of agonistic GABA A receptor modulators. *Am J Physiol*, 1996;**271**:E763–E772.

5. Rajagopal, K., P. Abbrecht, and B. Jabbari, Effects of medroxyorogesterone acetate in obstructive sleep apnea. *Chest*, 1986;**909**(6):815–821.

6. White, D., N. Douglas, C. Pickett, J. Weil, and C. Zwillich, Hypoxic ventilatory response during sleep in normal premenopausal women. *Am Rev Respir Dis*, 1982;**126**:530–553.

7. Brownell, L., P. West, and M. Kruger, Breathing during sleep on normal pregnant women. *Am Rev Respir Dis*, 1986;**133**:38–41.

8. Popovic, R.M. and D.P. White, Influence of gender on waking genioglossus electromyogram and upper airway resistance. *Am J Respir Crit Care Med*, 1995;**152**:725–731.

9. Leavitt, W.W. and G.C. Blaha, An estrogen-stimulated, progesterone-binding system in the hamster uterus and vagina. *Steroids*, 1972;**19**:263–274.

10. Pickett, C.K., J.G. Regensteiner, W.D. Woodard, et al., Progestin and estrogen reduce sleep-disordered breathing in postmenopausal women. *J Appl Physiol*, 1989;**66**:1656–1661.

11. Cistulli, P.A., D.J. Barnes, R.R. Grunstein, and C.E. Sullivan, Effect of short-term hormone replacement in the treatment of obstructive sleep apnea in postmenopausal women. *Thorax*, 1994;**49**:699–702.

12. Wesstrom, J., J. Ulfberg, and S. Nilsson, Sleep apnea and hormone replacement therapy: a pilot study and a literature review. *Acta Obstet Gynecol Scand*, 2005;**84**(1):54–57.

13. Lange, P., J. Parner, E. Prescott, et al., Exogenous female sex steroid hormones and risk of asthma and asthma-like symptoms: a cross sectional study of the general population. *Thorax*, 2001;**56**:613–616.

14. Tchernof, A. and E.T. Poehlman, Effect of menopause transition on body fatness and body fat distribution. *Obesity Res*, 1998;**6**:246–254.

15. Trinder, J., A. Kay, J. Kleiman, Gender differences in airway resistance during sleep. *J Appl Physiol*, 1997;**83** (6):1986–1997.

16. Thurnheer, R., P.K. Wraith, and N.J. Doughlas, Influence of age and gender on upper airway resistance in NREM and REM sleep. *J Appl Physiol*, 2001;**90**:981–988.

17. Mohsenin, V., Gender differences in the expression of sleep-disordered breathing: role of upper airway dimensions. *Chest*, 2001;**120**(5):1442–1447.

18. Pillar, G., A. Malhotra, R. Fogel, et al., Airway mechanics and ventilation in response to resistive loading during sleep. *Am J Respir Crit Care Med*, 2001;**163**:1627–1632.

19. D'Ambrosio, C., T. Bowman, and V. Mohsenin, Quality of life in patients with obstructive sleep apnea. Effect of nasal continuous positive airway pressure—a prospective study. *Chest*, 1999;**115**:123–129.

20. Guilleminault, C., R. Stoohs, Y. Kim, R. Chervin, J. Black, and A. Clerk, Upper airway sleep disordered breathing in women. *Ann Intern Med*, 1995;**122**:493–501.

21. Ambrogetti, A., L. Olson, and N. Saunders, Differences in the symptoms of men and women with obstructive sleep apnea. *Aust NZ J Med*, 1991;**21**:863–866.

22. Halvarson, D.J. and E.S. Porubsky, Obstructive sleep apnea in women. *Otolaryngol Head Neck Surg*, 1998;**119**(5):497–501.

23. Guilleminault, C., M.-A. Quera-Salva, M. Partinen, and A. Jamieson, Women and the obstructive sleep apnea syndrome. *Chest*, 1998;**93**:104–109.

24. Schellenberg, J.B., G. Maislin, and R.J. Schwab, Physical findings and the risk for obstructive sleep apnea. The importance of oropharyngeal structures. *Am J Respir Crit Care Med*, 2000;**162**:740–748.

25. Wilhoit, S.C. and P.M. Suratt, Obstructive sleep apnea in premenopausal women. A comparison with men and with postmenopausal women. *Chest*, 1987;**91**(5):654–658.

26. Redline, S. and K.P. Strohl, Recognition and consequences of obstructive sleep apnea hypopnea syndrome. *Clin Sleep Med*, 1998;**19**:1–19.

27. Nieto, F.J., T.B. Young, B.K. Lind, et al., Association of sleep-disordered breathing, sleep apnea, and hypertension in a large community-based study. *JAMA*, 2000;**283**:1829–1836.
28. Pepperd, P.E., T. Young, M. Plata, and J. Skatrud, Prospective study of the association between sleep-disordered breathing and hypertension. *N Engl J Med*, **342**:1378–1384.
29. Bassetti, C. and M.S. Aldrich, Sleep apnea in acute cerebrovascular diseases. Final report on 128 patients. *Sleep*, 1999;**22**:217–223.
30. Teran-Santos, J., A. Jimenez-Gomez, and J. Cordero-Guevara, The association between sleep apnea and the risk of traffic accidents. *N Engl J Med*, 1999;**340**:847–851.
31. Edwards, N., I. Wilcox, and C. Sullivan, Sleep apnea in women. *Thorax*, 1998;**53**:S12–S15 .
32. Charbonneau, M., T. Falcone, M. Cosio, and R. Levy, Obstructive sleep apnea during pregnancy: therapy and implications for fetal health. *Am Rev Respir Dis*, 1991;**144**:461–463.
33. Feinsilver, S.H. and G. Hertz, Respiration during sleep in pregnancy. *Clin Chest Med*, 1992;**13**:637–644.
34. Pilkington, S., F. Carli, M. Dakin, et al., Increase in Mallampati score during pregnancy. *Br J Anesth*, 1995;**74**:638–642.
35. Brownell, L., P. West, and M. Kryger, Breathing during sleep in normal pregnant women. *Am Rev Respir Dis*, **133**:38–41.
36. Loube, D.I., J.S. Pceta, M.C. Morales, M.D. Peacokc, and M.M. Mitler, Self reported snoring in pregnancy: association with fetal outcome. *Chest*, 1996;**109**:885–889.
37. Franklin, K.A., P.A .Holmgran, F. Jonsson, N. Poromaa, H. Stenlund, and E. Svanborg, Snoring, pregnancy-induced hypertension, and growth retardation of the fetus. *Chest*, 2000;**117**:137–141.
38. Maasilta, P., A. Bachour, K. Teramo, et al., Sleep-related disordered breathing during pregnancy in obese women. *Chest*, 2001;**120**:1448–1454.
39. Izci, B, R.L. Riha, S.E. Martin, et al., The upper airway in pregnancy and preeclampsia. *Am J Respir Crit Care Med*, 2003;**167**:137–140.
40. Vgontzas, A.N., R.S. Legro, E.O. Bixler, A. Grayev, A. Kales, and G.P.Chrousos, Polycystic ovarian syndrome is associated with obstructive sleep apnea and daytime sleepiness: role of insulin resistance. *J Clin Endocrinol Metab*, 2001;**86**:517–520.
41. Fogel, R.B., A. Malhotra, G. Pillar, S.D. Pittman, A. Dunaif, and D.P. White, Increased prevalence of obstructive sleep apnea syndrome in obese women with polycystic ovary syndrome. *J Clin Endocrinol Metab*, 2001;**86**:1175–1180.
42. Miller, C.M. and A.M. Husain, Should women with obstructive sleep apnea syndrome be screened for hypothyroidism? *Sleep Breath*, 2003;**7**(4):185–188.
43. Millman, R.P., C. Carlisle, S. McGarvey, S. Eveloff, and P. Levinson, Body fat distribution and sleep apnea severity in women. *Chest*, 1995;**107**:362–366.
44. Ware, J. R.H McBrayer, and J.A. Scott, Influence of sex and age on duration and frequency of sleep apnea events. *Sleep*, 2000;**23**:165–170.
45. Walker, R.P., R. Durazo-Arvizu, B. Wachter, and C. Gopalsami, Preoperative differences between male and female patients with sleep apnea. *Laryngoscope*, 2001;**111**(9):1501–1505.
46. O'Connor, C., K. Thornley, and P. Hanly, Gender differences in the polysomnographic features of obstructive sleep apnea. *Am J Respir Crit Care Med*, 2000;**161**:1465–1472.
47. Young, T., D. Rabago, A. Zgierska, D. Austin, and L. Finn, Objective and subjective sleep quality in premenopausal, perimenopausal, and postmenopausal women in the Wisconsin Sleep Cohort Study. *Sleep*, 2003;**26**(6):667–672.
48. Izci, B., S.E. Martin, K.C. Dundas, W.A. Liston, A.A. Calder, and N.J. Douglas, Sleep complaints: snoring and daytime sleepiness in pregnant and pre-eclamptic women. *Sleep Med*, 2005;**6**(2):163–169.
49. Smith, P.L., A.R. Gold, N. Schubert, et al., Weight loss in mildly to moderately obese patients with obstructive sleep apnea. *Ann Intern Med*, 1983;**103**:850–855.
50. Guilleeminault, C., R. Stoohs, A. Clerk, et al., From obstructive sleep apnea syndrome to upper airway resistance syndrome: consistency of daytime symptoms: *Sleep*, 1992;**15**(Suppl):S13–S16
51. Loube, D.I., P.C. Gay, K.P. Strohl, et al., Indications for positive airway pressure treatment of adult obstructive sleep apnea patients. A consensus statement. *Chest*, 1999;**115**:863–866.

52. Guilleminault, C., L. Palombini, D. Poyares, et al., Chronic insomnia, post menopausal women, and SDB, part 2: comparison of non drug treatment trials in normal breathing and UARS post menopausal women complaining of insomnia. *J Psychosom Res*, 2002;**53**:617–623.

53. Edwards, N., D.M. Blyton, T. Kirjavainen, G.J. Kesby, and C.E. Sullivan, Nasal continuous positive airway pressure reduces sleep-induced blood pressure increments in preeclampsia. *Am J Respir Crit Care Med*, 2000;**162**:252–257.

54. American Sleep Disorders Association, Practice parameters for the treatment of snoring and obstructive sleep apnea with oral appliances. *Sleep*, 1995;**18**(6):511–513.

55. Yoshida, K., Oral device therapy for the upper airway resistance syndrome patient. *J Prosthet Dent*, 2002;**87**:427–430.

56. Standard of Practice Committee of American Sleep Disorders Association, Practice parameters for the treatment of obstructive sleep apnea in adults: the efficacy of surgical modifications of the upper airway. *Sleep*, 1996;**19**:152–155.

11

Polycystic Ovary Syndrome and Obstructive Sleep Apnea

Mira Aubuchon

INTRODUCTION

Polycystic ovary syndrome (PCOS) is an extremely common disorder in women of reproductive age. Affected patients frequently complain of menstrual irregularities, symptoms of hyperandrogenism, and infertility. The entity was first characterized in 1935 by Stein and Leventhal *(1)*, who observed enlarged ovaries, obesity, hirsutism, and infertility associated with chronic anovulation *(2)*. Because PCOS is associated in the long term with diabetes, heart disease, and cancer *(1)*, accurate diagnosis and treatment are extremely important. In recent years, it has become increasingly evident that PCOS is also a significant risk factor for obstructive sleep apnea (OSA). OSA is characterized by sleep-disordered breathing (SDB) and can be a debilitating condition leading to serious health problems if not treated or diagnosed adequately.

DIAGNOSIS OF PCOS

PCOS is complex and consists of a variety of symptoms, but because the basic pathophysiological defect is unknown, there are no universally accepted criteria at present for its diagnosis *(1)*. In the United States, PCOS is defined by the 1990 National Institutes of Health (NIH)–National Institute of Child Health and Human Development Conference as chronic anovulation and androgen excess after other causes have been ruled out *(1)*. Ovarian morphological findings are not required, as not all women with PCOS have polycystic ovaries (PCO) by ultrasound *(2)*.

At the 2003 Rotterdam conference in Europe, the NIH criteria were expanded to include ultrasonographic PCO morphology because it was felt to be predictive of ovarian dysfunction *(3)*. The Rotterdam consensus determined ultrasonographic criteria for PCOS as at least one ovary containing more than 12 follicles 2–9 mm in diameter and/or ovarian volume of more than 10 mL *(3)*.

From: *Current Clinical Neurology: Sleep Disorders in Women: A Guide to Practical Management*
Edited by: H. P. Attarian © Humana Press Inc., Totowa, NJ

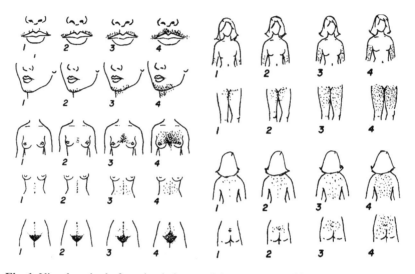

Fig. 1. Visual method of scoring hair growth in women, modified from the system originally reported by Ferriman and Gallwey in 1961. Each of the nine body areas depicted is
scored from 0 (absence of terminal hairs) to 4 (extensive terminal hair growth), and the
scores in each area are summed for a total hair growth score. Hair growth scores of 6–8 or
greater are generally considered to represent hirsutism. (From ref. *3a*.)

Chronic anovulation, although not strictly defined by either criterion, is generally described as six to eight spontaneous episodes of vaginal bleeding per year *(2)*.
Both require exclusion of related disorders such as congenital adrenal hyperplasia,
androgen-secreting tumors, Cushing's syndrome, and hyperprolactinemia *(2,3)*.

Clinical hyperandrogenemia is characterized by hirsutism and/or acne *(2,3)*.
Evaluation should focus on location of terminal hair on the upper lip, chin, lower
abdomen, and inner thighs, with a Ferriman-Gallwey score of more than 5 defining
hirsutism *(1)* (Fig. 1).

Biochemical evidence of hyperandrogenism may also be useful for diagnosis,
including elevated measurements of total and free testosterone, sex hormone-
binding globulin, androstenedione (A4), and dehydroepiandrosterone sulfate levels, although these may not be accurate in the presence of oral contraceptive pills.
Androgen measurements are best performed when clear hirsutism is not present,
with some clinicians measuring only total testosterone (abnormal being considered
>60 ng/dL) and 17-hydroxyprogesterone levels to rule out congenital adrenal
hyperplasia *(1)*. However, clinical assessment can be somewhat subjective, and normal biochemical ranges are not well established.

DIAGNOSIS OF OSA

OSA is a disorder resulting in episodes of either diminished or absent breathing
during sleep. It is characterized by intermittent partial or complete airway obstruc-

Table 1
Significant Factors Independently Predicting AHI ≥ 15
in Symptomatic Severely Obese Subjects[a]

Variables	OR for AHI ≥ 15 (95% CI)	p Value	Corrected OR for AHI ≥ 15 (95% CI)	Adjusted p value
BMI ≥ 45 (n = 51)	4.3 (1.7–11.1)	0.002	4.6 (1.1–20)	0.043
Age ≥ 38 yr (n = 58)	3.4 (1.3–92)	0.007	4.66 (1.0–22)	0.050
Observed sleep apnea (n = 37)	3.3 (1.4–8)	0.006	4.8 (1.2–18.9)	0.024
HbA$_{tc}$ ≥ 6% (n = 25)	5.9 (2.2–15.8)	< 0.001	4.5 (1.1–18.4)	0.036
Fasting plasma insulin ≥ 28 µmol/L (n = 23)	10.2 (3.4–30)	< 0.001	14.7 (2.9–74)	0.001
Male sex (n = 23)	5.2 (1.9–14.8)	0.001	7.3 (1.6–31.8)	0.008
Neck ≥ 43 cm (n = 52)[b]	10.2 (3.7–28)	< 0.001	13.2 (2.4–75)	0.004

[a]The six factors combined provide a BASHIM score Cox and Snell r^2 = 0.46.
[b]Neck circumference can replace male sex and BMI and with the remaining four factors provides similar predictive value (Cox and Snell r^2 = 0.46). (From ref. 9.)

tion that can lead to oxygen desaturation, blood pressure and heart rate changes, and interrupted sleep (4). The gold standard for diagnosis is overnight polysomnography (PSG), which records the electric potentials of the brain and heart, eye movements, muscle activity, respiratory effort, airflow, oxygen saturation, and leg movements throughout the night (5).

Apnea is defined as complete airflow cessation at the nose or mouth of 10 or more seconds, whereas a hypopnea refers to a 30–50% decrease in airflow for 10 or more seconds accompanied by oxygen desaturation of 2–4% or more (5). Severity is determined by the frequency of apnea and hypopnea events per hour of sleep (apnea–hypopnea index [AHI]) as measured by overnight PSG (4). AHI can be used interchangeably with the respiratory disturbance index (RDI) (5). OSA syndrome is a term used when PSG findings are accompanied by functional abnormalities such as excessive daytime sleepiness (EDS) (6).

Symptoms of OSA in adults include EDS, partner-witnessed apneic episodes, snoring, or nocturnal gasping (5). It is also important to elicit a medication history because OSA may be associated with the use of antidepressants or antihypertensives (7). However, EDS alone in obese patients may be a result of metabolic or circadian abnormalities rather than nocturnal sleep disturbances (8). When PSG was performed in 99 morbidly obese patients in Australia describing symptoms suggestive of OSA, the only symptom that predicted OSA and OSA severity was partner-observed sleep apnea (9; Table 1).

Physical exam may yield evidence of large neck circumference, pitting edema, hypertension, anatomical facial or oropharyngeal abnormalities, and increased weight, although one-third of OSA patients are nonobese (5). In addition to body mass index (BMI) of 45 kg/m^2 or more, the best clinical predictive measure for OSA was neck circumference followed by waist circumference (9; Table 1).

When laboratory evidence is combined with clinical features, glycosylated hemoglobin (HbA1c) greater than 6% and fasting plasma insulin greater than 28 μmol/L were most predictive, although high-density lipoprotein (HDL) less than 1.17 mmol/L and fasting plasma glucose greater than 5.6 mmol/L were also associated with OSA (9; Table 1).

The differential diagnosis for EDS includes idiopathic hypersomnia, narcolepsy, atypical depression, periodic leg movements during sleep, central sleep apnea, and insufficient sleep syndrome (5). Partner-witnessed nocturnal choking, gasping, coughing, or shortness of breath could be attributable to gastroesophageal reflux disease, nocturnal asthma, congestive heart failure, central sleep apnea, nocturnal panic attacks, or sleep-related laryngospasm (5).

The gold standard of objective measurement is PSG in a sleep laboratory because electrode dysfunction can be corrected and sleeping behavior can be observed (5). PSG can differentiate OSA from upper airway resistance syndrome (UARS) or idiopathic hypersomnia, in which patients suffer from EDS and occasionally heavy snoring but do not exhibit apneas or oxygen desaturation (11). The PSG typically includes monitors for electroencephalogram, electro-oculography, facial and lower extremity electromyography, electrocardiography, finger pulse oximeters, nasal and oral airflow thermistors, and thoracic and abdominal excursion strain gauges (12).

In 1999, the American Academy of Medicine Sleep Task Force standardized the severity of OSA using the AHI (6). A minimum AHI of 5 or more events per hour is needed for a diagnosis of mild OSA, whereas moderate and severe OSA are distinguished with AHI cutoffs of ≥ 15 and ≥ 30, respectively (6).

EPIDEMIOLOGY OF PCOS

PCOS is the most common cause of anovulation and hirsutism in women (13). Epidemiological data for PCOS are limited as a result of a lack of uniform diagnostic criteria as well as selection bias from using patients from PCOS referral centers (1). Guzick determined that the best prevalence study was performed in 1998 on an unselected population of 277 women 18–45 years of age in Alabama (1). The overall prevalence of PCOS in that study was 4%, with 4–4.7% in whites and 3.4% in African Americans, although the authors cited a possible overall prevalence range of 3.5–11.2% (14). The 11 women with PCOS ranged in age from 18 to 29 years (14). Guzick extrapolated these figures to 3 million current PCOS cases in the United States (1). In adults, obesity is clearly a risk factor for PCOS. The obesity rate for American women with PCOS is much higher than for the general population: 50–60% vs 30%, respectively (15). However, PCOS is also present in women of normal weight, suggesting that other factors may play a role. In the Alabama study, 4 of the 11 (36%) PCOS cases were obese, with a BMI of more than 30 kg/m², indicating that a significant number (64%) were nonobese (14). PCOS is the leading cause of hirsutism in adolescents, with a prevalence in the United Kingdom of 8–26% (10). Obesity is not as clearly a risk factor in this population (10). Predictors of PCOS in adolescents include history of low birthweight, onset of pubic hair prior to age 8, African American or Caribbean Hispanic ethnicity, and positive family history of PCOS in first-degree relatives *(10)*. There appears to be tendency for PCOS patients to cycle more regularly as they get older, which may be attributable to declining androgen levels, particularly for those 42–47 years of age *(16)*.

EPIDEMIOLOGY OF OSA

It is estimated that 1 in 5 adults has mild OSA and 1 in 15 has moderate-to-severe OSA *(4)*. In the OSA population, men outnumber women 8:1 *(4)*. However, the ratio in unselected populations falls to 2:1, indicating that women may be less likely to be diagnosed *(4)*. The main risk factors for OSA are male gender, obesity, and older age, but it also occurs in thin, younger women. In a Wisconsin-based population study of 602 state employees aged 30–60 years, mild OSA rates in women and men were 9 vs 24% and severe OSA rates 4 vs 9.1%, respectively *(17)*. It is estimated that 75–80% of OSA cases in the United States are undiagnosed, which is distressing in light of the effective treatment modalities available *(4)*. In another study involving 1000 women, the overall prevalence of moderate OSA (AHI >10 with daytime symptoms) was 1.2% and of severe OSA was 2.2% *(18)*.

Obesity seems to affect overall prevalence much more in men than in women. In the obese population with BMI of more than 40 kg/m^2, one study reported OSA prevalence rates of 7% of women and 76.9% of men *(19)*. A longitudinal study indicated that with each 10% gain (up to 20%) in weight, AHI increased by 30% and the risk for developing moderate to severe OSA increased sixfold *(20)*. It should be stressed, however, that OSA can and does occur in lean women *(21)*.

Data are conflicting in the United States on prevalence in African Americans vs Caucasians *(6)*. In two studies from Hong Kong, prevalence of OSA was 5% in men and 2% in women and was thought to be attributable to factors other than obesity *(6)*.

Severe OSA prevalence increases with age, reaching a plateau of 13% for men and 7% for women after age 65 *(4)* (Table 2). OSA prevalence rises with menopause to 29 vs 10.8% in the premenopause, based on 589 women sampled from the longitudinal Wisconsin Sleep Cohort study, even after controlling for BMI *(22)* (Fig. 2).

SEQUELAE OF PCOS

PCOS patients are often infertile and have a higher rate of endometrial cancer because of unopposed estrogen *(1)*. Metabolic risks imparted by PCOS include impaired glucose tolerance (IGT), diabetes mellitus (DM), lipid abnormalities, and preclinical atherosclerotic changes *(1)*.

Obese and nonobese PCOS patients have much higher rates of IGT and type 2 DM, as measured by 75-g oral glucose tolerance test, than non-PCOS similar weight controls and the general population *(23)* (Fig. 3).

Comparisons of lipid profiles of 195 PCOS patients and 62 controls showed that both lean and obese PCOS groups had higher total cholesterol and low-density lipoprotein (LDL) cholesterol than the lean and obese control groups, but only obese PCOS had higher triglycerides (TG) *(24)*. An unexpected finding, as yet unexplained, was the relatively higher HDL cholesterol levels in both weight groups of PCOS participants *(24)*.

Table 2
Prevalence of Obstructive Sleep Apnea (OSA) by Sex and Age Group:
Two US Population Studies

| | % (95% Confidence interval) | | | |
| | Mild or worse OSA[a] | | Moderate or worse OSA[b] | |
Age, years	Women	Men	Women	Men
	Wisconsin state employees (N = 691)			
30–39	6.5 (1.4–11.0)	17.0 (9.6–25.0)	4.4 (1.1–7.3)	6.2 (1.9–10.0)
40–49	8.7 (4.2–13.0)	25.0 (18.0–32.0)	3.7 (1.0–6.5)	11.0 (6.7–16.0)
50–59	16.0 (5.2–26.0)	31.0 (21.0–40.0)	4.0 (0–10.0)	9.1 (5.1–13.0)
	Southern Pennsylvania households (N = 1741)			
20–44	[c]	7.9 (5.0–12.0)	0.6 (0.2–2.0)	1.7 (0.6–4.4)
45–64	[c]	8.7 (4.2–13.0)	2.0 (1.0–4.0)	6.3 (4.2–8.8)
65–100	[c]	31.0 (21.0–42.0)	7.0 (4.0–12.0)	13.0 (7.3–23.0)

[a]All groups with apnea–hypoxia index of 5 or more events per hour.
[b]All groups with an apnea–hypoxia index of 15 or more events per hour in the Wisconsin study and all groups with an apnea–hypoxia index of 20 or more events per hour in the Pennsylvania study.
[c]Not provided.

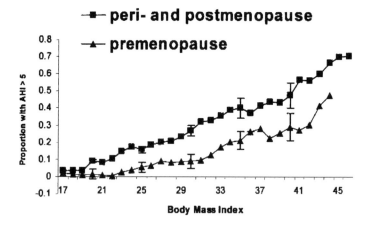

Fig. 2. Prevalence of sleep-disordered breathing indicated by an AHI of 5 or greater for premenopausal women and perimenopausal plus postmenopausal women by body mass index. Values represent a 5-unit moving average. (From ref. 22.)

PCOS participants 45 years of age or older have significantly greater ultrasonographic carotid intima-media wall thickness, which indicates premature subclinical carotid atherosclerosis, than controls of similar age and BMI (25). The findings imply that subclinical cardiovascular changes that can occur with aging seem to be augmented by PCOS (25). However, Spanish investigators determined that increases in markers associated with cardiovascular disease, such as C-reactive

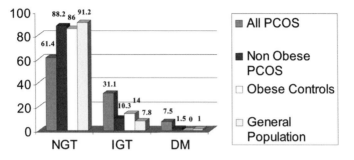

Fig. 3. Percent prevalence of glucose intolerance by Word Health Organization criteria. (Based on data from ref. *23*.)

protein, had the best statistical relationship to obesity, not presence of PCOS or insulin sensitivity *(26)*. Fortunately, mortality rates do not appear to be increased compared to the national averages, according to a retrospective study in the United Kingdom that examined hospital records and death certificates of 786 women with PCOS diagnosed between 1930 and 1979 *(27)*.

SEQUELAE OF OSA

OSA is associated with DM, hypertension, coronary artery disease (CAD), congestive heart failure, and stroke *(4)*. Other co-morbid conditions include problems with daytime functioning and motor vehicle crashes *(4)*. Mortality from untreated OSA is estimated at 2–10% and is attributed to vascular disease *(28)*.

Two studies determined that type 2 DM and insulin resistance (IR), measured by homeostasis model assessment, were associated with OSA in men independent of obesity *(29,30)*. In the Sleep Heart Health Study, however, a cross-sectional evaluation of 470 diabetic vs 4402 nondiabetic male and female individuals showed that increases in OSA in the diabetic group were no longer evident after controlling for body habitus and BMI *(31)*.

Evidence for a causal influence of OSA on hypertension was supported by the prospective 8-year Wisconsin Sleep Cohort Study, in which odds ratios for hypertension increased as AHI scores worsened, even after adjusting for age, gender, body habitus, smoking, and alcohol *(32)*. OSA is also an independent risk factor for CAD, according to a cross-sectional study of 6424 participants from the Sleep Health Heart Study who underwent home PSG *(33)*. The acute hypoxia, CO_2 retention, sympathetic activation, and increases in blood pressure that occur during OSA events may all contribute to eventual coronary vascular damage *(34)*.

Severe OSA also contributes to left ventricular (LV) dysfunction. A prospective study of 169 patients with severe OSA but without preexisting CAD found a 7.7% prevalence of LV systolic dysfunction that normalized with continuous positive airway pressure (CPAP) treatment *(35)*. OSA is probably a risk factor for cerebrovascular disease according to several prospective studies showing similarly high rates of OSA in both stroke and transient ischemic attack patients compared with controls *(36)*. Potential mechanisms include arterial hypertension and decreased cerebral blood flow *(36)*. Patients with OSA also show neurocognitive impairment, which may relate to hippocampal hypoxia *(37)*. Cognitive dysfunction can encompass learning and memory, attention, executive function, and motor skills *(28)*. This may account for the increased frequency of motor vehicle accidents found in this population, involving more than 800,000 drivers and 1400 deaths in 2000 alone *(38)*.

PATHOPHYSIOLOGY OF PCOS

The exact mechanism by which PCOS develops has yet to be determined. However, IR and hypothalamic–pituitary hormonal changes likely play a major role.

IR is a state in which high serum levels of insulin are needed to maintain normal glucose tolerance until pancreatic β-cells can no longer compensate, leading to glucose intolerance and type 2 DM *(39)*. Of patients with PCOS, 50 to 70% have some degree of IR, compared with 10–25% in the general population *(40)*.

IR can arise in visceral or intra-abdominal fat, such as that found in omentum or mesentery. Visceral fat has much higher cellularity, blood flow, and innervation compared to subcutaneous fat and is associated with increased free fatty acids *(41)*. Free fatty acids then lead to diminished hepatic insulin clearance and increased hepatic glucose production *(42)*. Although strongly associated with obesity, PCOS seems to be an independent risk factor for IR, based on a 1989 study by Dunaif, which showed levels of IR in lean PCOS patients that were similar to obese cycling controls *(42a)*. In patients with IR, insulin enhances luteinizing hormone (LH) action on these cells, leading to increased androgen secretion *(43)* (Fig. 4). Hyperandrogenemia is further exacerbated by the suppressive effects of insulin on sex hormone-binding globulin (SHBG) synthesis in the liver *(2)*. Insulin also enhances aromatase activity in granulosa cells, such that tonic low levels of estradiol are produced that feed back negatively on follicle-stimulating hormone (FSH) from the pituitary *(43)*, leading to arrested follicular growth and anovulation *(1)*. It remains a mystery, however, how the ovary remains sensitive to insulin in the face of systemic IR *(1)*. During the normal menstrual cycle, gonadotropin-releasing hormone (GnRH) is released from hypothalamic neurons in a precise pulsatile fashion, which leads to LH pulsatile release from the pituitary. Proper frequency and amplitude of gonadotropin pulses are crucial for hypothalamic–pituitary–ovarian regulation of the menstrual cycle. For as yet unexplained reasons, women with PCOS exhibit alterations of this neuroendocrine axis. In particular, they exhibit increased LH pulse frequency and amplitude, with overall increased LH serum levels *(1)*. The altered GnRH pulsatility is also thought to play a role in the diminished FSH levels seen in PCOS (1). The changes in LH pulsatility can be especially appreciated during sleep. Normally cycling women have sleep-related suspension of episodic LH pulsations, especially in the early follicular phase of the menstrual cycle *(44,45)*. In women with PCOS, however, increased frequency of LH pulsations is seen, independent of body mass index *(43,46,47)*. The increased pulse frequency of PCOS suggests an aberrant nocturnal pattern of GnRH secretion *(48,49)*. The reason for this is unclear.

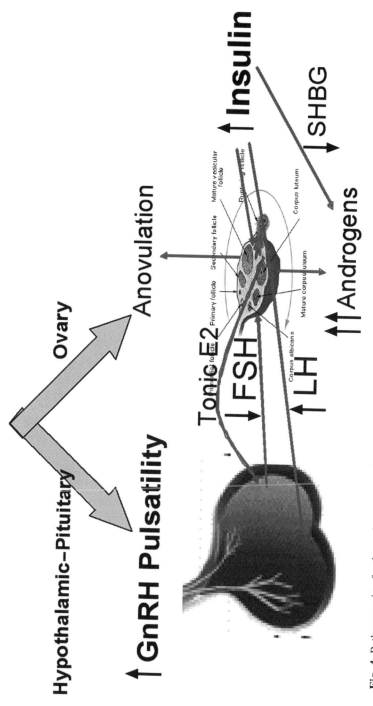

Fig. 4. Pathogenesis of polycystic ovary syndrome. (Author's own diagram based on text from refs. *1–3*.)

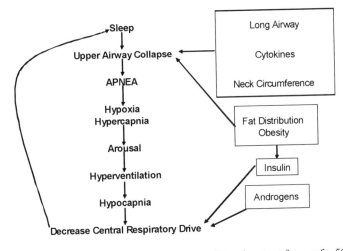

Fig. 5. Pathogenesis of obstructive sleep apnea. (Based on text from refs. *50* and *51*.)

PATHOPHYSIOLOGY OF OSA

The pathogenesis of OSA is also uncertain, but seems to involve interrelated mechanisms such as upper airway anatomy, pharyngeal muscle activity, body fat distribution, inflammation, IR, hyperandrogenism, and central respiratory control (Fig. 5). These mechanisms, once elucidated, may help to explain the role of gender differences and obesity in OSA.

During wakefulness, the pharyngeal muscles in an OSA patient compensate for a vulnerable airway's propensity to collapse, but activation of those muscles is lost during sleep *(50)*. Apnea causes hypoxia and hypercapnia, which eventually lead to nighttime arousal, at which time hyperventilation lowers CO_2 and subsequently reduces central respiratory drive to produce cessation of respiration *(50)*. This cycle of OSA repeats when the patient falls back asleep *(50)*.

Men have significantly longer airway lengths than women, even after controlling for body height *(51)*. Men's airways collapsed much more readily than women's, despite having significantly greater airway lumen area *(51)*. In addition, healthy men had increased pharyngeal volume and soft palate area, which could also contribute to increased risk of OSA in susceptible individuals *(51)*. Obesity is a well-known risk factor for OSA, but the distribution of subcutaneous body fat is more important than total body fat as predictor of OSA severity; in patients with OSA matched for BMI and waist-to-hip ratio (WHR), men had greater upper-body fat by subscapular and tricep skinfold measurements and higher AHIs than women *(52)*. Visceral body fat, independent of BMI, is even more predictive than subcutaneous fat for OSA severity *(53)* (Fig. 6).

Although greater neck circumference in men is thought to contribute to higher OSA rates, men still had higher OSA rates than women, even after controlling for BMI, age, and neck-to-height ratio *(54)*.

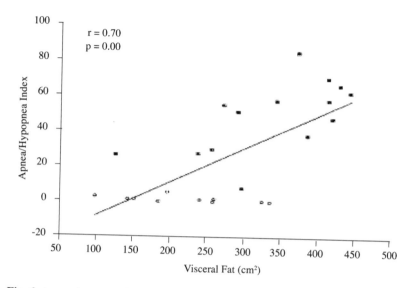

Fig. 6. Apnea–hypopnea index vs visceral fat in obstructive sleep apnea. (From ref. *53*.)

In nonapneic individuals, pharyngeal muscle activity—the genioglossus (GG) in particular—is maintained during sleep but decreases in individuals with OSA *(50)*. Abnormalities in GG fast-twitch muscle fibers have been demonstrated in both lean and obese OSA *(55)*. Pharyngeal tissues from OSA patients show significant interstitial and lymphocytic infiltration and decreased levels of an anti-inflammatory enzyme, all of which can lead to pharyngeal vasodilation and upper airway collapsibility *(56)*.

The systemic inflammatory markers tumor necrosis factor (TNF)-α and interleukin (IL)-6 are also significantly increased in men with OSA compared with controls *(57)*. These cytokines cause sleepiness and increases in BMI and are associated with OSA independent of obesity *(53,58)* (Fig. 7).

Gender differences appear in cytokine response to altered sleep. After finding that TNF-α, which is known to be directly linked to IR, was associated with OSA, Vgontzas et al. found that IR may also be associated with OSA independent of obesity *(53)*. When male obese apneics were compared with obese controls, the former had significantly higher fasting glucose and insulin levels and more visceral fat, which itself releases cytokines *(53)* (Table 3).

IR could reflect an effect of OSA, or it could be contributing to OSA development, because "insulin-dependent diabetes mellitus can lead to an overall depression in ventilatory control mechanisms" *(59)*. At this point its exact role in the pathogenesis of OSA is unclear.

Gender differences are also observed with respect to central ventilatory control, which may be accounted for by testosterone. Men require less reduction in CO_2 to induce apnea during non-rapid eye-movement sleep than women in either the fol-

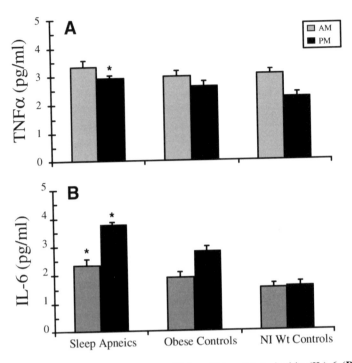

Fig. 7. Plasma tumor necrosis factor (TNF)-α **(A)** and interleukin (IL)-6 **(B)** in sleep apneics and body mass index (BMI)-matched obese and normal weight controls. (From ref. *53*.)

Table 3
Plasma Glucose and Insulin Levels in Sleep Apneics
and Obese Controls

	Sleep apneics ($n = 14$)	Obese controls ($n = 11$)
Glucose (µg/dL)	106.2 ± 4.1^a	85.4 ± 4.4
Insulin (µg/mL)	25.70 ± 4.22^b	14.55 ± 2.49

Data are presented as the mean ± SE. (From ref. *53*.)
[a]$p < 0.01$.
[b]$p > 0.05$.

licular or luteal phase of the menstrual cycle *(60)*. Eight healthy mid-reproductive age normally cycling nonobese nonapneic women were given transdermal testosterone for 10–12 days during the follicular phase, which resulted in male levels of testosterone greater than 130 ng/dL *(61)*. Response to hypocapnia determined at baseline and after testosterone administration showed an increase in CO_2 chemoresponsiveness with testosterone during non-rapid-eye-movement sleep, which increases the likelihood of developing apnea *(61)*. Obese men with OSA have decreased nocturnal LH and total testosterone secretion by mean and area under the curve compared with similar weight controls *(62)*. A review of the study

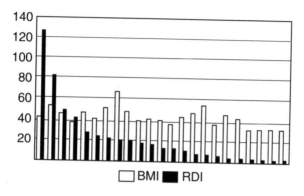

Fig. 8. Relationship of obesity (measured by BMI) to severity of obstructive sleep apnea syndrome (measured by RDI). Each pair of bars represents each individual subject. (From ref. *64*.)

concluded that although the sample size of five was small, the results suggest that OSA is associated with pituitary suppression of androgen production *(63)*. Although these results seem paradoxical, the relative hypoandrogenism may reflect an adaptive response to OSA rather than an etiology *(63)*.

OBSTRUCTIVE SLEEP APNEA AND POLYCYSTIC OVARY SYNDROME

Women with PCOS have a markedly increased OSA prevalence compared with the general female population. One study of 23 obese premenopausal women with PCOS found that 69.6% met criteria for symptomatic OSA *(64)* (Fig. 8). However, the severity of OSA by RDI did not necessarily depend on higher BMI *(64)* (Table 4). Another study reported that 44.4% of 18 obese women with PCOS had symptomatic OSA compared with 5.5% in weight- and aged-matched controls *(65)*. The severity of OSA by AHI in these PCOS patients was significantly correlated with WHR and with total testosterone, whereas for the control women severity correlated only with WHR *(65)* (Figs. 9 and 10).

Insulin sensitivity in PCOS women was associated with SDB, which included OSA and UARS severe enough to warrant treatment, for nine PCOS and three controls displaying SDB (66). SDB was best correlated with fasting insulin, even adjusted for BMI, and to a lesser extent with glucose:insulin ratio *(66)* (Table 5).

OSA shows a male gender predilection related to generalized and visceral obesity, elevated androgens, inflammatory mediators, IR, and upper-body and neck fat. This gender gap narrows, however, in women with PCOS. PCOS patients share many of these characteristics, which may explain their markedly increased risk of OSA compared with the general female population.

TREATMENT FOR OSA

Treatment for OSA is multifaceted. It can involve lifestyle changes, weight loss, mechanical assistance, and surgery, with possible roles being investigated for phar-

Table 4
Presence or Absence of Excessive Daytime
Sleepiness, OSAS, the BMI, and the RDI

Subject	BMI	RDI	Symptoms	OSA
1	42.1	126.7	Present	Yes
2	32.5	2.7	Absent	No
3	31.8	2.1	Absent	No
4	38.1	17.7	Present	Yes
5	46.6	3.7	Absent	No
6	45.6	49.7	Present	Yes
7	53.9	6.2	Present	Yes
8	43.5	10.4	Present	Yes
9	31.8	2.1	Absent	No
10	36.6	42.1	Present	Yes
11	35.8	10.7	Present	Yes
12	46.9	27.6	Present	Yes
13	43.3	3.1	Absent	No
14	36.5	6	Absent	No
15	40.4	16.6	Present	Yes
16	48.2	19.7	Present	Yes
17	50.0	21.6	Present	Yes
18	31.4	2.7	Absent	No
19	39.8	12.6	Present	Yes
20	40.9	23	Present	Yes
21	67	20.2	Present	Yes
22	47.5	6.7	Present	Yes
23	52.6	82.4	Present	Yes

From ref. *64*.

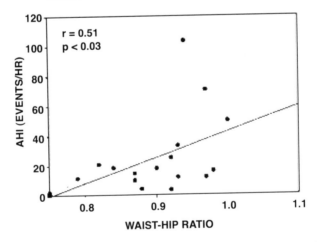

Fig. 9. Correlation between waist-to-hip ratio and sleep-disordered breathing in women with PCOS. (From ref. *65*.)

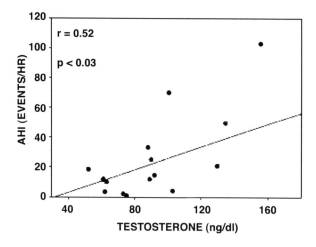

Fig. 10. Correlation between serum total testosterone and sleep-disordered breathing in women with PCOS. (From ref. *65*.)

Table 5
Biochemical Profiles of PCOS Women With and Without SDB

	SDB group	Non-SDB group	*p*
Free testosterone (nmol/L)	124.81 ± 44.52	118.11 ± 16.54	NS
Total testosterone (nmol/L)	276.20 ± 73.1	284.77 ± 26.41	NS
Glucose (nmol/L)	5.65 ± 0.31	5.48 ± 0.25	NS
Insulin (pmol/L)	306.48 ± 52.39	176.71 ± 18.53	0.01
Glucose/insulin ratio	0.02 ± 0.006	0.04 ± 0.003	0.05

From ref. *66*.

macological therapies. Treatment modalities may help not only SDB, but also associated visceral obesity, IR, and neuroendocrine abnormalities.

Lifestyle changes refer primarily to improving sleep hygiene by avoiding possible triggers of airway collapsibility and sleep-related arousals *(67)*. These triggers include alcohol, sedatives, and supine positioning, although outcomes of avoiding these triggers have not been measured *(67)*. Longitudinal assessment of weight changes and SDB indicated that even a 5% reduction of body weight resulted in a significant (14%) reduction in OSA severity by AHI *(20)*. Weight reduction interventions do produce fairly good improvement in OSA in the short term (6–12 months), but weight maintenance is more difficult *(68,69)*. Furthermore, even for patients who maintain their weight loss in the long term, OSA may persist or recur *(68,69)*.

Nasal CPAP is the most commonly accepted mechanical treatment for OSA. CPAP prevents negative inspiratory pressure in the upper airway and thus prevents pharyngeal collapse *(70)*. This modality requires wearing a mask over the nose that is held in place with chin straps *(5)*. The level of positive pressure is determined with PSG, because too little may be ineffective and too much may promote arousal,

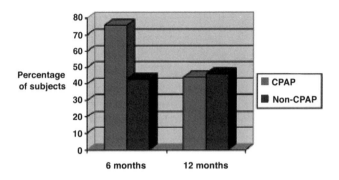

Fig. 11. Patients showing treatment success in CPAP and non-CPAP groups. At 6 months, 13 of 17 patients in the CPAP group and 6 of 14 in the non-CPAP group showed treatment success. At 24 months, 7 of 16 CPAP and 6 of 13 non-CPAP patients showed treatment success. (From ref. *68*.)

central sleep apnea, and even cardiac arrhythmias in susceptible patients *(5)*. Although the device effectively treats OSA in 80–90% of cases, patient compliance is often poor as a result of skin, eye, and nasal irritation.

Other forms of mechanical assistance include bilevel positive airway pressure, which provides different pressures during inspiration and expiration *(5)*, and oral devices to modify the position of upper airway structures, such as the tongue, to improve airway collapsibility and muscle function *(67)*.

CPAP and weight loss were both evaluated in a Finnish study in which 31 men received weight loss therapy over 2 years, half of whom were randomly selected to also receive CPAP during the first 6 months *(68)*. At the 6-month follow-up, the CPAP group had greater improvement in OSA relief than the non-CPAP group; however, this difference was not seen at the 2-year follow-up (Fig. 11) *(68)*. This indicates that CPAP works well while it is being used, but effects do not seem to persist once it is stopped *(68)*.

Visceral body fat, as measured by computed tomography, significantly decreased with CPAP treatment in a Japanese report of 12 mostly male, overweight OSA patients treated with more than 6 months of CPAP without body weight changes *(71)*. These patients also had improvements in HDL and LDL cholesterol *(71)*. Insulin sensitivity as measured by hyperinsulinemic euglycemic clamp may, without BMI reduction, improve with CPAP in non-insulin-dependent DM patients with moderate to severe OSA *(72)*, although this improvement was not seen in a more recent study *(73)*. Glucose tolerance does not appear to improve with CPAP in the absence of BMI reduction, as variously measured by insulin, fasting glucose, HbA1c, or oral glucose tolerance testing *(71–73)*.

CPAP seems to effect neuroendocrine changes, as well. OSA in men is associated with decreased serum secretion of insulin growth factor (IGF)-1, perhaps owing to changes in slow-wave sleep, as well as decreased SHBG and total testosterone *(74)*. In 43 obese men with OSA studied before and after 3 months of CPAP, IGF-1, total testosterone, and SHBG rose to normal levels without changes in body weight *(74)*.

The most common surgical procedure to treat OSA is uvulopalatopharyngoplasty (UPPP), which removes the uvula, portions of the soft palate, and redundant pharyngeal tissue, but is only successful in 40–50% of cases *(5)*. UPPP works best with isolated upper pharyngeal pathology, but usually fails if the obstruction is at the tongue base *(67)*. Laser-assisted uvulopalatoplasty compares favorably to UPPP in terms of success, but carries a higher risk of worsening the OSA if it fails *(67)*. Other options include midline glossectomy to trim an obstructive tongue, maxillary advancement, and procedures to correct craniofacial abnormalities *(5)*.

Limited information is available regarding pharmacological treatment of OSA. Estrogen alone or combined estrogen–progestin therapy has not been shown to be effective in treating OSA in postmenopausal women *(75)*. Three weeks of Etanercept, which blocks TNF-α and IL-6, significantly reduced daytime sleepiness and modestly reduced AHI in eight obese men in a randomized, double-blind, placebo-controlled, crossover pilot study *(58)*.

CONCLUSION

The combination of OSA and PCOS begs for more study, both from a public health point of view and to understand their probable interrelated pathophysiology. Studies evaluating these conditions before and after treatment would be particularly valuable in this regard, because most of the literature focuses on men. Because PCOS is common, these patients represent an important opportunity to improve the screening, prevention, and treatment of sleep disorders and their sequelae in women.

REFERENCES

1. Guzick, D.S., Polycystic ovary syndrome. *Obstet Gynecol*, 2004;**103**(1):181–193.
2. Legro, R.S., Diagnostic criteria in polycystic ovary syndrome. *Semin Reprod Med*, 2003;**21**(3):267–275.
3. Rotterdam ESHRE/ASRM-Sponsored PCOS Consensus Workshop Group. Revised 2003 consensus on diagnostic criteria and long-term health risks related to polycystic ovary syndrome (PCOS). *Hum Reprod*, 2004;**19**(1):41–47.
3a. Hatch, R., R.L. Rosenfield, M.H. Kim, and D. Tredway, Hirsutism: implications, etiology, and management. *Am J Obstet Gynecol*, 1981;**140**:815–830.
4. Young, T., J. Skatrud, and P.E. Peppard, Risk factors for obstructive sleep apnea in adults. *JAMA*, 2004;**291**(16):2013–2016.
5. Attarian, H.P. and A.N. Sabri, When to suspect obstructive sleep apnea syndrome. Symptoms may be subtle, but treatment is straightforward. *Postgrad Med*, 2002;**111**(3):70–76.
6. Young, T., P.E. Peppard, and D.J. Gottlieb, Epidemiology of obstructive sleep apnea: a population health perspective. *Am J Respir Crit Care Med*, 2002;**165**(9):1217–1239.
7. Farney, R.J., A. Lugo, R.L. Jensen, J.M. Walker, and T.V. Cloward, Simultaneous use of antidepressant and antihypertensive medications increases likelihood of diagnosis of obstructive sleep apnea syndrome. *Chest*, 2004;**125**(4):1279–1285.
8. Vgontzas, A.N., E.O. Bixler, T.L. Tan, D. Kantner, L.F. Martin, and A. Kales, Obesity without sleep apnea is associated with daytime sleepiness. *Arch Intern Med*, 1998;**158**(12):1333–1337.
9. Dixon, J.B., L.M. Schachter, and P.E. O'Brien, Predicting sleep apnea and excessive day sleepiness in the severely obese: indicators for polysomnography. *Chest*, 2003;**123**(4):1134–1141.
10. Driscoll, D.A., Polycystic ovary syndrome in adolescence. *Semin Reprod Med*, 2003;**21**(3):301–307.
11. Exar, E.N. and N.A. Collop, The upper airway resistance syndrome. *Chest*, 1999;**115**(4):1127–1139.
12. Seneviratne, U. and K. Puvanendran, Excessive daytime sleepiness in obstructive sleep apnea: prevalence, severity, and predictors. *Sleep Med*, 2004;**5**(4):339–343.

13. Franks, S., Polycystic ovary syndrome. *N Engl J Med*, 1995;**333**(13):853–861.
14. Knochenhauer, E.S., T.J. Key, M. Kahsar-Miller, W. Waggoner, L.R. Boots, and R. Azziz, Prevalence of the polycystic ovary syndrome in unselected black and white women of the southeastern United States: a prospective study. *J Clin Endocrinol Metab*, 1998;**83**(9):3078–3082.
15. Wright, C.E., J.V. Zborowski, E.O. Talbott, K. McHugh-Pemu, and A. Youk, Dietary intake, physical activity, and obesity in women with polycystic ovary syndrome. *Int J Obes Relat Metab Disord*, 2004;**28**(8):1026–1032.
16. Winters, S.J., E.O. Talbott, D.D. Guzick, J.V. Zborowski, and K.P. McHugh, Serum testosterone levels decrease in middle age in women with the polycystic ovary syndrome. *Fertil Steril*, 2000;**73**(4):724–729.
17. Young, T., M. Palta, J. Dempsey, J. Skatrud, S. Weber, and S. Badr, The occurrence of sleep-disordered breathing among middle-aged adults. *N Engl J Med*, 1993;**328**(17):1230–1235.
18. Bixler, E.O., A.N. Vgontzas, H.M. Lin, et al., Prevalence of sleep-disordered breathing in women: effects of gender. *Am J Respir Crit Care Med*, 2001;**163**(3 Pt 1):608–613.
19. Rajala, R., M. Partinen, T. Sane, R. Pelkonen, K. Huikuri, and A.M. Sappalainen, Obstructive sleep apnoea syndrome in morbidly obese patients. *J Intern Med*, 1991;**230**(2):125–129.
20. Peppard, P.E., T. Young, M. Palta, J. Dempsey, and J. Skatrud, Longitudinal study of moderate weight change and sleep-disordered breathing. *JAMA*, 2000;**284**(23):3015–3021.
21. Guilleminault, C., R. Stoohs, Y. Kim, R. Chervin, J. Black, and A. Clerk, Upper airway sleep-disordered breathing in women. *Ann Intern Med*, 1995;**122**(7):493–501.
22. Young, T., L. Finn, D. Austin, and A. Peterson, Menopausal status and sleep-disordered breathing in the Wisconsin Sleep Cohort Study. *Am J Respir Crit Care Med*, 2003;**167**(9):1181–1185.
23. Legro, R.S., A.R. Kunselman, W.C. Dodson, and A. Dunaif, Prevalence and predictors of risk for type 2 diabetes mellitus and impaired glucose tolerance in polycystic ovary syndrome: a prospective, controlled study in 254 affected women. *J Clin Endocrinol Metab*, 1999;**84**(1):165–169.
24. Legro, R.S., A.R. Kunselman, and A. Dunaif, Prevalence and predictors of dyslipidemia in women with polycystic ovary syndrome. *Am J Med*, 2001;**111**(8):607–613.
25. Talbott, E.O., D.S. Guzick, K. Sutton-Tyrrell, et al., Evidence for association between polycystic ovary syndrome and premature carotid atherosclerosis in middle-aged women. *Arterioscler Thromb Vasc Biol*, 2000;**20**(11):2414–2421.
26. Escobar-Morreale, H.F., G. Villuendas, J.I. Botella-Carretero, J. Sancho, J.L. San Millán, Obesity, and not insulin resistance, is the major determinant of serum inflammatory cardiovascular risk markers in pre-menopausal women. *Diabetologia*, 2003;**46**(5):625–633.
27. Pierpoint, T., P.M. McKeigue, A.J. Isaacs, S.H. Wild, and H.S. Jacobs, Mortality of women with polycystic ovary syndrome at long-term follow-up. *J Clin Epidemiol*, 1998;**51**(7):581–586.
28. Redline, S. and K.P. Strohl, Recognition and consequences of obstructive sleep apnea hypopnea syndrome. *Clin Chest Med*, 1998;**19**(1):1–19.
29. Elmasry, A., E. Lindberg, C. Berne, et al., Sleep-disordered breathing and glucose metabolism in hypertensive men: a population-based study. *J Intern Med*, 2001;**249**(2):153–161.
30. Coughlin, S.R., L. Mawdsley, J.A. Mugarza, P.M.A. Calverley, and J.P.H. Wilding, Obstructive sleep apnoea is independently associated with an increased prevalence of metabolic syndrome. *Eur Heart J*, 2004;**25**(9):735–741.
31. Resnick, H.E., S. Redline, E. Shahar, et al., Diabetes and sleep disturbances: findings from the Sleep Heart Health Study. *Diabetes Care*, 2003;**26**(3):702–709.
32. Peppard, P.E., T. Young, M. Palta, and J. Skatrud, Prospective study of the association between sleep-disordered breathing and hypertension. *N Engl J Med*, 2000;**342**(19):1378–1384.
33. Shahar, E., C.W. Whitney, S. Redline, et al., Sleep-disordered breathing and cardiovascular disease: cross-sectional results of the Sleep Heart Health Study. *Am J Respir Crit Care Med*, 2001;**163**(1):19–25.
34. Shamsuzzaman, A.S., B.J. Gersh, and V.K. Somers, Obstructive sleep apnea: implications for cardiac and vascular disease. *JAMA*, 2003;**290**(14):1906–1914.
35. Laaban, J.P., S. Pascal-Sebaoun, E. Bloch, E. Orvoën-Frija, J.M. Oppert, and G. Huchon, Left ventricular systolic dysfunction in patients with obstructive sleep apnea syndrome. *Chest*, 2002;**122**(4):1133–1138.

36. Neau, J.P., J. Paquereau, J.C. Meurice, J.J. Chavagnat, and R. Gil, Stroke and sleep apnoea: cause or consequence? *Sleep Med Rev*, 2002;**6**(6):457–469.
37. Bartlett, D.J., C. Rae, C.H. Thompson, et al., Hippocampal area metabolites relate to severity and cognitive function in obstructive sleep apnea. *Sleep Med*, 2004;**5**(6):593–596.
38. Sassani, A., L.J. Findley, M. Kryger, E. Goldlust, C. George, and T.M. Davidson, Reducing motor-vehicle collisions, costs, and fatalities by treating obstructive sleep apnea syndrome. *Sleep*, 2004;**27**(3):453–458.
39. Goldstein, B.J., Insulin resistance as the core defect in type 2 diabetes mellitus. *Am J Cardiol*, 2002;**90**(5A):3G–10G.
40. Ovalle, F. and R. Azziz, Insulin resistance, polycystic ovary syndrome, and type 2 diabetes mellitus. *Fertil Steril*, 2002;**77**(6):1095–1105.
41. Bjorntorp, P., The regulation of adipose tissue distribution in humans. *Int J Obes Relat Metab Disord*, 1996;**20**(4):291–302.
42. Jensen, M.D., J.A. Kanaley, J.E. Reed, and P.F. Sheedy, Measurement of abdominal and visceral fat with computed tomography and dual-energy x-ray absorptiometry. *Am J Clin Nutr*, 1995;**61**(2):274–278.
42a. Dunaif, A., K.R. Segal, W. Futterweit, and A. Dobrjawsky, Profound peripheral insulin resistance, independent of obesity, in polycystic ovarian syndrome. *Diabetes*, 1989;**38**:1165–1174.
43. Morales, A.J., G.A. Laughlin, T. Bützow, H. Maheshwari, G. Baumann, and S.S.C. Yen, Insulin, somatotropic, and luteinizing hormone axes in lean and obese women with polycystic ovary syndrome: common and distinct features. *J Clin Endocrinol Metab*, 1996;**81**(8):2854–2864.
44. Filicori, M., N. Santoro, G.R. Merriam, and W.F.C. Crowley, Characterization of the physiological pattern of episodic gonadotropin secretion throughout the human menstrual cycle. *J Clin Endocrinol Metab*, 1986;**62**(6):1136–1144.
45. Soules, M.R., R.A. Steiner, N.L. Cohen, W.J. Bremner, and D.K. Clifton, Nocturnal slowing of pulsatile luteinizing hormone secretion in women during the follicular phase of the menstrual cycle. *J Clin Endocrinol Metab*, 1985;**61**(1):43–49.
46. Apter, D., T. Bützow, G.A. Laughlin, and S.S.C. Yen, Accelerated 24-hour luteinizing hormone pulsatile activity in adolescent girls with ovarian hyperandrogenism: relevance to the developmental phase of polycystic ovarian syndrome. *J Clin Endocrinol Metab*, 1994;**79**(1):119–125.
47. Taylor, A.E., B. McCourt, K.A. Martin, et al., Determinants of abnormal gonadotropin secretion in clinically defined women with polycystic ovary syndrome. *J Clin Endocrinol Metab*, 1997;**82**(7):2248–2256.
48. Waldstreicher, J., N.F. Santoro, J.E. Hall, M. Filicori, and W.F. Crowley, Hyperfunction of the hypothalamic-pituitary axis in women with polycystic ovarian disease: indirect evidence for partial gonadotroph desensitization. *J Clin Endocrinol Metab*, 1988;**66**(1):165–172.
49. Zumoff, B., R. Freeman, S. Coupey, P. Saenger, M. Markowitz, and J. Kream, A chronobiologic abnormality in luteinizing hormone secretion in teenage girls with the polycystic-ovary syndrome. *N Engl J Med*, 1983;**309**(20):1206–1209.
50. Jordan, A.S., D.P. White, and R.B. Fogel, Recent advances in understanding the pathogenesis of obstructive sleep apnea. *Curr Opin Pulm Med*, 2003;**9**(6):459–464.
51. Malhotra, A., Y. Huang, R.B. Fogel, et al., The male predisposition to pharyngeal collapse: importance of airway length. *Am J Respir Crit Care Med*, 2002;**166**(10):1388–1395.
52. Millman, R.P., C.C Carlisle, S.T. McGarvey, S.E. Eveloff, and P.D. Levinson, Body fat distribution and sleep apnea severity in women. *Chest*, 1995;**107**(2):362–366.
53. Vgontzas, A.N., D.A. Papanicolaou, E.O. Bixler, et al., Sleep apnea and daytime sleepiness and fatigue: relation to visceral obesity, insulin resistance, and hypercytokinemia. *J Clin Endocrinol Metab*, 2000;**85**(3):1151–1158.
54. Dancey, D.R., P.J. Hanly, C. Soong, B. Lee, J. Shepard, and V. Hoffstein, Gender differences in sleep apnea: the role of neck circumference. *Chest*, 2003;**123**(5):1544–1550.
55. Carrera, M., F. Barbé, J. Sauleda, et al., Effects of obesity upon genioglossus structure and function in obstructive sleep apnoea. *Eur Respir J*, 2004;**23**(3):425–429.
56. Hatipoglu, U. and I. Rubinstein, Inflammation and obstructive sleep apnea syndrome pathogenesis: a working hypothesis. *Respiration*, 2003;**70**(6):665–671.

57. Vgontzas, A.N., D.A. Papanicolaou, E.O. Bixler, A. Kales, K. Tyson, and G.P. Chrousos, Elevation of plasma cytokines in disorders of excessive daytime sleepiness: role of sleep disturbance and obesity. *J Clin Endocrinol Metab*, 1997;**82**(5):1313–1316.

58. Vgontzas, A.N., E. Zoumakis, H.M. Lin, E.O. Bixler, G. Trakada, and G.P. Chrousos, Marked decrease in sleepiness in patients with sleep apnea by etanercept, a tumor necrosis factor-alpha antagonist. *J Clin Endocrinol Metab*, 2004;**89**(9):4409–4413.

59. Vgontzas, A.N., E.O. Bixler, and G.P. Chrousos, Metabolic disturbances in obesity versus sleep apnoea: the importance of visceral obesity and insulin resistance. *J Intern Med*, 2003;**254**(1):32–44.

60. Zhou, X.S., S. Shahabuddin, B.R. Zahn, M.A. Babcock, and M.S. Badr, Effect of gender on the development of hypocapnic apnea/hypopnea during NREM sleep. *J Appl Physiol*, 2000;**89**(1):192–199.

61. Zhou, X.S., J.A. Rowley, F. Demirovic, M.P. Diamond, and M.S. Badr, Effect of testosterone on the apneic threshold in women during NREM sleep. *J Appl Physiol*, 2003;**94**(1):101–107.

62. Luboshitzky, R., A. Aviv, A. Hefetz, et al., Decreased pituitary-gonadal secretion in men with obstructive sleep apnea. *J Clin Endocrinol Metab*, 2002;**87**(7):3394–3398.

63. McCowan, K.C. and A. Malhotra, The correlation between obstructive sleep apnea and low gonadotropin secretion in men. *Sleep Med*, 2003;**4**(1):83–84.

64. Gopal, M., S. Duntley, M. Uhles, and H. Attarian, The role of obesity in the increased prevalence of obstructive sleep apnea syndrome in patients with polycystic ovarian syndrome. *Sleep Med*, 2002;**3**(5):401–404.

65. Fogel, R.B., A. Malhotra, G. Pillar, S.D. Pittman, A. Dunaif, and D.P. White, Increased prevalence of obstructive sleep apnea syndrome in obese women with polycystic ovary syndrome. *J Clin Endocrinol Metab*, 2001;**86**(3):1175–1180.

66. Vgontzas, A.N., R.S. Legro, E.O. Bixler, A. Grayev, A. Kales, and G.P. Chrousos, Polycystic ovary syndrome is associated with obstructive sleep apnea and daytime sleepiness: role of insulin resistance. *J Clin Endocrinol Metab*, 2001;**86**(2):517–520.

67. Goldberg, R., Treatment of obstructive sleep apnea, other than with continuous positive airway pressure. *Curr Opin Pulm Med*, 2000;**6**(6):496–500.

68. Kajaste, S., P.E. Brander, T. Telakivi, M. Partinen, and P. Mustajoki, A cognitive-behavioral weight reduction program in the treatment of obstructive sleep apnea syndrome with or without initial nasal CPAP: a randomized study. *Sleep Med*, 2004;**5**(2):125–131.

69. Sampol, G., X. Muñoz, M.T. Sagalés, Long-term efficacy of dietary weight loss in sleep apnoea/hypopnoea syndrome. *Eur Respir J*, 1998;**12**(5):1156–1159.

70. Bahammam, A. and M. Kryger, Decision making in obstructive sleep-disordered breathing. Putting it all together. *Clin Chest Med*, 1998;**19**(1):87–97.

71. Chin, K., K. Shimizu, T. Nakamura, et al., Changes in intra-abdominal visceral fat and serum leptin levels in patients with obstructive sleep apnea syndrome following nasal continuous positive airway pressure therapy. *Circulation*, 1999;**100**(7):706–712.

72. Brooks, B., P.A. Cistulli, M. Borkman, et al., Obstructive sleep apnea in obese noninsulin-dependent diabetic patients: effect of continuous positive airway pressure treatment on insulin responsiveness. *J Clin Endocrinol Metab*, 1994;**79**(6):1681–1685.

73. Smurra, M., P. Philip, J. Taillard, C. Guilleminault, B. Bioulac, and H. Gin, CPAP treatment does not affect glucose-insulin metabolism in sleep apneic patients. *Sleep Med*, 2001;**2**(3):207–213.

74. Grunstein, R.R., D.J. Handelsman, S.J. Lawrence, C. Blackwell, I.D. Caterson, and C.E. Sullivan, Neuroendocrine dysfunction in sleep apnea: reversal by continuous positive airways pressure therapy. *J Clin Endocrinol Metab*, 1989;**68**(2):352–358.

75. Polo-Kantola, P., E. Rauhala, H. Helenius, R. Erkkola, K. Irjala, and O. Polo, Breathing during sleep in menopause: a randomized, controlled, crossover trial with estrogen therapy. *Obstet Gynecol*, 2003;**102**(1):68–75.

12

Women and Excessive Daytime Sleepiness

Hrayr P. Attarian

INTRODUCTION

This chapter discusses excessive daytime sleepiness (EDS) related to primary sleep disorders other than obstructive sleep apnea syndrome (OSAS) and restless legs syndrome (RLS) and EDS secondary to other medical problems—the secondary hypersomnias.

Several studies over the years have demonstrated that sleep complaints in general, and EDS in particular, tend to be more prevalent among women. More recently, some evidence has suggested that this is partly owing to women being more sleep deprived (1). Further research demonstrates that women who care for families are more likely to suffer from EDS than those living alone, although being married and having a family is protective against sleep deprivation in men (2). This suggests that one of the causes of more prevalent insufficient sleep in women is more extensive work and home care responsibilities (2). Women also nap less during the day than men do despite having similar total sleep time (TST) at night and similar sleep efficiency (3), thus curtailing their TST further. Another variable that may partially contribute to the higher prevalence of excessive sleepiness in women is that most sleep disorders are underdiagnosed. One of the screening tools most commonly used for EDS, and therefore sleep disorders, is the Epworth Sleepiness Scale (ESS) (Table 1). The ESS is the most commonly used subjective sleepiness assessment test. It is a simple, self-administered questionnaire, that provides a measurement of the subject's general level of daytime sleepiness, wherein patients rate the chances that they would doze off or fall asleep in eight different, commonly encountered, daily life situations (4).

A recent study demonstrated that using the ESS to detect subjective sleepiness is more likely to identify men with sleepiness. Because the ESS is more strongly related to other subjective measures in men, it may be a more sensitive measure of subjective sleepiness in men than in women. Findings indicate that men and women answer questions about sleepiness differently (5). A third factor is hormonal changes, their impact on sleep in women, and subsequent EDS. This gender difference in the prevalence of EDS is not present among prepubertal children (6) but seems to be consistently reported in adults. (*See* other chapters in this volume for detailed descriptions of hormonal variables and their impact on sleep.)

From: *Current Clinical Neurology: Sleep Disorders in Women: A Guide to Practical Management*
Edited by: H. P. Attarian © Humana Press Inc., Totowa, NJ

Table 1
Epworth Sleepiness Scale

0 = no chance of dozing 1 = slight chance of dozing 2 = moderate chance of dozing 3 = high chance of dozing	Score of 9 or higher indicative of sleepiness
Situation	Chance of dozing
Sitting and reading	0 1 2 3
Watching TV	0 1 2 3
Sitting inactive in a public place (e.g., a theater or a meeting)	0 1 2 3
As a passenger ina car for an hour without a break	0 1 2 3
Lying down to rest in the afternoon when circumstances permit	0 1 2 3
Sitting and talking to someone	0 1 2 3
Sitting quietly after a lunch without alcohol	0 1 2 3
In a car, while stopped for a few minutes in traffic	0 1 2 3

DIAGNOSTIC TESTS

Polysomnogram

The polysomnogram (PSG) is a polygraph of electroencephalographic (EEG) findings, eye movements, electromyography readings—the three basic stage-scoring parameters—as well as oxygen saturation, limb movements, airflow, eclectrocardiogram, and chest and abdominal movements taken during sleep, usually for the entire night.

Multiple Sleep Latency Test

The multiple sleep latency test (MSLT) is a well-validated measurement of the tendency to fall asleep during normal waking hours. It consists of four or five opportunities, at 2-hour intervals throughout the day, to take a 15- to 20-minute nap. A mean sleep latency of 5 minutes or less is significant for hypersomnia, and 10 minutes or more is normal.

Maintenance of Wakefulness Test

The maintenance of wakefulness test (MWT) determines the ability to remain awake while sitting in a quiet, darkened room. The test consists of four 20- or 40-minute trials conducted four times at 2-hour intervals commencing 2 hours after awakening from a night of sleep. A mean sleep latency of less than 10.9 minutes for the MWT 20 and less than 19.4 minutes for MWT 40 is significant for hypersomnia (7,8).

PERIMENSTRUAL HYPERSOMNIA

A rarely described but distinct entity is a periodic hypersomnia associated with the menstrual cycle. This is usually noted during the first few years after menarche. The EDS generally lasts 1–2 weeks after ovulation, with sudden resolution occur-

Table 2
Diagnostic Criteria: Menstrual-Associated Sleep Disorder

A. The patient has a complaint of insomnia or episodes of excessive sleepiness.
B. The complaint of insomina or excessive sleepiness is temporarily associated with the menopause.
C. The disorder is present for at least 3 months.
D. Polysomnographic monitoring demonstrates both of the following:

　1. Reduced sleep efficiency and reduced total sleep time, with frequent awakenings during the symptomatic time.
　2. A sleep latency of less than 10 minutes on the multiple sleep latency test obtained during the time that symptoms of excessive sleepiness are present.

E. Other medical or mental disorders, except premenstrual syndrome, can be present.
F. No other sleep disorder accounts for the symptom.

Note: The particular type of sleep disorder (i.e., premenstrual insomnia, premenstrual hypersomnia, or menopausal insomnia) can be stated on axis A (e.g., menstrual-associated sleep disorder–premenstrual insomina type). If the patient meets the criteria for a mental diagnosis of premenstrual syndrome, state and code premenstrual syndrome on axis A.
Minimal criteria: A plus B plus C.

ring at the time of menses. This condition is listed in the International Classification of Sleep Disorders as a *proposed sleep disorder (9)* (Table 2).

The first case in the medical literature discussing this distinct entity was published in 1975 by Billiard and colleagues *(10).* They described a 13-year-old girl with recurring episodes of periodic excessive sleepiness with each menstruation. During episodes of hypersomnia, the subject slept for an average time of 14 hours and 19 minutes per 24 hours. They also showed a significantly reduced level of performance when evaluated by the Wilkinson Addition Test (a performance test in which the subjects add numbers for 1 hour, often used, in concert with other tests, to measure the impact of sleep loss). Looking for hormonal abnormalities did not reveal any striking findings. Based on the close relationship between the episodes of hypersomnia and the end of menstruation, they suggested that progesterone might have a role in its pathogenesis. The hypersomnia is this case was successfully treated with oral contraceptives to block ovulation *(10).* Papy et al. *(11)* followed another subject with menstrual-related hypersomnia for 8 years. Serial EEGs during the period of excessive sleepiness did not reveal any abnormalities. Her events initially occurred approx 5–6 days after menstruation and later occurred during ovulation. Again, hormonal abnormalities were not found and oral contraception eliminated the events *(11).* Sachs et al. *(12)* also reported a case in 1982 of menstrual-related hypersomnia in a 16-year-old girl followed for 3 years after a hospital stay of 31 days. Neurological and gynecological exams were normal and as before. Serum levels of reproductive hormones were normal. Cerebrospinal fluid (CSF) concentrations of homovanillic acid and 5-hydroxyindolacetic acid were lower in her hypersomniac than in her symptom-free phases. As in the previous two cases, sleep periods occurred only in connection with ovulation. Inhibition of ovulation with the oral contraceptive pill (OCP) led to a resolution of the hypersomnia. When treatment was discontinued, ovulation and periodic hypersomnia reoccurred regularly. Reinstitution of the OCP again controlled the symptoms. The recurrence of the sleepiness and ovulation when off OCPs and its resolution with the resumption of the OCP was reproduced twice during the 3 years *(12)*.

A case of an older (42 years) woman with the same symptoms was reported in 1993 by Bamford *(13)*. This subject's menstrual cycles stopped while taking metoclopramide, but stopping the cycles did not improve the EDS; the periods of EDS became more erratic. High serum prolactin levels were found to coincide with the subject's periods of sleepiness. Unlike the previous cases, hormone replacement therapy did not control the periods of somnolence. Low-dose methylphenidate provided successful symptomatic relief *(13)*. None of these cases had any other medical or psychiatric symptoms associated with the EDS. Perimenstrual hypersomnia has also been reported during the luteal phase in some women with severe premenstrual symptoms, as well as opposed to premenstrual insomnia during the same phase in women with mild premenstrual symptoms *(14)*.

Pathophysiology

Bamford *(13)* postulated, based on the high prolactin levels coinciding with the episodes of somnolence, that it is likely that the pathophysiology of menstrual-related hypersomnia involves the dopaminergic and monoaminergic neurotransmitter systems. This has been also theorized to be the underlying cause of Kleine-Levin syndrome (KLS), another disorder characterized by episodic hypersomnia. KLS is a rare disorder occurring most often in adolescent males characterized by episodic hypersomnia and altered behavior *(15)*.

Diagnosis

MSLT and PSG, administered in a standardized fashion during and after the symptomatic period, usually make the diagnosis. These tests should be performed no earlier than the second night after the onset of a symptomatic episode and the following day to reveal maximal hypersomnolence and more than 2 weeks after a symptomatic episode to represent the asymptomatic interval *(16)*.

Treatment

Perimenstrual hypersomnia can be treated using stimulants or hormones. Stimulants are usually given during the symptomatic phase. The preferred stimulant, because of it favorable adverse-effect profile and low risk of addiction, is modafinil. Hormonal treatments such as OCPs and hormone replacement therapy have also been shown to be effective.

NARCOLEPSY

Narcolepsy (*see* Table 3) is a neurological disorder characterized by a tetrad of EDS, cataplexy, sleep paralysis, and hypnagogic hallucinations. Men and women are equally affected. Usually it is of gradual onset, with symptoms typically starting during the second or third decade of life. However, case reports exist that detail childhood onset, and some patients are not diagnosed until middle age *(17,18)*.

Table 3
Diagnostic Criteria: Narcolepsy

A. The patient has a complaint of excessive sleepiness or sudden muscle weakness.
B. Recurrent daytime naps or lapses into sleep occur almost daily for at least 3 months.
C. Sudden bilateral loss of postural muscle tone occurs in association with intense emotion (cataplexy).
D. Associated features include:
    1. Sleep paralysis
    2. Hypnagogic hallucinations
    3. Automatic behaviors
    4. Disrupted major sleep episode
E. Polysomnography demonstrates one or more of the following:
    1. Sleep latency less than 10 minutes
    2. REM sleep latency less than 20 minutes
    3. An MSLT that demonstrates a mean sleep latency of less than 5 minutes
    4. Two or more sleep-onset REM periods
F. HLS typing demonstrates DQB1*0602 or DR2 positivity.
G. No medical or mental disorder accounts for the symptoms.
H. Other sleep disorders (e.g., periodic limb movement disorder or central sleep apnea syndrome) may be present but are not the primary cause of the symptoms.

Minimal criteria: B plus C, or A plus D plus E plus G.

EDS is the *sine qua non* of narcolepsy. Like the sleepiness characteristic of other sleep disorders, the EDS of narcolepsy presents with an increased propensity to fall asleep, nod, or doze easily in relaxed or sedentary situations or a need to exert extra effort to avoid sleeping in these situations *(19)*. EDS of narcolepsy no different from that found in other sleep disorders. The "sleep attacks" are not instantaneous lapses into sleep, as is often thought by the general public, but are similar to episodes of profound sleepiness experienced by those with marked sleep deprivation or other severe sleep disorders *(19)*. Cataplexy, a unique feature of narcolepsy, is the partial or complete loss of bilateral muscle tone in response to strong emotion. Reduced muscle tone may be minimal, occur in a few muscle groups, and cause minimal symptoms such as bilateral ptosis, head drooping, slurred speech, or dropping things from the hand. It may be so severe that total body paralysis occurs, resulting in complete collapse.

Cataplectic events usually last from a few seconds to 2 or 3 minutes but occasionally continue longer *(19)*. Respiratory and oculomotor muscles are not affected. Cataplexy rarely precedes the onset of excessive sleepiness but may develop simultaneously with sleepiness or with a delay ranging from 1 to 30 years.

Hypnagogic (hypnopompic) hallucinations are vivid perceptual experiences that occur at sleep onset (hypnagogic) or at sleep offset (hypnopompic). Sleep paralysis is a transient, generalized inability to move or to speak during the transition between sleep and wakefulness. The experiences are often frightening. Disrupted nocturnal sleep with frequent awakenings is common. Some patients with otherwise typical features of narcolepsy do not have cataplexy, a condition referred to as monosymptomatic narcolepsy.

Pathophysiology

A specific human leukocyte antigen (HLA) haplotype that includes HLA-DR1501 (formerly called DR15 or DR2) and HLA-DQB1-0602 (formerly DQ1 or DQ6) has been associated with narcolepsy. The DQB1-0602 may be the HLA-associated narcolepsy susceptibility gene *(20,21)*. Recent discoveries suggest that two hypothalamic peptides, hypocretin I and II, also called orexin A and B *(22)*, are important in the pathophysiology of narcolepsy *(23)*. Narcolepsy in dogs is caused by a deletion in the hypocretin 2-receptor gene *(24)*, whereas rapid eye-movement (REM) sleep episodes while awake and cataplexy are observed in hypocretin knock-out mice *(25)*. In the hypothalamus of patients with narcolepsy, hypocretin-producing cells are reduced by 85–95% *(26)*. CSF content of hypocretin is undetectable in most patients with narcolepsy *(27)*. Serum levels, however, are normal, indicating the brain locality of the disorder. Certain genetic forms of narcolepsy with cataplexy do not depend on the hypocretin pathway and in which patients have normal CSF hypocretin levels *(28)*.

Epidemiology

The prevalence is roughly 0.047% *(29)*.

Treatment

No cause-specific treatment is available for narcolepsy. The main treatment methods are geared toward controlling the different symptoms.

EDS is usually treated with modafinil or any of the other stimulant medications. Modafinil is a novel wake-promoting agent that is chemically and pharmacologically unique and distinct from the other stimulants. It has a low potential for abuse *(30)*, is a first-line therapy for EDS associated with narcolepsy, and is recognized as standard patient care *(31)*. Modafinil is not a dopamine receptor agonist *(32,33)* and does not promote widespread activation of the central nervous system *(34)*. It promotes wakefulness through the selective modulation of hypothalamo–cortical pathways involved in the physiological regulation of sleep and wakefulness *(35,36)*. The dose of modafinil is usually 200–600 mg per day in one to three divided doses.

Cataplexy has traditionally been treated with tricyclic antidepressants or fluoxetine. More recently, a specific medication, sodium oxybate, has been approved for this purpose. There is evidence supporting the long-term efficacy of sodium oxybate for the treatment of cataplexy. In contrast with antidepressant drug therapy, there is no evidence of rebound cataplexy upon abrupt discontinuation of treatment *(37)*. Sodium oxybate is γ-hydroxybutyrate, a 4-carbon fatty acid found in mammalian hypothalamus, basal ganglia, and archicortex *(38)*. It has been used as an anesthetic for many years in Europe.

The dosage for cataplexy is 4.5–9 g taken in two divided doses at night (one dose at bedtime and one dose in the middle of the major sleep period, about 3 hours after the first dose). Sodium oxybate and the antidepressants have also been shown effective in treating the fragmentation of nighttime sleep, hypnic hallucinations, and the sleep paralysis associated with narcolepsy.

Table 4
Diagnostic Criteria: Idiopathic Hypersomnia

A. The patient has a complaint of prolonged sleep episodes, excessive sleepiness, or excessibely deep sleep.

B. The patient has a prolonged nocturnal sleep period or frequent daily sleep episodes.

C. The onset is insidious and typically occurs before age 25.

D. The complaint is present for at least 6 months.

E. The onset does not occur within 18 months of head trauma.

F. Polysomnography demonstates one or more of the following:

    1. A sleep period that is normal or prolonged in duration

    2. Sleep latency less than 10 minutes

    3. Normal REM sleep latency

    4. A less-than-10-minute sleep latency on MSLT

    5. Fewer than two sleep-onset REM periods

G. No medical or mental disorder is present that could account for the symptom.

H. The symptoms do not meet the diagnostic criteria of any other sleep disorder causing excessive sleepiness (e.g., narcolepsy, obstructive sleep apnea syndrome, or post-traumatic hypersomnia).

Minimal criteria: A plus B plus C plus D.

IDIOPATHIC HYPERSOMNIA

Idiopathic hypersomnia (IH; *see* Table 4) is a recently identified clinically heterogeneous entity characterized by prolonged nocturnal sleep, great difficulty waking up, and EDS with nonrefreshing daytime naps lasting from one to several hours *(39)*. Its pathophysiology is much less understood than that of narcolepsy because of a lack of animal models *(39)*. There have been reports that, unlike in narcolepsy, the levels of CSF hypocretin in patients with IH are normal to high *(40)*. CSF levels of leptin, however, are low in both subjects with narcolepsy and those with IH *(41)*. The prevalence of IH is not well defined for the above-mentioned reasons and because the lack of widely recognized laboratory tests has led to overdiagnosis of the condition. Since its discovery in the late 1970s, however, the reported prevalence has varied from approx 2–5 to 30–60 per 100,000 *(42)*. (*See* Table 5.) It is more common in women, with a female to male ratio of 1.8:1, and tends to be more common in Caucasians than in African Americans *(42)*. Another difference between IH and narcolepsy is that IH is sometimes self-limiting and the symptoms of excessive sleepiness can resolve on their own *(42)*.

There are at least two forms of this disorder: (a) a polysymptomatic form, characterized by EDS, nocturnal sleep of abnormally long duration, and signs of sleep drunkenness on awakening, and (b) a monosymptomatic form that manifests only by EDS *(43)*. There are also variants associated with head trauma (posttraumatic) and systemic viral infections (postinfectious).

Treatment

No systemic, controlled trials have been performed in the treatment of idiopathic hypersomnia. Modafinil, however, looks promising in combating the EDS associated with this condition *(39)*.

Table 5
Clinical Features of Narcolepsy vs Clinical Features of Idiopathic Hypersomnia

Narcolepsy	Idiopathic hypersomnia
Onset generally in adolescence	Onset generally in midlife
Associated symptoms of cataplexy, hypnic hallucinations, and sleep paralysis	No associated symptoms
No antecedent head trauma or illness	May have antecedent head trauma or viral illness
Never remits	May resolve spontaneously
HLA-linked	Not HLA linked
F = M	F > M

Table 6
Medications Associated With EDS

Analgesics
Antiasthmatic agents
Anticonvulsants
Antidepressants
Antihistamines
Antihypertensives
Antiparkinsonian agents
Antipsychotic agents
Benzodiazepines
Antiemetics
Withdrawal from stimulants

SECONDARY HYPERSOMNIAS

The most common cause of secondary hypersomnia (not caused by a sleep disorder) is medication-adverse effects. A detailed discussion of all medications that can cause hypersomnia is beyond the scope of this chapter, but certain characteristics are common to most of these medications and pharmacological agents. Most of these drugs tend to be highly lipophilic, and they affect, dopaminergic, cholinergic, or histaminergic receptors. In addition to direct action, the use of certain medications and drugs can result in EDS by disturbing sleep architecture or by producing it as a symptom of withdrawal. Table 6 outlines the different classes of medications associated with EDS.

In addition to iatrogenic secondary hypersomnia, two common medical conditions are associated with EDS: hypothyroidism and major depression (unipolar and bipolar).

HYPOTHYROIDISM AND EXCESSIVE DAYTIME SLEEPINESS

Autoimmune hypothyroidism is more common in women. The mean annual incidence rate female to male ratio is 4:1. Subclinical hypothyroidism is twice as common in women than in men *(44)*. Tiredness is reported as a very prominent symptom of hypothyroidism, although there are no studies in the medical literature that look specifically at objective daytime somnolence measures in patients with hypothyroidism. There is solid evidence, however, for the increased prevalence of OSAS in patients with hypothyroidism *(45–47)*. Apart from being a risk factor for OSAS, hypothyroidism's role in EDS remains to be elucidated. The tiredness reported may represent fatigue or EDS or both. Hypothyroidism being more common in women makes this potential cause of secondary EDS another diagnosis that must be kept in mind while working up female patients with the complaint of tiredeness.

UNIPOLAR AND BIPOLAR DEPRESSION

Hypersomnia can be a symptom of depression, especially in women. Khan et al. *(48)* explored gender differences in the symptoms of major depression in male–female twin pairs. Female twins reported experiencing significantly more fatigue, hypersomnia, and psychomotor retardation during the most severe major depressive episodes, whereas male twins reported more insomnia and agitation *(48)*. In addition, depression is twofold more prevalent in women and depressive episodes more common in women with bipolar illness *(49)*. Given the above factors, although a diagnosis of exclusion, depression should be relatively high on the differential diagnosis list for female patients complaining of fatigue and EDS. Patients complaining of psychiatric hypersomnia tend to have more disrupted sleep at night and on objective measures of EDS tend to score in the normal range despite profound subjective sleepiness. This is in contrast to patients with primary hypersomnia, who tend to have normal sleep at night and are profoundly sleepy both on objective and subjective measures of sleepiness *(50)*.

Treatment

In secondary hypersomnias, the treatment is geared toward treating the underlying cause or eliminating the offending medication whenever possible.

CONCLUSION

EDS is a prevalent problem in developed societies. Women tend to complain more about EDS than men. This gender difference may result from greater sleep deprivation, hormonal factors, and the higher incidence of some primary and secondary sleep disorders in women.

REFERENCES

1. Liu, X., M. Uchiyama, K. Kim, et al., Sleep loss and daytime sleepiness in the general adult population of Japan. *Psychiatry Res*, 2000;**93**(1):1–11.
2. Doi, Y. and M. Minowa, Gender differences in excessive daytime sleepiness among Japanese workers. *Soc Sci Med*, 2003;**56**(4):883–894.
3. Lichstein, K.L., H.H. Durrence, B.W. Riedel, D.J. Taylor, and A.J. Bush, *Epidemiology of Sleep*. Mahwah, NJ: Lawrence Erlbaum Associates, 2004:238.
4. Johns, M. and B. Hocking, Daytime sleepiness and sleep habits of Australian workers. *Sleep*, 1997;**20**(10):844–849.
5. Baldwin, C.M., V.K. Kapur, C.J. Holberg, C. Rosen, and F.J. Nieto, Associations between gender and measures of daytime somnolence in the Sleep Heart Health Study. *Sleep*, 2004;**27**(2):305–311.

6. Liu, X., Z. Sun, M. Uchiyama, K. Shibui, K. Kim, and M. Okawa, Prevalence and correlates of sleep problems in Chinese schoolchildren. *Sleep*, 2000;**23**(8):1053–1062.

7. Doghramji, K., M.M. Mitler, R.B. Sangal, et al., A normative study of the maintenance of wakefulness test (MWT). *Electroencephalogr Clin Neurophysiol*, 1997;**103**(5):554–562.

8. Mitler, M.M., K. Doghramji, and C. Shapiro, The maintenance of wakefulness test: normative data by age. *J Psychosom Res*, 2000;**49**(5):363–365.

9. American Academy of Sleep Medicine.*The International Classification of Sleep Disorders, revised. Diagnostic and Coding Manual.* Chicago: American Academy of Sleep Medicine, 2001.

10. Billiard, M., C. Guilleminault, and W.C. Dement, A menstruation-linked periodic hypersomnia. Kleine-Levin syndrome or new clinical entity? *Neurology*, 1975;**25**(5):436–443.

11. Papy, J.J., B. Conte-Devolx, J. Sormani, R. Porto, and V. Guillame, [The periodic hypersomnia and megaphagia syndrome in a young female, correlated with menstrual cycle (author's transl)]. *Rev Electroencephalogr Neurophysiol Clin*, 1982;**12**(1):54–61.

12. Sachs, C., H.E. Persson, and K. Hagenfeldt, Menstruation-related periodic hypersomnia: a case study with successful treatment. *Neurology*, 1982;**32**(12):1376–1379.

13. Bamford, C.R., Menstrual-associated sleep disorder: an unusual hypersomniac variant associated with both menstruation and amenorrhea with a possible link to prolactin and metoclopramide. *Sleep*, 1993;**16**(5):484–486.

14. Manber, R. and R.R. Bootzin, Sleep and the menstrual cycle. *Health Psychol*, 1997;**16**(3):209–214.

15. Lemire, I., [Review of Kleine-Levin syndrome: toward an integrated approach]. *Can J Psychiatry*, 1993;**38**(4):277–284.

16. Rosenow, F., P. Kotagal, B.H. Cohen, C. Green, and E. Wyllie, Multiple sleep latency test and polysomnography in diagnosing Kleine-Levin syndrome and periodic hypersomnia. *J Clin Neurophysiol*, 2000;**17**(5):519–522.

17. Rye, D.B., B. Dihenia, J.D. Weissman, C.M. Epstein, and D.L. Bliwise, Presentation of narcolepsy after 40. *Neurology*, 1998;**50**(2):459–465.

18. Wise, M.S., Childhood narcolepsy. *Neurology*, 1998;**50**(2 Suppl 1):S37–S42.

19. Black, J.E., S.N. Brooks, and S. Nishino, Narcolepsy and syndromes of primary excessive daytime somnolence. *Semin Neurol*, 2004;**24**(3):271–282.

20. Ellis, M.C., A.H. Hetisimer, D.A. Ruddy, et al., HLA class II haplotype and sequence analysis support a role for DQ in narcolepsy. *Immunogenetics*, 1997;**46**(5):410–417.

21. Mignot, E., A. Kimura, A. Lattermann, et al., Extensive HLA class II studies in 58 non-DRB1*15 (DR2) narcoleptic patients with cataplexy. *Tissue Antigens*, 1997;**49**(4):329–341.

22. Sakurai, T., A. Amemiya, M. Ishii, et al., Orexins and orexin receptors: a family of hypothalamic neuropeptides and G protein-coupled receptors that regulate feeding behavior. *Cell*, 1998;**92**(4):573–585.

23. Kanbayashi, T., Y. Inoue, S. Chiba, et al., CSF hypocretin-1 (orexin-A) concentrations in narcolepsy with and without cataplexy and idiopathic hypersomnia. *J Sleep Res*, 2002;**11**(1):91–93.

24. Lin, L., J. Faraco, R. Li, et al., The sleep disorder canine narcolepsy is caused by a mutation in the hypocretin (orexin) receptor 2 gene. *Cell*, 1999;**98**(3):365–376.

25. Chemelli, R.M., J.T. Willie, C.M. Sinton, et al., Narcolepsy in orexin knockout mice: molecular genetics of sleep regulation. *Cell,* 1999;**98**(4):437–451.

26. Thannickal, T.C., R.Y. Moore, R. Nienhuis, et al., Reduced number of hypocretin neurons in human narcolepsy. *Neuron*, 2000;**27**(3):469–474.

27. Nishino, S., B. Ripley, S. Overeem, G.J. Lammers, and E. Mignot, Hypocretin (orexin) deficiency in human narcolepsy. *Lancet*, 2000;**355**(9197):39–40.

28. Khatami, R., S. Maret, E. Werth, et al., Monozygotic twins concordant for narcolepsy-cataplexy without any detectable abnormality in the hypocretin (orexin) pathway. *Lancet*, 2004;**363**(9416):1199–1200.

29. Ohayon, M.M., M. Caulet, P. Philip, C. Guilleminault, and R.G Priest, How sleep and mental disorders are related to complaints of daytime sleepiness. *Arch Intern Med*, 1997;**157**(22):2645–2652.

30. Thorpy, M.J., J.R. Schwartz, R. Kovacevic-Ristanovic, and R. Hayduk, Initiating treatment with modafinil for control of excessive daytime sleepiness in patients switching from methylphenidate: an open-label safety study assessing three strategies. *Psychopharmacology (Berl)*, 2003;**167**(4):380–385.

31. Littner, M., S.F. Johnson, W.V. McCall, et al., Practice parameters for the treatment of narcolepsy: an update for 2000. *Sleep*, 2001;**24**(4):451–466.

32. Akaoka, H., B. Roussel, J.S. Lin, G. Chouvet, and M. Jouvet, Effect of modafinil and amphetamine on the rat catecholaminergic neuron activity. *Neurosci Lett*, 1991;**123**(1):20–22.

33. Ferraro, L., T. Antonelli, W.T. O'Connor, S. Tanganelli, F.A. Rambert, and K. Fuxe, Modafinil: an antinarcoleptic drug with a different neurochemical profile to d-amphetamine and dopamine uptake blockers. *Biol Psychiatry*, 1997;**42**(12):1181–1183.

34. Engber, T.M., E.J. Koury, S.A. Dennis, M.S. Miller, C. Contreras, and R.V. Bhat, Differential patterns of regional c-Fos induction in the rat brain by amphetamine and the novel wakefulness-promoting agent modafinil. *Neurosci Lett*, 1998;**241**(2–3):95–98.

35. Lin, J.S., Y. Hou, and M. Jouvet, Potential brain neuronal targets for amphetamine-, methylphenidate-, and modafinil-induced wakefulness, evidenced by c-fos immunocytochemistry in the cat. *Proc Natl Acad Sci USA*, 1996;**93**(24):14128–1433.

36. Scammell, T.E., I.V. Estabrooke, M.T. McCarthy, et al., Hypothalamic arousal regions are activated during modafinil-induced wakefulness. *J Neurosci*, 2000;**20**(22):8620–8628.

37. U.S. Xyrem Multicenter Study Group, Sodium oxybate demonstrates long-term efficacy for the treatment of cataplexy in patients with narcolepsy. *Sleep Med*, 2004;**5**(2):119–123.

38. Scrima, L., P.G. Hartman, F.H. Johnson Jr., E.E. Thomas, and F.C. Hiller, The effects of gamma-hydroxybutyrate on the sleep of narcolepsy patients: a double-blind study. *Sleep*, 1990;**13**(6):479–490.

39. Billiard, M. and Y. Dauvilliers, Idiopathic hypersomnia. *Sleep Med Rev*, 2001;**5**(5):349–358.

40. Dauvilliers, Y., C.R. Baumann, B. Carlander, et al., CSF hypocretin-1 levels in narcolepsy, Kleine-Levin syndrome, and other hypersomnias and neurological conditions. *J Neurol Neurosurg Psychiatry*, 2003;**74**(12):1667–1673.

41. Bassetti, C., M. Gugger, M. Bischof, et al., The narcoleptic borderland: a multimodal diagnostic approach including cerebrospinal fluid levels of hypocretin-1 (orexin A). *Sleep Med*, 2003;**4**(1):7–12.

42. Bassetti, C. and M.S. Aldrich, Idiopathic hypersomnia. A series of 42 patients. *Brain*, 1997;**120**(Pt 8):1423–1435.

43. Billiard, M., Idiopathic hypersomnia. *Neurol Clin*, 1996;**14**(3):573–582.

44. Jameson, L.J. and A.P. Weetman, Disorders of the thyroid gland. In: *Harrison's Principles of Internal Medicine* (D.L. Kasper, et al., eds.). Hightstown, NJ: McGraw-Hill, 2004:2104–2127.

45. Lin, C.C., K.W. Tsan, and P.J. Chen, The relationship between sleep apnea syndrome and hypothyroidism. *Chest*, 1992;**102**(6):1663–1667.

46. Miller, C.M. and A.M. Husain, Should women with obstructive sleep apnea syndrome be screened for hypothyroidism? *Sleep Breath*, 2003;**7**(4):185–188.

47. Skjodt, N.M., R. Atkar, and P.A. Easton, Screening for hypothyroidism in sleep apnea. *Am J Respir Crit Care Med*, 1999;**160**(2):732–735.

48. Khan, A.A., C.O. Gardner, C.A. Prescott, and K.S. Kendler, Gender differences in the symptoms of major depression in opposite-sex dizygotic twin pairs. *Am J Psychiatry*, 2002;**159**(8):1427–1429.

49. Sadock, B.J. and V.A. Sadock, Mood disorders. In: *Kaplan and Sadock's Synopsis of Psychiatry: Behavioral Sciences/Clinical Psychiatry* (B.J. Sadock and V.A. Sadock, eds.). Philadelphia: Lippincott Williams & Wilkins, 2002:534–572.

50. Vgontzas, A.N., E.O., Bixler, A. Kales, C. Criley, and A. Vela-Bueno, Differences in nocturnal and daytime sleep between primary and psychiatric hypersomnia: diagnostic and treatment implications. *Psychosom Med*, 2000;**62**(2):220–226.

13
Parasomnias From a Woman's Health Perspective

Carlos H. Schenck and Mark W. Mahowald

INTRODUCTION

Parasomnias are defined as undesirable physical events or experiences that occur during entry into sleep, within sleep, or during arousals from sleep *(1)*. Parasomnias encompass abnormal movements, behaviors, emotions, perceptions, dreaming, and autonomic nervous system functioning that can emerge in relation to any sleep stage at any time of the night. Parasomnias can affect people of any age—infants, newborns, and even fetuses (as described in the documentary *Sleep Runners: The Stories Behind Everyday Parasomnias [2]*). It is believed that the kicking of a fetus *in utero* is a manifestation of "spontaneous motility patterns," that is, the most primitive form of motor activation—without concurrent inhibition—during primordial sleep *(3)*. This developmentally normal motor activity, when exaggerated in intensity and duration, could alter or disrupt the sleep of the "bed partner" (the mother), causing an insomnia in the mother induced by parasomnia behavior in her fetus *(1)*.

Parasomnias are clinical disorders that result in injuries, sleep disruption, adverse health effects, and psychological or interpersonal distress affecting a person and his or her bed partner or roommate. In fact, the new sleep disorders nosology *(1)* has formally introduced the diagnostic category *environmental sleep disorder* to acknowledge how a sleep disturbance in one bed partner (e.g., snoring, leg jerking, general restlessness, sleep terrors, sleepwalking, sleep violence, sleep-related eating, sleeptalking) can cause a sleep disturbance in the bed partner.

Parasomnias often involve problematic release of our basic drives, or deepest instinctual urges, which can become inappropriately activated and co-mingled during our sleep, often with bizarre, frightening, and harmful consequences. Appetitive urges, such as feeding, sex, and sleep itself, can become pathologically linked night after night. Locomotion and aggression are other basic drives that often emerge with parasomnias.

Parasomnias can be categorized as primary parasomnias (disorders of sleep *per se*) or as secondary parasomnias (disorders of other organ systems that manifest themselves during sleep) *(4,5)*. Primary parasomnias now comprise 12 diagnostic

From: *Current Clinical Neurology: Sleep Disorders in Women: A Guide to Practical Management*
Edited by: H. P. Attarian © Humana Press Inc., Totowa, NJ

categories across rapid eye-movement (REM) and non-REM sleep *(1)*. This chapter focuses on parasomnias of particular relevance to females.

Secondary parasomnias can be subdivided according to the organ system involved, such as central nervous system (seizures, headaches), cardiopulmonary system (cardiac arrhythmias; nocturnal angina pectoris, nocturnal asthma, etc.), and gastrointestinal system (gastroesophageal reflux, etc.). Also, various sleep disorders can trigger a secondary parasomnia, such as obstructive sleep apnea (OSA)-induced arousals precipitating an episode of sleepwalking.

During the past two decades, a growing body of work on the parasomnias has been published in peer-reviewed medical journals. As a result, our understanding of this fascinating branch of medicine and its underlying science has been expanded and deepened. New disorders have been identified, and known disorders are now recognized to occur more frequently, across a broader age group, and with more serious consequences than previously recognized. Furthermore, striking gender differences exist across many of the parasomnias, which is a theme that is emphasized in this chapter. A strong genetic basis has been identified for some of the parasomnias, and it is common for multiple parasomnias to be present within the same family or for a person to be afflicted with multiple parasomnias. Finally, most parasomnias can be substantially if not fully controlled with specific therapies once the correct diagnosis is established.

The authors of this chapter served as chairmen of the parasomnias committee for the *International Classification of Sleep Disorders-2* (ICSD-2) *(1)* and therefore are in a good position to share with the readers the latest findings on the parasomnias, including evaluation, diagnosis, co-morbidities, differential diagnosis, and treatment. We focus on the following aspects of women's health: (a) women are especially vulnerable to developing certain parasomnias; (b) women can be adversely affected by parasomnias that affect men equally; (c) women can be adversely affected by aggressive and violent parasomnias preferentially emerging in men; (d) parasomnias can emerge premenstrually in some susceptible women; (e) parasomnias can pose various risks during pregnancy. (Six primary [experiential, sensory, motor] parasomnias listed in ICSD-2 are either beyond the scope of this chapter or quite rare: nightmare disorder, isolated sleep paralysis, sleep-related hallucinations, sleep enuresis, nocturnal groaning, and exploding head syndrome.)

CLINICAL EVALUATION OF PARASOMNIAS

Specific screening questions for parasomnias include the following:

1. Do you or your bed partner believe that you move your arms, legs, or body too much or have unusual and disturbing behaviors during sleep?
2. Do you move while dreaming, as if you are simultaneously attempting to act out the dream?
3. Have you ever hurt yourself or your bed partner during sleep?
4. Do you sleepwalk or have night terrors with shouting or loud screaming?
5. Do you eat, drink, or have sex without full awareness during the night?
6. Do you wake up in the morning with food in your mouth, or feel bloated, have no desire to eat breakfast, or see a mess with food that you created in the kitchen or in the bed?
7. Are you gaining weight inexplicably and wondering if it is from eating during the night?

8. Are you told that you engage in abnormal sexual behaviors with yourself or your bed partner during sleep, such as prolonged and/or violent masturbation, loud or objectionable sexual vocalizations, or (inappropriate) sexual contact with your bed partner?
9. Do your legs feel restless or uncomfortable and/or jump around, or even force you to get up and walk around when you are sleepy, which makes it hard to fall asleep?
10. Do you have episodes of sudden muscle paralysis as you are falling asleep or waking up? Are these episodes sometimes accompanied by visual, auditory, or tactile hallucinations?
11. Do you have episodes of arising during the night after having fallen asleep in which you wander around town, travel long distances, or act like another person with a different personality without remembering what you did and are later told about it?
12. Do you have loud and prolonged groaning during sleep that you may not be aware of, but that disturbs the sleep of others?
13. Do you have body rocking, head rolling, or head banging while being drowsy or during sleep?
14. Do you scratch yourself often during sleep, usually without being aware of it, and draw blood, have scabs marks, and otherwise injure your skin? (Same question for nail biting and hair pulling.)

Anyone who answers "yes" to one or more of the above questions may have a parasomnia and should proceed with the following steps:

1. Talk with people in your family and/or those who sleep in your vicinity to get their input about your sleep. What have they noticed?
2. "Look hard in the mirror" and be honest with yourself to identify any bad habits that could be adversely affecting your sleep. This topic is called sleep hygiene, and many books are available covering all aspects of proper sleep hygiene. Some obvious considerations would be: How regular or irregular is your schedule for falling asleep and waking up? Are you getting enough sleep? (Do you wake up rested or unrefreshed?) What is your pattern and timing for consuming alcohol and caffeine? Do you drink too much of either? Is there too much stress, and might you be having trouble handling it? Do you have physical symptoms or a medical or psychiatric disorder that could be affecting your sleep? Are medications or over-the-counter drugs affecting your sleep? Many of these are commonsense questions, but we all can have blind spots about ourselves or may be too busy to take stock of our situation. That is why seeking the input of others who know about your sleep is important. However, on the other hand, don't unnecessarily blame yourself for having a persistent sleep problem, such as a parasomnia, if you could not identify any major issues with your sleep hygiene or if in fact you did clean up your act, but the sleep problems continued. Then you need to go on to the next step in the process.
3. Make an appointment to see your doctor to discuss these sleep issues, to have him or her examine you, order the appropriate tests, and perhaps adjust the dose of a medication that you may be taking, or even consider a medication change.
4. If none of the above measures helps to solve your parasomnia and/or other sleep complaint, then your physician should refer you to a physician at an accredited sleep-disorders center who is experienced in evaluating and treating parasomnias and who could order polysomnographic monitoring.

The evaluation of complex, disruptive, and violent sleep-related behaviors should include the following *(6)*:

1. Clinical sleep–wake interview and examinations: the bed partner is urged to attend the interview. Past and current medical records are reviewed, along with a patient-completed questionnaire that covers the following areas: sleep–wake, medical, and psychi-

atric history, and caffeine/alcohol/chemical use and abuse history; review of systems (i.e., review of any current physical and mental–emotional symptoms); past or current history of abuse (physical, sexual, verbal–emotional); and family medical, sleep, and psychiatric history.
2. Screening psychological tests (e.g., Beck Depression and Anxiety Inventories, Minnesota Multiphasic Personality Inventory, Symptom Checklist–90, Dissociative Experiences Scale) and, whenever indicated, a psychiatric interview.
3. Extensive overnight polysomnographic (PSG) monitoring at a hospital-based sleep laboratory, with continuous, time-synchronized (to the PSG tracing) audiovisual recording. PSG involves the recording of eye movements (electro-oculogram), brain wave activity (EEG) employing a full conventional EEG montage; muscle tone and muscle twitch activity (electromyograms), electrocardiogram, and nasal–oral airflow with full respiratory effort monitoring.

FEMALE-PREDOMINANT PARASOMNIAS
Sleep-Related Eating Disorder
Clinical Findings

The following comments were made by the index patient in a series of 38 cases reported by our sleep center: "I have buttered pop cans and then tried to eat them...I will take the big container of salt—not the salt shaker—and I'll pour it in my hand and I'll eat it just like that. Why do I eat salt sandwiches? That's a biggie... I have sat at the kitchen table eating pancakes at two o'clock in the morning with no clothes on...How primitive can one get? Leftover casseroles—it's awful."

The hallmark of sleep-related eating disorder (SRED) is involuntary ("out-of-control") eating and drinking during nighttime sleep that usually occur during partial arousals from sleep, with spotty recall the next morning. However, a broad range of consciousness and of subsequent recall can be present *(1,7–10)*.

Problems associated with recurrent episodes of SRED include the following: the consumption of peculiar forms or odd combinations of food or of inedible or toxic substances; insomnia from sleep disruption; sleep-related injury; morning anorexia (lack of hunger) and abdominal distention; and adverse health consequences (e.g., weight gain/obesity).

Most affected people report a nightly frequency of eating, including multiple times nightly. The episodes of eating can occur during any time of the night. Highly caloric foods are eaten with preference (e.g., sweets, pasta, peanut butter, milkshakes). Fruits and vegetables are ignored. The foods preferentially consumed with SRED are not typically consumed with any preference during the day. Alcohol is rarely consumed at night—even in those who enjoy drinking alcohol or in former alcoholics. Also, there is virtually never any awareness of hunger or thirst during episodes of SRED. If an individual is interfered with during an episode (e.g., a spouse trying to redirect one back to bed to prevent any eating), the usual response is irritability and agitation.

Sometimes the episodes of eating are experienced as food-related enactment of a dream. One woman dreamed that she was preparing to host an elaborate dinner party, and when the food she had cooked during the night was placed on the dining room table the next morning, she awakened dressed in an evening gown and was surprised and irritated that no guest had arrived—until she suddenly realized that she had "done it again" in her sleep. To adapt a line from a famous poem by Samuel Taylor Coleridge: the feast was set, the guests were not met.

Simple foods or entire hot or cold meals can be prepared, even cooked, and then eaten, often quite sloppily. Food is often brought back to bed, where another mess is made. One husband, who finally resigned himself to his wife's nightly sleepeating, asked her: "Can't you at least keep the crumbs on your side of the bed?" Another woman would commonly awaken in the morning and see "the ketchup line on the floor leading from the kitchen to my bed." Yet another woman, a single mother, out of desperation paid her teenage children to sleep in sleeping bags in the kitchen at night, so that when she went there every night to raid the refrigerator they would block her passage to the food and direct her back to bed. When she became increasingly irritated by this repeated denial of her midnight snacking, she ended up paying her children even more money to return to their rooms to sleep, allowing her once again unlimited access to the refrigerator. An Australian tabloid once had a headline that described a night-eating lady who awakened one morning "glued to her bed" after she had brought some caramel-laden chocolate bars back to bed from the pantry, rolled over them during sleep, and by morning had become stuck to the melted mess, and screamed when she couldn't move.

A preliminary study utilizing a self-report questionnaire found a prevalence of SRED (defined as eating during semi-awakenings from sleep at least once weekly) of nearly 5% *(11)*. This included a prevalence of 4.6% in an unselected university student group. This study suggests that there are many people with SRED in our society. Confirmatory studies across different clinical and nonclinical population groups are clearly needed.

SRED is a female-predominant condition, with approximately two-thirds to three-fourths of published cases being female. The age of onset is usually in the late teens or early 20s, but a very broad range exists—including onset during infancy. The average duration of sleep-related eating prior to clinical presentation at our sleep center is 10–15 years, which indicates that this is often a relentless, longstanding disorder.

Although sleep-related eating can be a spontaneous or idiopathic disorder, it often is associated with a primary, underlying sleep disorder or other clinical condition. For example, sleepwalking is the most commonly associated sleep disorder, although once eating becomes part of the behavioral repertoire of sleepwalking, it quickly becomes the predominant, if not the exclusive, sleepwalking behavior. What is impressive about this scenario is that individuals with a longstanding history of displaying a broad range of sleepwalking behaviors will shortly cease to engage in these customary sleepwalking behaviors once the eating appears and becomes the dominant or exclusive behavior.

Other sleep disorders that can be closely associated with SRED include restless legs syndrome, OSA, and circadian rhythm disorders (such as irregular sleep–wake pattern). Medication-induced (amnestic) sleep-related eating disorder has been reported with the hypnotic agents zolpidem (Ambien) *(12,13)*, triazolam (Halcion) *(8)*, and various medications used to treat major psychiatric disorders (e.g., lithium carbonate for bipolar mood disorder and anticholingeric antidepressants and antipsychotics) *(8)*.

Onset of SRED can also occur with cessation of cigarette smoking, with cessation of alcohol and substance abuse (especially cocaine and amphetamine), with acute stress (usually involving major separation reactions), after daytime dieting, and with onset of narcolepsy, migraine headaches, and various other conditions. SRED at times can be associated with daytime eating disorders (such as bulimia nervosa [BN] or binge-eating disorder [BED]) and with a nocturnal dissociative disorder (e.g., multiple personality disorder, with one of the "alter" personalities being a nocturnal eater).

The onset can be insidious and sporadic, or it can be precipitous and fulminant, with rapid development of nightly episodes of eating. The clinical course is usually unremitting, with episodes often occurring on a nightly or multiple-times-nightly basis. A family history of sleep-related eating disorder is not uncommon.

Serious complications can occur as a result of the typically indiscriminate nocturnal eating: excessive weight gain and obesity; compromise in the control of diabetes mellitus (type 1 or type 2), hypercholesterolemia, or hypertriglyceridemia; tooth decay; risk of consuming foods to which one is allergic; overnight fasting prior to next-day surgery; etc. Furthermore, secondary depressive disorders may emerge from longstanding personal dejection and a sense of failure resulting from the inability to control the nocturnal eating.

Despite the broad range of predisposing and precipitating factors for SRED, the relatively homogeneous set of clinical features suggests the presence of a final common pathway. Although there are prominent features of both a sleep disorder and an eating disorder, its relatively homogeneous presentation supports its classification as a separate diagnostic entity. Also, more than half of the patients have a history of parasomnia (usually sleepwalking) that preceded the onset of nocturnal eating, which indicates that the presence of a parasomnia is a major risk factor for the development of SRED. On the other hand, the female predominance is more consistent with eating disorders than with sleepwalking, restless legs syndrome or periodic limb movement disorder, which do not have a gender predominance. Thus it appears that two basic drive states—sleeping and eating—are pathologically intertwined in the unique diagnostic entity of sleep-related eating disorder.

The episodes of eating always occur after an interval of sleep, and usually during partial arousals from sleep, with reduced alertness and awareness, impaired judgment, and diminished subsequent recall. However, the episodes of eating can also emerge from sleep with nearly complete unawareness and total subsequent amnesia. A minority of episodes may occur with nearly complete awareness and clear subsequent recall. Also, there can be variability of awareness and subsequent recall within one night and across the course of this disorder in individual patients.

Adverse consequences of sleep-related eating (other than the involuntary nature of the eating) include at least one category from the following group:

1. Eating peculiar forms or combinations of food (e.g., frozen pizzas; raw bacon; peanut butter, salt, and sugar sandwiches; cat food sandwiches) and inedible or toxic sub-

stances (e.g., cigarettes, coffee grounds, glue, nail polish, ammonia-containing cleaning compounds).

2. Insomnia related to sleep disruption from repeated episodes of eating, with daytime sleep-deprivation symptoms: tiredness, fatigue, irritability, moodiness, interpersonal problems, reduced attention span, diminished memory, and sub-par work or school performance.

3. Sleep-related injury: cutting oneself from carelessly cutting food or opening cans, and so on; internal or external burns from consuming or spilling hot or scalding foods or beverages; poisoning and internal injuries from ingesting toxic substances.

4. Dangerous behaviors performed while seeking food: for example, driving a car while half-asleep or starting a fire in the kitchen while engaged in sleep-related cooking prior to eating.

5. Morning anorexia, often with bloating and no desire to eat breakfast.

6. Adverse health consequences from recurrent binge-eating of excessive quantities of high-caloric foods; excessive weight gain/obesity; destabilization (or precipitation) of diabetes mellitus (type 1 or 2); hypertriglyceridemia; hypercholesterolemia; tooth damage and decay.

Differential Diagnoses

There are two main differential diagnostic considerations for abnormal nocturnal eating other than SRED: (a) nocturnal BN or BED (i.e., extensions of a daytime eating disorder) and (b) night-eating syndrome (NES) *(14)*.

If inappropriate compensatory behavior in order to prevent weight gain from nocturnal eating is present—such as self-induced vomiting or misuse of enemas, laxatives, diuretics, or other medications—eating disorder should be diagnosed (BN, BED, anorexia nervosa [AN]). However, patients with longstanding SRED and excessive weight gain may eventually fast during the daytime and/or engage in excessive exercise to prevent further weight gain and obesity.

If a history of excessive eating between dinner and sleep onset is present, the diagnosis would probably be a different eating disorder—NES—which is not a parasomnia, but rather a disorder of wakefulness. Sometimes patients with SRED will eat dinner or have a substantial second dinner shortly before going to bed at night in a futile attempt to suppress the compulsion to eat after subsequently arousing from sleep.

BN, BED, and NES are described here to distinguish them from SRED.

BN and AN binge/purge subtype involve purging followed bingeing, which never occurs with SRED. Also, bingeing during SRED generally occurs during a state of partial consciousness or unconsciousness with either spotty subsequent recall or no recall whatsoever for the bingeing episode(s). In contrast, bingeing with BN and AN occurs during full wakefulness and with complete subsequent recall. People with BN and AN—but not with SRED—are excessively influenced by the (mis)perceptions of their body weight and shape, and they openly acknowledge being preoccupied with ongoing thoughts about food. BED involves consuming large quantities of food very rapidly with a concomitant feeling of shame, but no subsequent purging takes place. However, BED rarely occurs at night, and there is usually no history of sleep disruption or parasomnia.

NES may at times overlap with SRED in individual patients, but in general these are two separate conditions. NES involves overeating during full wakefulness either in the evening between dinner and bedtime and/or during full awakenings during the nocturnal sleep period, and there is always full recall of the eating the next day. During these nocturnal awakenings, it is very difficult to return to sleep without eating. Therefore, NES is often associated with sleep-maintenance insomnia (and sleep-onset insomnia), and not with a parasomnia, whereas the opposite is true for SRED, which is a parasomnia with eating typically occurring during partial arousals from sleep (often in patients with a history of sleepwalking or other primary sleep disorder, such as restless legs syndrome), and compromised recall for the eating the next day. SRED appears to be considerably more female-predominant than NES. Both SRED and NES share common features, such as the foods consumed at night ("comfort foods," i.e., high in fat and carbohydrates), and lack of hunger for breakfast in the morning. NES seem to have a considerably higher risk for depression and "neurotic" traits than SRED, although some overlap exists in this area between these two conditions. Although the prevalence of NES has not been established, just as the prevalence for SRED has not been established, a conservative estimate is 1.5%.

Treatment of SRED

Treatment is at first directed at controlling any underlying sleep disorder or discontinuing any medication that is suspected to be causing or promoting the SRED. For example, in patients with SRED presumably induced by OSA, treatment of the OSA with nasal continuous positive airway pressure (nCPAP) may also control abnormal nocturnal eating. In patients with SRED associated with restless legs syndrome, treatment with a "dopamine-enhancing" medication, at times combined with another medication(s), can control both sleep problems.

SRED can be a challenging parasomnia to control. Our sleep center has identified successful treatments, such as dopaminergic (and supplemental) therapy, to help control SRED *(7,8)*. A promising new treatment in SRED cases associated with atypical sleepwalking or that are otherwise unexplained (idiopathic), and in certain other cases, consists of the (appetite-suppressing) anticonvulsant topiramate taken at bedtime *(15)*.

Sleep-Related Dissociative Disorders

Clinical Findings

Sleep-related (or nocturnal) dissociative disorders (DDs) comprise the only true psychiatric parasomnia. However, this category of parasomnia emerges during well-established wakefulness after periods of sleep *(1,16)*. Sleep-related DDs can emerge at any time during the night from well-developed wakefulness—either at the transition from wakefulness to sleep or within several minutes after an awakening from any stage of sleep. This is very different from sleepwalking or night terrors, which emerge immediately during precipitous arousals from non-REM sleep. It is also very different from REM sleep behavior disorder, which emerges during REM sleep.

Nocturnal DDs comprise a sleep-related variant of DDs, which are defined in the fourth edition of the *Diagnostic and Statistical Manual of Psychiatric Disorders* (DSM-IV), published by the American Psychiatric Association, as follows:

"The essential feature...is a disruption in the usually integrated functions of consciousness, memory, identity, or perception of the environment."

Of the five listed diagnostic categories contained within the DD section of DSM-IV, three categories to date have been documented with nocturnal DDs: Dissociative identity disorder (formerly called multiple personality disorder), dissociative fugue, and dissociative disorder not otherwise specified.

Most patients with nocturnal DDs also have corresponding daytime DDs and also have past and/or current histories of physical and/or sexual abuse. Posttraumatic stress disorder, major mood disorders, severe anxiety disorders, multiple suicide attempts, self-mutilating behaviors, and repeated psychiatric hospitalizations are also common. Nevertheless, a nocturnal DD can at times (seemingly) occur in isolation, without a daytime component.

During the sleep period, patients with nocturnal dissociation can scream; walk or run around in a frenzied manner; engage in self-mutilating behaviors (including genital and body slashing with a knife; burning oneself; head banging; hair pulling) and other violent behaviors, including acts of violence—and attempted homicidal acts—toward the bed partner.

The episodes of nocturnal dissociation can be elaborate and last several minutes to an hour or longer and often involve behaviors that represent reenactments of previous physical or sexual abuse scenarios. This activity may occur with perceived dreaming, which is actually a dissociated wakeful memory of past abuse. Sexualized behavior (e.g., pelvic thrusting) can occur and be paired with defensive behavior (e.g., warding off or hitting an attacker) and with congruent verbalization (e.g., telling the attacker to stop or go away). Other dissociative episodes may occur as confusional states, with or without elaborate behaviors, which are not associated with perceived dreaming. A postassault headache can be reexperienced during nocturnal dissociation. One patient was reported with at least two episodes of nocturnal fugues in which she awakened from sleep and drove her car to an airport, where she purchased a ticket and flew to a distant city, where shortly after arrival she "came to" and realized she had just finished another dissociative episode.

Nocturnal DDs are highly female-predominant. Age of onset ranges from childhood to early-mid-adulthood. Onset can be abrupt and fulminant, or it can be gradual and sporadic. The course is usually chronic and severe, with episodes often occurring several times weekly or multiple times nightly. Complications include repeated injuries to oneself and/or one's bed partner while the person is in a dissociative state, including bruises, fractures, lacerations, and burn wounds. Skin and genital infections from self-mutilation can also occur. A past and/or current history of physical, sexual, or verbal–emotional abuse, along with a severe and chronic history of psychiatric disorders, constitute the major predisposing and precipitating factors.

Polysomnographic Findings

At least eight cases have been documented (four from our sleep center) involving 11 episodes of nocturnal dissociation recorded during polysomnographic monitoring. EEG (brain-wave) wakefulness was maintained before, during, and after each episode.

Treatment

Specialized psychiatric treatments, both inpatient and outpatient, offer the best chance of helping severely afflicted patients. DDs are among the most difficult psychiatric disorders to control, and chronic, relapsing histories are common.

GENDER-NEUTRAL PARASOMNIAS

Non-REM Sleep Parasomnias: Sleepwalking, Night (Sleep) Terrors, and Confusional Arousals

Sleepwalking and sleep terrors typically arise from the delta- or slow-wave stage of deep non-REM sleep *(1)*. Sleepwalking and sleep terrors primarily affect children, but we now know that many adults can also be affected. In fact, not only have many adults not outgrown their sleepwalking and sleep terrors, but in one of our published studies, one-third developed sleepwalking and sleep terrors after puberty and often well into adulthood. Even some people in their 60s can suddenly develop sleepwalking and sleep terrors.

Sleepwalking is characterized by complex, automatic behaviors, such as leaving the bed, wandering about aimlessly or semi-purposely, carrying objects nonsensically from one place to another, rearranging furniture, engaging in inappropriate eating or sexual activity, urinating in closets or into waste baskets, running around, going outdoors, jumping into a lake or river—and sometimes driving an automobile. The eyes are usually wide open and have a glassy or peculiar stare, and there may be some mumbling or talking, including prolonged talking that may be punctuated by shouting or loud swearing. Not surprisingly, communication with a sleepwalker is usually limited or impossible.

Frenzied or aggressive behavior, the wielding of weapons (knives, guns, baseball bats), or the calm suspension of judgment (e.g., going out a bedroom window or wandering far outdoors on a winter's night) can result in inadvertent injury or death to oneself or others *(6,17)*.

Sleepwalking episodes usually emerge 15–120 minutes after sleep onset, but they can occur throughout the entire sleep period in adults. The duration of each episode can vary widely.

Sleep terrors are characterized by sudden, loud, terrified screaming, with wide dilation of the pupils, rapid heart rate and breathing, and profuse sweating *(1)*. The person may sit up rapidly while shouting or screaming and engage in frenzied activity and become injured *(6)*. Sleep terror episodes usually appear as early in the sleep period as sleepwalking, although episodes of sleepwalking and sleep terrors in adults can occur at any time of the night.

Childhood sleepwalking and sleep terrors are characterized by complete amnesia of the events. In adult sleepwalking and sleep terrors, there can be subsequent recall of the events and also recall of dreaming during the events that usually involves being threatened by an imminent danger, such as a menacing intruder, a fire, or the ceiling caving in. Sometimes there can be plot development within dreams during sleepwalking and sleep terrors. The distinction between sleep terrors and agitated sleepwalking in adults is often blurred, because terrified screaming can be intermixed with angry shouting in a person who is alternately seeking safety and fighting a perceived attacker. Therefore, at our center we often diagnose adults with mixed "sleepwalking/sleep terrors."

Much more interaction with the actual environment takes place with sleepwalking and sleep terrors than with REM sleep behavior disorder (RBD), because the eyes are open during episodes of sleepwalking and sleep terrors, whereas they are usually closed with RBD while the person is attending to his or her dream environment and is oblivious to the real world.

The prevalence of sleepwalking has been estimated to be as high as 17% in childhood (peaking at age 4–8 years), and recent data indicate a higher prevalence in adults (4%) than previously recognized. The prevalence of sleep terrors ranges from 1–6.5% in children and 2.3–2.6% across the 15- to 64-year age span, before dropping to 1%. A familial-genetic basis for sleepwalking and sleep terrors is well established. Noninjurious sleepwalking has no gender preference, but injurious sleepwalking is more male predominant. There is no distinct gender difference in sleep terrors.

Confusional arousals comprise another category of disorder of arousal and represent partial manifestations of sleepwalking and sleep terrors *(1)*. Confusional arousals can last for variable intervals of time, including prolonged episodes with irritability and anger. Confusional arousals are especially prevalent among children and adults younger than 35 years. The prevalence rate in children 3–13 years of age in one large population-based study was 17.3%. The prevalence among adults older than 15 years of age is 2.9–4.2%. Genetic factors are the most important predisposing factors, but rotating shift work, night shift work, other sleep disorders (hypersomnia, insomnia, circadian), sleep insuffiency, stress, and anxiety, bipolar, and depressive disorders are other recognized predisposing factors. Precipitating factors include recovery from sleep deprivation, alcohol consumption, OSA, periodic limb movements of sleep, psychotropic medication use, drug abuse, and forced awakenings.

Sleep inertia—the inability to promptly and properly transition oneself both physically and mentally from sleep to wakefulness—is commonly present with confusional arousals. A variant of confusional arousals consists of severe morning sleep inertia, in which the affected individual is unable to transition from sleep to wakefulness in a timely fashion, resulting in adverse consequences at school, work and with interpersonal relationships *(1)*. Also, sleep-related abnormal sexual behavior is a recently recognized variant of confusional arousals, with published reports referring to this phenomenon as "sleepsex," "sexsomnia," or "atypical sexual behavior during sleep" *(1,18–21)*. Behaviors during sleep include loud sexual vocalizations, prolonged and/or violent masturbation, sexual molestation and assaults of minors or adults (including spouses), and initiation of sexual intercourse irrespective of the menstrual status of the bed partner (unlike during wakefulness). The presence of snoring during nocturnal sexual activity has clearly indicated that the person was asleep. Some cases have also included other parasomnia activity, such as sleep-related eating and sleep-related driving. Morning amnesia for the nocturnal sexual behavior has been present in all reported cases. Polysomnographic monitoring has usually documented evidence supporting the diagnosis of a disorder of arousal (mainly confusional arousals and/or sleepwalking).

Finally, repetitive nocturnal scratching, nail-biting, and hair-pulling can be regarded as other variants of confusional arousals and consist of frequent (often nightly) repetitive scratching that can be so vigorous as to draw blood, resulting in multiple scabs, skin sores, and infections. At times the focus of the repetitive scratching is the peri-anal region. Gender distribution appears to be equal. Treatment may consist of wearing gloves to bed (often wrapped in tape to make them more difficult to remove during sleep) as well as medications effective in controlling other disorders of arousal.

Polysomnographic Findings in Sleepwalking, Sleep Terrors, and Confusional Arousals

Episodes of sleepwalking and sleep terrors arise abruptly during arousals from any stage of non-REM sleep, most commonly from delta (slow-wave) non-REM sleep. During an episode, the brain wave activity (EEG) can show either the persistence of sleep, the admixture of sleep and wakefulness, or complete wakefulness. There is often an impressive dissociation—a major discordance—between a fully awake brain wave pattern and the very "spacey" appearance and confused behavior of the sleepwalker (or person in the midst of a sleep terror).

Episodes of sleepwalking and sleep terrors can be triggered by sleep deprivation, alcohol use or abuse, stress, fever, menstruation, pregnancy, medical and psychiatric disorders, and various medications. The contemporary medical literature on adult sleepwalking and sleep terrors indicates that most cases are not causally associated with a psychological problem or a psychiatric disorder, although stress can play a promoting role. Nevertheless, at least half of adult patients with sleepwalking and sleep terrors have a history of depression and/or anxiety.

Treatment of Sleepwalking, Sleep Terrors, and Confusional Arousals

Treatment is often not necessary (especially in childhood cases), other than identifying and minimizing any identified risk factors and maximizing the safety of the bedroom. If a child or an adult has left the bed, he or she should be calmly redirected back to bed, avoiding any intervention that could agitate the individual.

Teaching a patient to practice self-hypnosis *(22)* or other relaxation techniques at bedtime can be effective in milder cases of adult or childhood sleepwalking and sleep terrors. A psychologist or other clinician can tailor the self-hypnosis and relaxation instructions to suit the individual needs and wishes of each affected person. Use of night lights, motion sensors, door alarms, and other safety devices should always be considered. In cases involving sleep-related injury (usually in adults), treatment with bedtime medication is usually necessary and can be life-saving.

Almost any benzodiazepine agent taken 30–75 minutes before bedtime is usually effective. At our sleep center, we usually prescribe clonazepam at a dose of 0.5–1.0 mg. Long-term, nightly benzodiazepine treatment of adult sleep terrors and sleepwalking and of other parasomnias has been found to be safe and remarkably effective, with a low incidence of side effects, misuse, or abuse *(23)*. These data should reassure patients, their families, sleep specialists, and primary physicians. Various other medications can be used (e.g., imipramine and paroxetine), although fewer numbers of patients have been reported with these treatments. Of great importance is the finding that treatment and control of any concurrent psychiatric disorder does not usually control sleepwalking and sleep terrors, even if both conditions began concurrently.

We have identified successful treatments of severe morning sleep inertia, primarily consisting of administration of sustained-release (SR) methylphenidate and/or bupropion-SR taken immediately before the onset of nocturnal sleep *(24)*.

Treatment of abnormal sleep-related sexual behaviors primarily consists of treating the underlying disorder, namely confusional arousals and sleepwalking: bedtime administration of clonazepam has been reported to be effective *(19)*, as has nCPAP therapy (if OSA is present, presumably enhancing the confusional arousals and/or sleepwalking with abnormal sexual behaviors). Also, the physician should consider referral of the patient and partner to a psychologist or psychiatrist for one of two reasons (or both): (a) to explore the marital/interpersonal relationship as a contributing factor to the sexual parasomnia and (b) to deal with the adverse consequences (personal and interpersonal) of the sexual parasomnia.

MALE-PREDOMINANT PARASOMNIA: REM SLEEP BEHAVIOR DISORDER

REM sleep in mammals involves a highly energized state of brain activity, with continuous and intermittent activity (called "tonic"and "phasic") occurring across a range of physiological functions. REM sleep has two major synonyms: "active sleep," because of the high level of brain activity during REM sleep, and "paradoxical sleep," because of the nearly complete suppression of muscle tone despite the high level of brain activity. This generalized muscle paralysis (REM-atonia) is one of the three defining features of mammalian REM sleep, besides rapid eye movements and an activated brain-wave (EEG) pattern virtually identical to the EEG of wakefulness.

The loss of the customary paradox of REM sleep in RBD carries serious clinical consequences, since sleep is no longer safe when the acting-out of dreams becomes possible.

Clinical Findings

There is a distinct clinical profile in the longstanding (chronic) form of RBD *(1,25)*. Chronic RBD has a striking older male predominance, with an average age of onset in the early fifties, and with males comprising more than 85% of patients. Nevertheless, females and virtually all age groups can be identified with RBD. A hallmark of RBD in about 90% of patients is the acting out of distinctly altered dreams that have become more vivid, intense, action-packed, confrontational, and violent. In other words, people with RBD do not act out their customary dreams, but rather act out dreams that are altered in a stereotypical, abnormal fashion. Most or all people with RBD have the same types of disturbed dreams that are then acted out. The typical RBD dream scenario involves being threatened or attacked by unfamiliar people, animals, or insects, and then fighting the attacker to protect oneself or a loved one from being harmed. Therefore, RBD is a dream disorder almost as much as it is a behavior disorder arising from REM sleep.

Dream-enacting behaviors observed by the bed partners and documented during sleep lab monitoring include the following: talking, yelling, swearing, gesturing, grabbing, arm flailing, punching, kicking, sitting, jumping out of bed, crawling, and running. Before eventually seeking help at a sleep-disorders center, patients with RBD often have had to protect themselves while sleeping and have resorted to such measures as retiring for the night to a sleeping bag, padded waterbed, barricade of pillows, or mattress placed on the floor or tying themselves to their beds or bedposts with belts, ropes, or dog leashes.

The wives of men with RBD are often battered during their husband's violent dream-enacting behaviors, and their faces, arms, and torsos can become bruised. Not uncommonly, physicians and nurses question whether willful domestic abuse has taken place. Nevertheless, it is evident to these wives that their husbands are asleep and dreaming while they engage in their aggressive and violent nocturnal behavior. Furthermore, in most cases the wives remain in bed with their husbands in order to protect their husbands from hurting themselves. Also, no case of marital separation or divorce has been reported with RBD, probably because most couples affected by RBD had been married for decades before its onset, and the wives knew that their husbands were gentle men without a propensity for aggression or violence during their waking lives. In contrast, marital discord directly related to RBD has been reported in a recently married young adult couple, which resolved when the RBD was eventually controlled with appropriate treatment *(26)*.

More than half of RBD cases are closely associated with brain disorders *(25)*. The brain disorders are predominantly neurodegenerative conditions, such as Parkinson's disease and related conditions, narcolepsy, and stroke, but a large number of brain disorders have been found with RBD. In fact, RBD may be the first sign of a neurological disorder whose other ("classic") manifestations may not emerge until several years or decades after the onset of RBD. For example, we now know from our sleep center's ongoing research that about two-thirds of men over the age of 50 years with RBD will eventually develop Parkinson's disease (PD) or a related condition, such as multiple system atrophy or Lewy body dementia, at a mean interval of 13 years, but with the range extending from 2 to 29 years *(27,28)*. This is fascinating, and also ominous, in that a distinct change in a person's dreams (a form of consciousness), and then the acting-out of those dreams, can be the harbinger of a full-fledged brain disorder that is decades from manifesting itself. Thus, routine neurological evaluations are indicated in the long-term management of RBD.

The prevalence of RBD is unknown, but is estimated to be as high as 0.5% in the elderly population *(1)*. It is possible that just as many females have RBD as men, but with less violence (a general trend in male–female comparisons), so that their more attenuated or "quiet" form of RBD does not cause problems, remains mainly unnoticed, and thus does not require medical intervention. A genetic or familial basis for RBD at present seems unlikely.

The course of RBD is usually progressive; spontaneous remissions are very rare. There is also an acute or sudden-onset form of RBD that emerges during withdrawal from alcohol or drug abuse and with various medication intoxication states, and acute withdrawal states. The behavioral and dream abnormalities in acute RBD are virtually identical to those in chronic RBD.

Psychiatric disorders are rarely associated with RBD. This is important to emphasize, since the symptoms of RBD can seem so "psychiatric"—with the acting-out of violent dreams, with screaming and shouting profanities. On the other hand, psychotropic medications used to treat psychiatric disorders can induce or aggravate RBD. This is an important new focus for future RBD research. Certain antidepressant medications appear to be especially likely to cause or aggravate RBD, or its precursor, preclinical RBD (i.e., polysomnographic abnormalities without a clinical parasomnia history to date)—selective serotonin reuptake inhibitors (fluoxetine [Prozac], sertraline [Zoloft], citalopram [Celexa], etc.), venlafaxine (Effexor), mirtazapine [Remeron], and others, such as tricyclic antidepressants and monoamine oxidase inhibitors *(29)*. However, bupropion (Wellbutrin) may actually protect against RBD because of its dopaminergic neurotransmitter profile, and no case of RBD or preclinical RBD caused or aggravated by bupropion has been reported (or would be expected to be reported) after more than 10 years of widespread use. As such, a patient with RBD who develops a clinical depression would be a prime candidate for bupropion therapy as the initial pharmacological consideration.

Diagnosis

The diagnosis requires formal sleep laboratory (i.e., polysomnographic) monitoring in conjunction with clinical evaluations *(1)*. The diagnostic criteria include (a) increased muscle tone and/or increased muscle twitching during REM sleep, (b) abnormal behaviors documented during REM sleep and/or a history of injurious or disruptive sleep behaviors, and (c) absence of epileptic brain-wave activity during REM sleep.

Treatment

RBD can be successfully controlled in about 90% of treated patients. Clonazepam is the treatment of choice, with the typical effective bedtime dose being 0.5–1.0 mg (occasionally higher). The long-term efficacy and safety of nightly clonazepam treatment of RBD has been well established *(23)*. Clonazepam appears to suppress the abnormal phasic muscle twitching and behavioral release during REM sleep, rather than restore the normal muscle paralysis (REM atonia) of REM sleep. More recently, the natural hormone melatonin (produced by the pineal gland in the center of the brain) administered at bedtime has been shown to be effective in RBD at doses ranging from 3 to 15 mg *(25)*. The mechanism of therapeutic action for melatonin is unknown. Some patients with RBD seem to respond best to a combination of clonazepam and melatonin, especially those with (advanced) neurodegenerative disorders. It is important to note that RBD cannot be "cured" but is rather controlled—provided that the medication(s) is taken faithfully every night.

Therefore, people must be diligent about taking their medication along on any trip, even a brief one, since any recurrence of RBD carries the risk of major injury to oneself and a loved one. Finally, maximizing the safety of the sleeping environment should always be encouraged (e.g., keep sharp objects away from the bedside).

PARASOMNIAS ASSOCIATED WITH OSA AND ITS TREATMENT

Parasomnias and OSA can interact in a number of adverse ways *(1,5)*:

1. OSA-induced arousals from REM sleep with dream-related complex or violent behaviors can resemble REM sleep behavior disorder: pseudo-RBD.
2. OSA-induced confusional arousals from non-REM sleep can be associated with recurrent abnormal sexual behaviors (sexsomnia), with both OSA and sexsomnia ultimately being controlled with nCPAP therapy of the OSA.
3. OSA-induced arousals from non-REM sleep with complex, agitated, or violent behaviors can resemble sleepwalking and/or sleep terrors.
4. nCPAP therapy of OSA may prompt a major slow-wave sleep "rebound" and the emergence of sleepwalking or sleep terrors.
5. Untreated sleepwalking or sleep terrors, with recurrent sleep disruption, can undermine nCPAP therapy of OSA, because of the repeated or prolonged removal of the CPAP mask.
6. OSA-induced confusional arousals from non-REM or REM sleep can be associated with involuntary SRED, which can eventually induce excessive weight gain, which, in turn, may aggravate OSA. Thus, a vicious cycle of persistent nocturnal eating, progressive weight gain, aggravation of OSA, and so on, is established.
7. SRED can induce weight gain, which may then result in the clinical emergence of OSA. (Overweight status and frank obesity are major risk factors for OSA.)
8. OSA may induce complex or violent epileptic seizures as a result of the brain insult resulting from hypoxia.
9. OSA (with precipitous decrease of available oxygen) can induce nocturnal cerebral anoxic attacks punctuated by vigorous behaviors.

PARASOMNIAS WITH DREAM-ENACTING BEHAVIORS

RBD is not the only parasomnia associated with dream-enacting behaviors *(25)*. It is therefore necessary for patients (and their bed partners) who complain of a dream-enacting disorder to have a careful interview with an experienced sleep clinician that is followed by extensive overnight PSG monitoring at an accredited sleep laboratory with a sleep technologist in continuous attendance. A history of dream-enacting behaviors should not prompt the reflexive and premature diagnosis of RBD and its treatment. As already alluded to, various parasomnias other than RBD can manifest with attempted dream enactment, such as sleepwalking, sleep terrors, parasomnia overlap disorder, sleep-related eating disorder, OSA, nocturnal DDs, nocturnal seizures, rhythmic movement disorders, and malingering.

Premenstrual Sleepwalking and Sleep Terrors

We have reported on two cases of exclusively premenstrual sleep terrors and injurious sleepwalking *(30)*. The first case involved a 17-year-old female who presented with a 6-year history of exclusively premenstrual sleep terrors and sleepwalking, associated with recurrent injury, which had begun 1 year after menarche. During the four nights preceding each menses, she would scream and run from her bed. There was no associated psychiatric history. A PSG study 3 days before the onset of menses confirmed the diagnosis of sleepwalking. Treatment with self-hypnosis practiced at bedtime was rapidly effective, with benefit maintained for more than 2 years. The second case involved a 46-year-old female who had a 5-year history of sleep terrors and sleepwalking, with recurrent injury, which initially was not menstrually related, but commencing 8 months prior to referral she developed an exclusively premenstrual parasomnia. Therefore, clinicians should inquire about any strong premenstrual association, or exacerbation, of sleepwalking or sleep terrors in their patients.

PARASOMNIAS DURING PREGNANCY

Only one epidemiological study has been published on this topic *(31)*, which consisted of 325 mothers in Finland completing five parasomnia-related questionnaires that covered the 3 months before they became pregnant; each of the three trimesters of pregnancy; and the 3 months after delivering their babies. The questionnaires included structured questions on the presence of sleeptalking and sleepwalking (lumped together), sleep starts, hypnagogic hallucinations, sleep paralysis, nightmares, sleep bruxism, and nocturnal enuresis. However, the following parasomnias or parasomnia symptoms were not covered in this questionnaire: sleep terrors, sleep-related eating disorder (or NES), restless legs syndrome, dream-enacting behaviors, and sleep violence. Also, the lumping together of sleepwalking and sleeptalking was another methodological limitation in this study. A methodological strength was the participation of a spouse or bed partner in helping answer the questionnaire in 93.5% of the cases. The main results were as follows: The total number of parasomnias declined during pregnancy, particularly in the primipara group compared to the multipara group, with the difference maintained until the third trimester. Sleep paralysis was the only parasomnia that increased during later pregnancy, even though it decreased during the first trimester.

At least two cases have been reported of either sleepwalking or sleep terrors becoming exacerbated during pregnancy *(32,33)*. Also, pregnant women who have an active parasomnia with complex, vigorous, or violent behaviors, or who are sleeping with husbands having an active parasomnia with aggression or violence, such as RBD or agitated sleepwalking/sleep terrors, are at risk for sleep-related injury, along with their unborn child. One book on parasomnias containing more than 60 clinical stories told by patients and their families provides diverse examples of the hazards associated with pregnancy and active parasomnias, along with the dangers to nonpregnant women who have agitated sleepwalking and sleep terrors or who sleep with men who have RBD or agitated sleepwalking and sleep terrors *(34)*.

CONCLUSION

Parasomnias encompass an array of recurrent, peculiar, dangerous, and distressing behaviors and altered experiences that can adversely affect women in diverse ways. Fortunately, parasomnias are often scientifically explainable and are usually treatable. An experienced sleep-disorders center, with the availability of sleep laboratory monitoring, is a valuable resource for the evaluation and treatment of parasomnias.

REFERENCES

1. American Academy of Sleep Science. *International Classification of Sleep Disorders*, 2nd ed: Diagnostic and Coding Manual. Westchester, IL: Author, 2005.
2. *Sleep Runners: The Stories Behind Everyday Parasomnias* (DVD). St. Paul, MN: Slow-Wave Films, LLC (www.sleeprunners.com), 2004.
3. Corner, M.A., Ontogeny of brain sleep mechanisms. In: *Brain Mechanisms of Sleep* (D.J. McGinty, R. Drucker-Colin, A. Morrison, and P.L. Parmeggiani, eds.). New York: Raven Press, 1985:175–197.
4. Mahowald, M.W. and M.G. Ettinger, Things that go bump in the night—the parasomnias revisited. *J Clin Neurophysiol*, 1990;**7**:119–143.
5. Mahowald M.W. and Schenck C.H., Parasomnias including the restless legs syndrome. *Clin Chest Med*, 1998;**19**:183–202.
6. Schenck C.H., D.M. Milner, T.D. Hurwitz, S.R. Bundlie, and M.W. Mahowald, A polysomnographic and clinical report on sleep-related injury in 100 adult patients. *Am J Psychiatry*, 1989;**146**:1166–1173.
7. Schenck C.H., T.D. Hurwitz, S.R. Bundlie, and M.W. Mahowald, Sleep-related eating disorders: polysomnographic correlates of a heterogeneous syndrome distinct from daytime eating disorders. *Sleep*, 1991;**14**:419–431.
8. Schenck C.H., T.D. Hurwitz, K.A. O'Connor, and M.W. Mahowald, Additional categories of sleep-related eating disorders and the current status of treatment. *Sleep*, 1993;**16**:457–466.
9. Schenck C.H. and M.W. Mahowald, Review of nocturnal sleep-related eating disorders. *Intl J Eating Disord*, 1994;**15**:343–356.
10. Winkelman, J.W., Clinical and polysomnographic features of sleep-related eating disorder. *J Clin Psychiatry*, 1998;**59**:14–19.
11. Winkelman, J.W., D.B. Herzog, and M. Fava, The prevalence of sleep-related eating disorder in psychiatric and non-psychiatric populations. *Psychol Med*, 1999;**29**:461–1466.
12. Morgenthaler, T.I. and M.H. Silber, Amnestic sleep-related eating disorder associated with zolpidem. *Sleep Med*, 2002;**3**:323–327.
13. Schenck, C.H., D.A. Connoy, M. Castellanos, et al., Zolpidem-induced sleep-related eating disorder (SRED) in 19 patients. *Sleep*, 2005;**28**:A259.
14. Birketvedt, G.S., J. Florholmen, J. Sundsfjord, et al.,Behavioral and neuroendocrine characteristics of the night-eating syndrome. *JAMA*, 1999;**282**:657–663.
15. Winkelman, J.W., Treatment of nocturnal eating syndrome and sleep-related eating disorder with topiramate. *Sleep Med*, 2003;**4**:243–246.
16. Schenck, C.H., D.M .Milner, T.D. Hurwitz, S.R. Bundlie, and M.W. Mahowald, Dissociative disorders presenting as somnambulism: video and clinical documentation (8 cases). *Dissociation*, 1989;**2**:194–204.
17. Mahowald, M.W., C.H. Schenck, M. Goldner, V. Bachelder, and M. Cramer-Bornemann, Parasomnia pseudo-suicide. *J Forens Sci*, 2003;**48**:1158–1162.
18. Rosenfeld, D.S. and A.J. Elhajjar, Sleepsex: a variant of sleepwalking. *Arch Sex Behav*, 1998;**27**:269–278.
19. Guilleminault, C., A. Moscovitch, K. Yuen, and D. Poyares, Atypical sexual behavior during sleep. *Psychosom Med*, 2002;**64**:328–336.
20. Shapiro, C.M., N.N. Trajanovic, and J.P. Fedoroff, Sexsomnia—a new parasomnia? *Can J Psychiatry*, 2003;**48**:311–317.
21. Mangan, M.A. A phenomenology of problematic sexual behavior occurring in sleep. *Arch Sex Behav*, 2004;**33**:287–293.

22. Hurwitz, T.D, M.W. Mahowald, C.H. Schenck, J.L. Schluter, and S.R. Bundlie,A retrospective outcome study and review of hypnosis as treatment of adults with sleepwalking and sleep terror.*J Nerv Mental Dis*, 1991;**179**:228–233.
23. Schenck, C.H. and M.W. Mahowald, Long-term, nightly benzodiazepine treatment of injurious parasomnias and other disorders of disrupted nocturnal sleep in 170 adults. *Am J Med*, 1996;**100**:333–337.
24. Schenck, C.H. and M.W. Mahowald, Treatment of severe morning sleep inertia (SI) with bedtime sustained-release (SR) methylphenidate, bupropion-SR, or other activating agents. *Sleep*, 2003;**26**(Suppl.):A75–A76.
25. Schenck, C.H. and M.W. Mahowald, REM sleep behavior disorder: clinical, developmental, and neuroscience perspectives 16 years after its formal identification. *Sleep*, 2002;**25**:120–138.
26. Yeh, S.-B. and C.H. Schenck, A case of marital discord and secondary depression with attempted suicide resulting from REM sleep behavior disorder in a 35 year-old woman. *Sleep Med*, 2004;**5**:151–154.
27. Schenck, C.H., S.R. Bundlie, and M.W. Mahowald, Delayed emergence of a parkinsonian disorder in 38% of 29 older males initially diagnosed with idiopathic REM sleep behavior disorder. *Neurology*, 1996;**46**:388–393.
28. Schenck, C.H., S.R. Bundlie, and M.W. Mahowald, REM behavior disorder (RBD): delayed emergence of parkinsonism and/or dementia in 65% of older men initially diagnosed with idiopathic RBD, and an analysis of the minimum & maximum tonic and/or phasic electromyographic abnormalities found during REM sleep. *Sleep*, 2003;**26**(Suppl.):A316.
29. Mahowald, M.W. and C.H. Schenck, REM sleep parasomnias. In: *Principles and Practice of Sleep Medicine*, 4th ed. (M.H. Kryger, T. Roth, and W.C. Dement, eds.). Philadelphia: Elsevier Saunders, 2005:897–916.
30. Schenck, C.H. and M.W. Mahowald, Two cases of premenstrual sleep terrors and injurious sleep-walking. *J Psychosom Obstet Gynecol*, 1995;**16**:79–84.
31. Hedman C., T. Pohjasvaara, U. Tolonen, A. S almivaara, and V.V. Myllyla, Parasomnias decline during pregnancy. *Acta Neurol Scand*, 2002;**105**:209–214.
32. Snyder, S., Unusual case of sleep terror in a pregnant patient. *Am J Psychiatry*, 1986;**143**:391.
33. Berlin, R.M., Sleepwalking disorder during pregnancy: a case report. *Sleep*, 1988;**11**:98–300.
34. Schenck, C.H., *Paradox Lost: Midnight in the Battleground of Sleep and Dreams*. Minneapolis, MN: Extreme-Nights, LLC (www.parasomnias-rbd.com), 2005.

IV Pregnancy

14

Restless Legs Syndrome in Pregnancy

Keith J. Nagle

INTRODUCTION

Restless legs syndrome (RLS) is characterized by limb akathisia that is maximal in the evening while at rest and transiently relieved by movement. The prevalence and severity of RLS increase with age. Women older than 65 have an RLS prevalence of 19%, whereas in nonpregnant women younger than 30 years of age it is only 5% (1). However, gestational RLS (gRLS) is strikingly common, with nearly 25% of pregnant women affected (see below). The association of RLS with pregnancy has been noted since the term was first coined by Ekbom in 1945. RLS is a clinical diagnosis. Its four cardinal clinical features were reviewed in Chapter 8. Further details regarding diagnosis are well described by the International RLS Study Group (2,3).

A sister condition to RLS is periodic limb movements of sleep (PLMS). PLMS occur during sleep and consist of episodes of flexion at the hips, knees, and feet lasting 0.5 to 5 seconds and recurring every 5 to 90 seconds (4). These movements will often lead to sleep fragmentation. Approximately 70% of persons with RLS have PLMS. However, not everyone found to have PLMS on polysomnography will have RLS (3). The conditions are therefore closely related but distinct.

Morbidity related to gRLS has not been well characterized. In a large cross-sectional questionnaire survey, Suzuki et al. (5) found that women with gRLS reported difficulty initiating and maintaining sleep and experience early morning awakening and excessive daytime somnolence. There was also a small but significant shortening of sleep hours (5). The detrimental effects of RLS–PLMS alone or combined with other sleep conditions common to pregnancy likely lead to considerable difficulties with daytime somnolence, mood, and quality of life.

EPIDEMIOLOGICAL CONSIDERATIONS

The prevalence of RLS in the general population is 5–10% and increases with age (6). Studies have reported an increased prevalence of RLS during pregnancy ranging from 11 to 30%. The findings of these studies are presented in Table 1. Variations in the prevalence rate are explained in part by differences in case definition, assessment method, the month during pregnancy in which symptoms were assessed, maternal age, and genetic inhomogenieties between study populations (7).

From: *Current Clinical Neurology: Sleep Disorders in Women: A Guide to Practical Management*
Edited by: H. P. Attarian © Humana Press Inc., Totowa, NJ

Table 1
RLS Prevalence During Pregnancy

First author/country	Publication year	Sample	Prevalence (%)
Ekbom/Sweden	1945	486	11
Jolivet/France	1953	100	27
Ekbom/Sweden	1970	202	12
Goodman/England	1988	500	19
Hedman/Finland	2002	325	30
Suzuki/Japan	2003	16,528	20
Manconi/Italy	2004	606	26

Adapted from ref. *7.*

The most rigorous study on this topic is that of Manconi et al. Of their sample of 642 consecutive pregnancies taken from an Italian obstetric clinic, 9.9% had pre-existing RLS and 16.7% were incident cases. Nearly 15% of their cases had RLS symptoms more than 3 days a week. Small but statistically significant factors associated with the development of gRLS were prior gRLS, maternal age, increased maternal weight prior to pregnancy, low hemoglobin, and mean corpuscular volume.

There is a steady rise in RLS symptoms during pregnancy, exceeding 5% by the fifth month. The peak incidence of RLS during pregnancy occurs during the sixth month. The condition is most severe during months 7 and 8. There is a rapid decline in RLS symptoms by 1 month postpartum. Goodman et al. noted a more than 50% decrease in gRLS by 1 week postdelivery. The illness may persist in a small subset of new-onset RLS cases *(5,8–10).*

ETIOLOGY OF RLS IN PREGNANCY

RLS is considered to be idiopathic if no secondary cause other than family history is identified. Thus far two pedigrees of familial RLS have led to the identification of a different autosomal dominant gene in each family. The presence of other gene loci related to RLS is suspected, but their discovery awaits further study. Several environmental modifiers likely affect the penetration, age of incidence, and severity of this syndrome.

A number of secondary causes of RLS have been identified, including pregnancy. Women with a family history of RLS experience a worsening of symptoms during pregnancy far more often than those without: 19 vs 3%, respectively *(11).* How the gravid state affects the incidence and severity of RLS is unclear.

A number of observations support the concept that RLS is a consequence of or is exacerbated by iron deficiency *(12).* Some suggest that a disorder in the homeostasis of iron in the central nervous system results in a decrease in dopamine production in the basal ganglia. In persons with RLS and normal systemic iron stores, an iron deficiency limited to the central nervous system has been suggested. This theory is supported by studies of the cerebrospinal fluid finding low ferritin and increased transferrin, low iron concentration of the substantia nigra and putamen on magnetic resonance iron quantification studies that have been confirmed by autopsy studies, and decreased D2 receptors on single photon emission computed tomography and positron emission tomography studies *(13,14)*.

Iron deficiency is common during pregnancy. An increased risk of gRLS in women with diminished iron stores (low ferritin and increased total iron-binding capacity) has been reported. Furthermore, iron supplementation is said to improve symptoms *(4)*. A recent study of women just prior to term observed a significant decrease in hemoglobin and mean corpuscular volume in women with gRLS relative to a control group *(15)*. Ferritin levels were not reported. No studies on central nervous system iron metabolism in gRLS have been reported. The replenishment of iron stores during the postpartum period takes 3 months. The striking improvement in gRLS at delivery is therefore a difficult observation to reconcile with the iron-deficiency hypothesis of gRLS.

It is tempting to attribute the occurrence of gRLS to the marked hormonal changes of pregnancy *(15,16)*. Prolactin levels are greatly elevated during pregnancy. This hormone is noted to have antidopaminergic properties, providing a potential mechanism of gRLS. However, prolactin levels continue to be elevated in the postpartum period in women who breast-feed. Estrogen and progesterone levels progressively rise during pregnancy and then dramatically fall at term. However, some women report a decrease in gRLS up to 2 weeks prior to delivery *(8)*. An improvement of symptoms prior to birth would argue against hormonal changes as the prime etiology. Furthermore, there are no controlled studies suggesting a variation in RLS during the menstrual cycle when cyclic changes in estrogen and progesterone are also present. Nevertheless, a relationship between hormonal factors and gRLS remains intriguing.

Some authors suggest that gRLS is related to altered neuronal function resulting from a local pressure or a traction effect on the proximal nerves and spinal cord An alteration in a subcortical sensorimotor oscillator has been suggested *(9)*. A number of cases of RLS have been described to occur coincident with or as a late feature of acute nerve and spinal cord injury. That a local affect on the thoracolumbar spinal cord or lumbosacral plexus might lead to an emergence of gRLS symptoms remains plausible *(9)*.

The etiology of gRLS remains unknown. This ignorance is of concern in light of the increase in RLS observed in multiparous women later in life. Berger et al. recently revealed a startling correlation of RLS prevalence with parity *(1)*. Nulliparous women and men under the age of 64 had a similar prevalence of RLS. However, women with one child had a near-doubling of RLS prevalence. There is an apparent dosage effect, with an increase in prevalence in women with three or more pregnancies. Also of interest is the finding that women with gRLS are more likely to re-present with RLS later in life *(17)*. These observations support the idea that the gravid state exacerbates a latent predisposition to this syndrome and that this effect is long lasting.

CLINICAL PRESENTATION OF gRLS

Those affected with gRLS seldom present to the clinician volunteering that they have the cardinal symptoms of RLS. More often a difficulty with initiating sleep or recurrent nocturnal awakenings is reported. A number of other conditions can lead to limb discomfort and sleep fragmentation in the third trimester, including abdominal distension, arthritis, insomnia, low back pain, muscle cramps, nocturia, and peripheral neuropathy. The clinician will likely have to specifically ask questions probing for RLS features to make a diagnosis. Adherence to the cardinal features of RLS typically allows differentiation of mimickers of this diagnosis.

No confirmatory test is needed to diagnose RLS. However, it is reasonable to exclude secondary causes in addition to pregnancy. Assessment for anemia and serum ferritin and iron-binding capacity should be obtained. Screens for diabetes and hypothyroidism are also considerations. Renal insufficiency can also produce RLS, and a creatinine and blood urea nitrogen level can address this concern. The presence of intact sensation, strength, and deep tendon reflexes of the proximal and distal limbs will help to exclude neuropathy.

TREATMENT OPTIONS FOR gRLS

The concern of possible teratogenic effects of medications severely limits pharmacological treatment options for RLS during pregnancy. Nearly all medications to treat RLS are US Food And Drug Administration pregnancy category C or greater, indicating fetal adverse effects in animal studies and a lack of human fetal outcome studies. Two exceptions are the category B agent pergolide and nonchronic use of oxycodone. However, the human data on pergolide during pregnancy are limited. There are also increasing reports of cardiac valvular fibrosis, a high incidence of side effects, and a likely negative effect on lactation with this agent. In addition, dopa-agonists suppress prolactin levels and may interfere with lactation. Narcotic use in pregnancy can lead to a neonatal withdrawal syndrome, making oxycodone a difficult agent to use in this circumstance. There are no reports of a pregnancy occurring during ropinirole use (personal communication, GlaxoSmithKline Inc., May 2005). The use of antiseizure agents (gabapentin, carbamazepine) may be associated with a number of side effects, including neonatal sedation and poor feeding. However, the often feared risk of spina bifida is not a concern when these agents are used in the third trimester of pregnancy, a time when gRLS symptoms are at their worst. If medication is considered in severe gRLS, use of the lowest possible dose and frequency is recommended.

Iron and folate supplementation have been shown to be efficacious *(9,18,19)*. Supplementation is suggested even if levels are not low. Earley *(18)* recommends 325 mg of ferrous sulfate three times daily. Increased absorption occurs if iron is taken on an empty stomach and supplemented with 100 mg of vitamin C. Abdominal pain and constipation are common side effects. Folate supplementation is already present in prenatal multivitamins, with most containing 0.8 mg. An additional 1 mg twice daily could be considered.

A safer approach is to review medications and limit those known to exacerbate RLS if possible. The leader among these agents is caffeine, which should be avoided in gRLS. Other medication categories known to exacerbate RLS are antiemetics, antihistamines, antipsychotics, neuroleptics, selective serotonin reuptake inhibitors, alcohol, and nicotine.

The complexities of medication use in the gravid state offer an excellent opportunity to maximize nonpharmacological options. Although few studies have assessed its efficacy or degree of benefit, many authors have suggested exercise including active stretching near bedtime, massage, and hot or cold baths. Mild to moderate exercise in the early evening, but not heavy exercise, is also reported to be of benefit. Poor sleep hygiene including sleep deprivation can aggravate RLS. Review of sleep hygiene and education is likely to lead to at least partial symptom improvement.

It should be emphasized that many patients report a great sense of relief upon hearing that their symptom complex is not the result of a psychiatric disorder of some progressive neurological condition. Accurate diagnosis and patient counseling may provide significant relief to the patient. It is important to review with patients that those with moderate to severe RLS are, for all intents and purposes, chronically sleep deprived. If symptoms of excessive daytime sleepiness are present, a discussion about driving safety and safety related to the operating of heavy machinery should be considered. Daytime naps, particularly in the morning hours when RLS symptoms are at their minimum, may be a helpful short-term strategy.

CONCLUSION

gRLS is a common and often unrecognized symptom constellation that produces discomfort, sleep fragmentation, and fatigue. The etiology of gRLS remains undetermined. When discovered, other conditions that can produce gRLS should be investigated, including diabetes, iron deficiency, hypothyroidism, renal insufficiency, and neuropathy. A number of pharmacological therapies are available, although their use in pregnancy poses many obstacles. Iron and folate supplementation should be implemented. A review of concurrent medications and limiting agents that may exaggerate RLS may often produce improvement. Nonpharmacological strategies are the mainstay of treatment. Although most women will have resolution of RLS symptoms in the weeks immediately prior to or following birth, there is an increased risk of symptom recurrence with future pregnancies or later in life.

REFERENCES

1. Berger, K., J. Luedemann, C. Trenkwalder, U. John, and C. Kessler, Sex and the risk of restless legs syndrome in the general population. *Arch Intern Med*, 2004;**164**(2):196–202.
2. Allen, R.P., E. Mignot, B. Ripley, S. Nishino, and C.J. Earley, Increased CSF hypocretin-1 (orexin-A) in restless legs syndrome. *Neurology*, 2002;**59**(4):639–641.
3. Walters, A.S., Toward a better definition of the restless legs syndrome. The International Restless Legs Syndrome Study Group. *Mov Disord*, 1995;**10**(5):634–642.
4. Chesson, A.L., Jr., M. Wise, D. Davila, et al., Practice parameters for the treatment of restless legs syndrome and periodic limb movement disorder. An American Academy of Sleep Medicine Report. Standards of Practice Committee of the American Academy of Sleep Medicine. *Sleep*, 1999;**22**(7):961–968.
5. Suzuki, K., T. Ohida, T. Sove, et al., The prevalence of restless legs syndrome among pregnant women in Japan and the relationship between restless legs syndrome and sleep problems. *Sleep*, 2003;**6**(6):673–677.
6. Lavigne, G.J. and J.Y. Montplaisir, Restless legs syndrome and sleep bruxism: prevalence and association among Canadians. *Sleep*, 1994;**17**(8):739–743.

7. Manconi, M. and L. Ferini-Strambi, Restless legs syndrome among pregnant women. *Sleep*, 2004;**27**(2):350–351.

8. Goodman, J.D., C. Brodie, and G.A. Ayida, Restless leg syndrome in pregnancy. *BMJ*, 1988;**297**(6656):1101–1102.

9. Lee, K.A., M.E. Zaffke, and K. Baratte-Beebe, Restless legs syndrome and sleep disturbance during pregnancy: the role of folate and iron. *J Womens Health Gend Based Med*, 2001;**10**(4):335–341.

10. Manconi, M., V. Govoni, A. De Vito, et al., Restless legs syndrome and pregnancy. *Neurology*, 2004;**63**(6):1065–1069.

11. Winkelmann, J., T.C. Wetter, V. Collado-Seidel, et al., Clinical characteristics and frequency of the hereditary restless legs syndrome in a population of 300 patients. *Sleep*, 2000;**23**(5):597–602.

12. Earley, C.J., R.P. Allen, J.L. Beard, and J.R. Connor, Insight into the pathophysiology of restless legs syndrome. *J Neurosci Res*, 2000;**62**(5):623–628.

13. Hening, W.A., R.P. Allen, C.J. Earley, D.L. Picchietti, and M. Silber, An update on the dopaminergic treatment of restless legs syndrome and periodic limb movement disorder. *Sleep*, 2004;**27**(3):560–583.

14. Hening, W.A., Treatment of restless legs syndrome. *Neurol Rev*, 2005;2(Suppl):11–17.

15. Manconi, M., V. Govoni, A. De Vito, et al., Pregnancy as a risk factor for restless legs syndrome. *Sleep Med*, 2004;**5**(3):305–308.

16. Pien, G.W. and R.J. Schwab, Sleep disorders during pregnancy. *Sleep*, 2004;**27**(7):1405–1417.

17. Montplaisir, J., S. Boucher, G. Poirier, G. Lavigne, O. Lapierre, and P. Lesperance, Clinical, polysomnographic, and genetic characteristics of restless legs syndrome: a study of 133 patients diagnosed with new standard criteria. *Mov Disord*, 1997;**12**(1):61–65.

18. Earley, C.J., Clinical practice. Restless legs syndrome. *N Engl J Med*, 2003;**348**(21):2103–2109.

19. Botez, M.I. and B. Lambert, Folate deficiency and restless-legs syndrome in pregnancy. *N Engl J Med*, 1977;**297**(12):670.

15
Evaluating Insomnia During Pregnancy and Postpartum

Kathryn A. Lee and Aaron B. Caughey

INTRODUCTION

Most women (78%) report that their sleep is worse during pregnancy than at any other time in their lives (1). Reasons for poor sleep vary by trimester, but sleep problems begin early in the first trimester with complaints of urinary frequency as progesterone level rises and creatinine clearance increases (2–4). Pregnant women who are obese are at higher risk for obstructive sleep apnea (OSA). The hypoxia associated with OSA may contribute to maternal hypertension and intrauterine growth retardation (IUGR). Furthermore, women with snoring and daytime sleepiness are at higher risk for developing pre-eclampsia (5). Anemia associated with pregnancy places women at increased risk for restless legs syndrome (RLS), and insufficient amounts of sleep during the third trimester may place women at increased risk for longer labors and cesarean births (6).

Sleep continues to be disrupted for new mothers during the postpartum period, regardless of type of infant feeding, location of infant, or extent of support with infant care at night. Postpartum depression may be difficult to distinguish from chronic sleep deprivation. Chronic postpartum sleep loss places women and their families at risk for accidents if they are driving or caring for their infants while excessively sleepy. Coping with a difficult infant while sleep deprived can place the infant at risk for physical abuse. This chapter reviews the expected changes in sleep that occur during pregnancy and postpartum and highlights particular issues of concern to guide clinical assessment with the goal of minimizing risk for adverse maternal health outcomes associated with insomnia.

INSOMNIA DURING PREGNANCY

In addition to feeling nauseated, early symptoms of pregnancy include fatigue and sleep disturbance. As early as the 10th week of pregnancy, 10–15% of women report disturbed sleep caused by nausea, backaches, or urinary frequency (2,7). In

From: *Current Clinical Neurology: Sleep Disorders in Women: A Guide to Practical Management*
Edited by: H. P. Attarian et al. © Humana Press Inc., Totowa, NJ

the second trimester, fetal movements and heartburn may begin to disrupt sleep, but sleep and daytime fatigue and mood improve for most women once the nausea disappears and they adapt to the hormonal changes. In the third trimester, the majority of women (65–80%) report symptoms such as urinary frequency, backaches, shortness of breath, leg cramps, itchy skin, and vivid, frightening dreams, or nightmares *(2,7,8)*. The content of dreams may change over the course of pregnancy, but both women and their male partners recall more dreams and different themes as the pregnancy progresses *(9)*. This may be a result of waking up more often, leading to a higher likelihood of dream recall. Women with a prior pregnancy loss often report disturbing dreams during their subsequent pregnancy, but the themes of these dreams do not differ from those of women experiencing their first pregnancy *(10)*.

During the third trimester, most women report two to three awakenings during the night and about 7.5 hours of sleep, but some report sleeping as little as 3 or 4 hours *(11,12)*. Older women (>30 years) report sleeping less than younger women, but this may be secondary to having other children in the household *(13)*. Nulliparas are at higher risk than multiparas for sleep deprivation during pregnancy, possibly because they have no prior experience with pregnancy. When multiparas become pregnant, they are more likely to spend extra time in bed at night and plan for extra sleep, regardless of whether or not they have other children who are sleeping through the night *(4)*.

Pregnant women are unlikely to complain of difficulty falling asleep (initiation insomnia) because they have an accumulated sleep loss from their frequent awakenings during the night and falling asleep is not at all problematic. They are more likely to report maintenance insomnia as a result of discomfort or frequent urination. With more objective measures, such as wrist actigraphy or polysomnography, pregnant women sleep about 7 hours (30 minutes less sleep than they self-report), and brief awakenings over the course of the night can reach a total of 45–60 minutes *(2,6,7,14)*. Table 1 compares the common reasons for awakenings in the third and first trimesters.

Clinical Summary

Over the course of pregnancy, women gradually lose about 1 hour of sleep each night as a result of many brief awakenings. Nulliparas are more likely to continue habitual bedtime and wake time, whereas multiparas are more likely to extend time in bed by an hour. Complaints of maintenance insomnia are common, but complaints of initiation insomnia are rare during pregnancy and should be further evaluated for possible causes such as anxiety and fears about labor and delivery, marital discord, or environmental factors. Any complaint about difficulty falling asleep should also include an evaluation for RLS, as discussed in detail in the next section. Table 2 summarizes six key points for the clinical assessment of pregnancy-related insomnia.

Leg Sensations That Disrupt Sleep

Twenty-seven to 36% of women consistently report the sensation of jerking legs at sleep onset across preconception, pregnancy, and postpartum *(15)*. This seldom

Table 1
Reasons for Nighttime Awakenings During Pregnancy (%)

	First trimester (2–14 weeks gestation)	Third trimester (28–42 weeks gestation)
Urination	51	47
Leg cramps	13	73
Joint pain	4	23
Bed partner	9	12
Dreams/nightmares	3	5
Anxiety	3	1
Fetal movement	0	5

Table 2
Insomnia During Pregnancy: Clinical Assessment Points

1. Sleep loss of about 1 hour per night is typical during pregnancy owing to frequent awakenings.
2. Nulliparas are at higher risk of insufficient sleep when compared with multiparas.
3. Complaint of initiation insomnia is rare during pregnancy and requires clinical evaluation for anxiety about labor and delivery, marital discord, depression, or feeling unsafe.
4. Women with initiation insomnia are not likely to experience excessive daytime sleepiness, but may complain of daytime fatigue and depressed mood.
5. Any complaint of initiation insomnia should include and evaluation for restless legs syndrome. These women are likely to experience excessive daytime sleepiness as well as daytime fatigue and depressed mood.
6. Women with a prior history of initiation insomnia are likely to report improvement during pregnancy because of the soporific and relaxing effects of higher progesterone levels.

interferes with sleep onset. Sudden awakening from sleep because of severe muscle cramps occurs in approx 10% of women before and after pregnancy, but the prevalence increases to 13% in the first trimester, 49% in the second trimester, and 73% in the third trimester *(15)*. Whether leg cramps are associated with periodic leg movements during sleep is not known, but women with a multiple gestation (twins or triplets) are more likely to have periodic leg movements during sleep than women with a singleton pregnancy *(8,13)*.

Initiation insomnia during pregnancy is most likely a result of RLS associated with iron-deficiency anemia, a common condition of pregnancy. Lower serum ferritin and folate levels at preconception, even within normal limits, are thought to contribute to this disorder *(15)*. The incidence of RLS reaches a peak of 19–22% by the third trimester and typically resolves with the birth of the infant *(16)*. It does not appear to vary by age *(13)*, but women with multiple gestations are more likely to experience RLS and periodic leg movements during sleep *(17)*. The wide range in incidence may be associated with either varying criteria for threshold frequency of self-reports during a typical week or month or parity, because multiparas are more likely to have RLS with subsequent pregnancies *(18)*.

Many women are unlikely to talk to their health care provider about their restless legs *(18)*, either because they do not want medication, they know it will disappear after delivery, or they feel that clinicians will think they are crazy or neurotic. Some women, on the other hand, characterize their symptoms as "pure torture" or "worse than delivering a 15-lb baby" and describe "worms crawling inside their veins" or "ants crawling up and down inside their legs." Some are so tortured that they vow never to become pregnant again. RLS typically begins in the evening before bedtime. Momentary relief comes with standing and walking, but as soon as the woman reclines, the sensation reappears.

In addition to experiencing restless legs at bedtime, sleep onset is significantly delayed and mood is more depressed *(15)*. Women who experience RLS in one pregnancy are more likely to experience it with subsequent pregnancies, but it can be totally absent between pregnancies *(13,19)*. RLS is often treated with opioids or dopamine agonists that many women and clinicians are loathe to use during pregnancy or lactation (Table 3). More acceptable remedies for pregnant women include walking, leg massage, or warm baths. In addition, reducing caffeine intake and increasing foods and dietary supplements of iron and folate should be encouraged even prior to pregnancy.

Clinical Summary

Women who are planning a pregnancy should be advised to begin taking prenatal vitamins with iron and folate for a number of reasons, including preventing neural tube defects. Dietary foods enriched with folate, such as breads and cereals, should be encouraged. To promote absorption of iron and folate, women should also be advised to take adequate amounts of vitamin C and eliminate caffeine and alcohol. Pregnant women at risk for anemia and women in the low range of normal serum levels for ferritin and folate should be asked about unusual leg sensations they might be experiencing in the evening while trying to fall asleep. If they are experiencing excessive daytime sleepiness as a result of their RLS and initiation insomnia, a referral to an accredited sleep disorders center should be considered.

Snoring and Obesity Risk Factors for Maintenance Insomnia

In addition to observable weight gain taking place over the course of pregnancy, women also increase blood volume by 2–3 L and overall body fluid volume by about 7 L. Higher fluid volume and increased estrogen secretion from the placenta are likely to result in complaints of nasal congestion and swelling of the extremities *(21)*. Congestion, upper body weight gain, and snoring are common complaints during pregnancy. However, these factors can place some women at higher risk for OSA while at the same time putting the fetus as risk for repeated hypoxia, placental insufficiency, and IUGR.

During pregnancy, shortness of breath (dyspnea) results from increased minute ventilation and is common during the last trimester, particularly when the gravid uterus reduces functional residual capacity. Women often find it more comfortable and easier to breathe sleeping with the head elevated, which also helps with complaints of heartburn and sleep disturbance caused by esophageal reflux. Oxygen saturation remains stable during sleep in nonobese women *(22,23)*. If a pregnant woman lies on her back, however, the gravid uterus can compress her vena cava

Table 3
Medication Risk During Pregnancy and Lactation[a]

	Class B	Class C	Class D	Contraindicated (X)
Antidepressants	Sertraline	Fluoxetine Paroxetine Trazodone Venlafaxine	Amitriptyline Imipramine	
Dopaminergics		Carbamazepine Carbidopa Levodopa		
Hypnotics	Diphenhydramine Zolpidem	Clonazepam Zaleplon	Alcohol (ethanol) Alprazolam Diazepam Lorazepam Midazolam Secobarbital	Flurazepam Temazepam Triazolam
Opioids	Meperidine Oxymorphone	Codeine Morphine		
Stimulants	Caffeine Pemoline	Dextroamphetamine Methamphetamine Mazindol Modafinil		

Class A (fetal harm is remote).
Class B (no risk in animals studies but no human studies, or risk in animals documented but no risk to fetus in controlled human studies).
Class C (animal studies document teratogenic effects but no studies in women or animals).
Class D (risk to fetus is present but use in pregnancy may outweigh risk of serious danger or disease to mother).
Class X (studies demonstrate high risk to fetus; drug is contraindicated regardless of risk to mother).
[a]Dosages should begin with half of the lowest recommended dosage owing to increased sensitivity during pregnancy; lactating women should consider alternatives to breastfeeding since long-term effects on the newborn's growth and neurodevelopment remain unknown. (From ref. 20.)

(supine hypotensive syndrome) *(21)*, and the fetus is at risk of hypoxemia due to utero-placental insufficiency.

In addition to increased minute ventilation and dyspnea, 10–30% of women report onset of snoring during pregnancy, compared to fewer than 5% who snored before conception *(13,24)*. Recent evidence from Scottish women indicates that these rates may be even higher than previously reported (32% in nonpregnant age-matched controls and 55% during pregnancy), particularly if the bed partner is also asked about a woman's snoring *(5)*. Snoring is at one end of the continuum of sleep-disordered breathing (SDB), while obstructive apneic events are at the more severe end of the continuum. SDB in pregnancy may be associated with a higher rate of fetal and newborn complications such as IUGR and low birthweight *(25,26)*. Because of the fragmented sleep associated with OSA, daytime sleepiness is often apparent, and women should be cautioned against performing hazardous jobs or driving and advised to schedule naptime during the day.

Pre-Eclampsia

Gestational hypertension, pre-eclampsia, Hemolysis-Elevated Liver enzymes–Low Platelet count (HELLP) syndrome, and eclampsia comprise the spectrum of a disorder associated with endothelial cell dysfunction (27), which occurs in about 5–10% of pregnancies. This collection of disorders is characterized by high blood pressure (28), but there may also be limited airflow during sleep because of pharyngeal edema. Pre-eclampsia is also associated with increased incidence of periodic leg movements during sleep. Women with pre-eclampsia may have significantly larger neck circumference compared to healthy pregnant women, and depending on body mass index, 75–85% of those with pre-eclampsia report snoring (5,28). Because pre-eclampsia is associated with restricted airflow, frequent arousals from sleep are common (29), and women with this type of maintenance insomnia may complain more about excessive daytime sleepiness (EDS) than about arousals from snoring and apnea. They are likely to complain of sudden awakenings with sensations of choking, coughing, or suffocating.

Clinical Summary

Snoring in a common phenomenon during pregnancy, but obstructive sleep apnea is rare. Women who complain of EDS in association with bed partner reports of snoring or apneic events need further evaluation to rule out obstructive sleep apnea. Women with excessive weight gain or women with pre-eclampsia are at higher risk for SDB, and both they and their fetuses can benefit from timely intervention, typically with nasal continuous positive airway pressure (CPAP), until the birth.

Nasal CPAP may improve sleep, reduce daytime sleepiness, and lower blood pressure in pregnant women with SDB. For those who may be unresponsive to current treatment for pre-eclampsia, nasal CPAP may be a worthwhile intervention to explore in a further attempt to prolong gestation until the fetus is viable. Although CPAP may not change the time spent in deep sleep or rapid eye-movement (REM) sleep stages, it may reduce nocturnal hypoxic episodes, improve placental perfusion, and extend gestation closer to full term. CPAP does not appear to have any adverse effects on the mother or fetus (28,30).

LABOR AND DELIVERY

It is well documented that sleep quality diminishes as pregnancy moves closer to term (40–42 weeks gestation). In one recent study, women who slept less than 6 hours at night during the few weeks prior to delivery had, on average, about 12 hours longer labor and were 4.5 times more likely to have a cesarean delivery than women who slept more than 7 hours (6). In the early stages of labor, when contractions do not seem to be regular and progressing, morphine sulfate or barbiturates have been commonly administered to induce sleep and reduce uterine contractions. The laboring woman often may awaken during active labor (31). The amount of sleep prior

Table 4
Implications of Sleep Loss for Labor and Delivery: Clinical Assessment Points

1. Sleep loss of about 1 hour during the night is typical during the third trimester.
2. Nulliparas who average less than 6 hours/hight are likely to have a length of labor that is 10 hours greater than nulliparas who sleep more than 7 hours/night.
3. Nulliparas who average less than 6 hours of sleep/night are more likely to have a cesarean birth than nulliparas who sleep more than 7 hours/night.
4. Labor contractions often improve after women awaken from pharmacotherapeutic-induced sleep.

to beginning labor and the sleep loss that occurs as a result of being in active labor during the night has more of an effect on early postpartum "baby blues" and emotional distress than the sleep loss that occurs during early postpartum recovery *(32)*.

During active labor, prolactin levels, which are high throughout pregnancy, begin to fall and reach a nadir about 2 hours before delivery. During a normal vaginal delivery, prolactin levels spike for 4–6 hours and then return to a normal circadian pattern *(33)*. Women who have emergency cesarean deliveries do not have the prolactin increase that normally occurs about 30 minutes after the onset of breast-feeding during the first few days postpartum *(33)*. How these labor and delivery factors affect mother and infant sleep remains unknown. Table 4 summarizes four key points for the clinical assessment of sleep for labor and delivery implications.

POSTPARTUM INSOMNIA

Sleep disruption continues from the day of delivery through the first 3 months postpartum and is particularly problematic for primiparas (74%) and for women after cesarean births (73%) compared to vaginal births (57%) *(34)*. After delivery, and until the infant is sleeping through the night, a new mother's sleep is disrupted by infant care needs.

When new mothers have their infants in the same room on their first postpartum night after vaginal delivery, they have lower sleep efficiency (74 ± 16.6%) and shorter REM latency (70.8 ± 23.2 minutes), but no differences in the amount of deep sleep (stages 3 and 4) or REM sleep compared to healthy controls *(35)*. Sleep efficiency averages about 90% during a healthy pregnancy. During the first few months of postpartum recovery, however, sleep efficiency falls to about 77% in novice mothers and about 84% in experienced mothers *(4)*. New first-time mothers in Japan, who often share a futon with their infants, have sleep efficiency comparable to Caucasian multiparas *(36)*. Regardless of parity, deep sleep (stages 3 and 4) is increased and light sleep (stages 1 and 2) is decreased during the first 3 postpartum months *(4,36–38)*. Table 5 summarizes eight key points for the clinical assessment of sleep associated with postpartum insomnia.

Lactation and Breast-Feeding

Mothers' perceptions of their sleep quality do not appear to be associated with type of infant feeding *(39,40)*. Lactating women do have higher basal levels of pro-

Table 5
Insomnia During Postpartum: Clinical Assessment Points

1. Pregnant women should discuss plans for infant sleeping arrangements.
2. Women who experience more changes in their sleep from pregnancy to postpartum may be at higher risk for postpartum depression.
3. Postpartum women should be assessed for sleep deprivation prior to assuming major depression.
4. New parents should be cautioned that chronic sleep loss places them at increased risk for accidents and errors of omission, such as forgetting to get their infants out of a car left in the hot sun or not following directions for mixing infant formula or infant medication dosages.
5. Infant sleeping arrangements should be evaluated.
6. Breast-feeding should be encouraged to promote deep sleep stages.
7. Proper excercise and light exposure should be emphasized for postpartum mothers.
8. Mothers should be queried about their infant's temperament, and any difficult infant temperament should be evaluated in relation to mother's and father's coping strategies and risk for infant abuse.

lactin and bursts of prolactin secretion at the onset of each breast-feeding event, regardless of when sleep occurs. Within 24 hours of weaning, prolactin levels return to low basal levels and to the circadian sleep-associated patterns found in healthy women *(41,42)*. There is little difference in REM sleep, but lactating women have more deep sleep (stages 3–4), less light sleep (stages 1 and 2), and fewer arousals compared to nonlactating postpartum women *(43)*. There may be a gradual decrease in REM sleep for formula-feeding compared to breast-feeding mothers *(44)*.

Co-Sleeping During the Postpartum Period

Adult parents in western cultures such as the United States are likely to value independence and, beginning at birth, find it more desirable to have the infant sleep alone in a separate room and bed *(45)*. A variety of co-sleeping (sleeping together) practices exist throughout the world and range from mother and baby sharing the same bed (bed-sharing) to mother and baby sleeping in the same room (room-sharing). Advantages of bed-sharing include facilitating breast-feeding and maternal–infant bonding, despite concerns about risk of smothering the infant from heavy blankets or obese parents or concerns about sudden infant death syndrome related to a softer adult mattress surface *(46)*. Postpartum mothers may have more arousals when bed-sharing with their infant, but sleep efficiency does not appear to be affected when sleeping-alone nights are compared to bed-sharing nights *(47)*.

Bed-sharing in the United States has increased from 6 to 13% during the past 10 years *(48)*, and current research would indicate that about 22% of families are bed-sharing at 1 month postpartum and only 13% continue to bed-share by 6 months postpartum *(49)*. There are some reports that bed-sharing promotes breast-feeding *(49,50)*, but the practice does not appear to be associated with breast-feeding, cultural values, or crowded households *(51)*. Bed-sharing may be more common for young single mothers with lower incomes and less education, but in our recent study about 40% of affluent new parents reported bed-sharing during the first month after delivery regardless of ethnicity or education, and the practice of bed-sharing decreased to about 20% by 3 months postpartum *(52)*. Only 7% of these couples indicated that they planned to bed-share after the baby was born, and, therefore, it is unlikely that many new parents are counseled about the health risks of bed-sharing.

New mothers are less likely to return to work in the early weeks of postpartum recovery and, therefore, have the opportunity to nap during the daytime and lessen the effects of sleep loss at night owing to infant care and fragmented sleep. New fathers, on the other hand, often return to work, but still experience substantial sleep loss during the night and have no opportunity for a scheduled nap during the day *(14)*. Both new mothers and new fathers should be assessed for EDS regardless of who is doing the primary infant care during the night.

Postpartum Depression

There is a 10–20% incidence of a major depressive episode at some point in a woman's life. The rate during the childbearing years is about 10–20% as well, but pharmacological treatment during pregnancy or lactation is of particular concern as a result of the potential growth and development risks to the infant. In an Italian sample of primiparous women, more than 30% were still complaining of sleep loss and fatigue at 15 months postpartum, and more than 50% were reporting depressive symptoms *(53)*. In a longitudinal study of women on the east coast of the United States, researchers excluded women who were depressed in the third trimester and followed 37 women for 15 months postpartum. Ten (26%) had significant depressive symptoms at 3–4 weeks postpartum, but only two women continued to have depressive symptoms at 12–15 months postpartum. With self-report sleep diaries, their total sleep time changed very little over the course of the study, but the 10 depressed mothers had more total sleep time, with later rise times and longer naps, during their third trimester; they also had more disrupted nighttime sleep, later rise times, and naps during the day when assessed at 3–4 weeks postpartum *(11)*. The new mothers at higher risk for postpartum depression may be the ones who experience more of a change in their sleep patterns between pregnancy and postpartum. Regardless of the documented associations between sleep and mood, it may be difficult for new mothers, family members, or clinicians to distinguish the signs and symptoms of chronic postpartum sleep deprivation from the signs and symptoms of depression.

An earlier onset of the first REM period after falling asleep and more REM sleep during the night is often seen in adults with major depressive episodes. Compared to healthy new mothers, postpartum women with depressive symptoms have significantly shorter REM latency as well, but they also average 1 hour less total sleep and about 12% lower sleep efficiency *(54)*. Because of the substantial sleep loss associated with caring for a new infant, most mothers easily fall asleep once they turn out the light. Particularly important hallmarks of postpartum depression include a new mother's complaint of not being able to fall asleep easily at bedtime (initiation insomnia) *(55)* as well as a low serum prolactin level *(56)*.

Nonpharmacological treatment options for women with postpartum depression can include late partial sleep deprivation, in which a new mother would sleep only until about 2 AM *(57)* to limit her amount of REM sleep or bright light therapy in the morning, which may take up to 4 weeks to be effective *(58)*. Pharmacological treatment options for women with insomnia or postpartum depression are presented in Table 3 along with their associated risk to the fetus or newborn *(20)*.

Difficult Infant Temperament and Maternal Insomnia

A new mother often measures success in her motherhood role by the growth and developmental stages reached by her infant, particularly the point at which the infant begins to sleep through the night. Many first-time mothers have the misconception that "sleeping through the night" means continuous sleep from 8 PM to 8 AM, whereas most clinicians interpret sleeping through the night as the point at which an infant no longer awakens in the middle of the night for a feeding 2–4 hours within the previous feeding. This point in time may fluctuate from night to night for many weeks before it becomes the infant's routine sleep pattern. That infant, however, may still be feeding late at night and again in the early morning hours, allowing parents only 5–6 hours of uninterrupted sleep when they may require 7–8 hours to feel rested. Even at 1 year, 20–30% of infants continue to have disrupted sleep during the night *(59)*. Parents who report fussy, irritable "colicky" infant temperament also describe the infant as a poor sleeper.

Even when assessed in the newborn nursery after delivery, there is wide variation in infant sleep, depending on gestational age and birthweight, type of delivery, and type of feeding. First-born infants sleep less than infants born to multiparous mothers, and infants from cesarean births have more active sleep (REM) than infants delivered vaginally *(59)*. A newborn's sleep pattern does not appear to vary by gender, maternal age, or socioeconomic status.

Despite the wide variation in recorded sleep, newborns in the nursery still sleep more during the 12-hour night (7 PM to 6:59 AM) than during the 12-hour day (7 AM to 6:59 PM), but there are many awakenings during the night that may or may not require parental intervention. If the new mother or father is sensitive to sleep loss and not coping well, there is a high risk for physical abuse of an infant who is difficult to settle at bedtime or during the night. Over time, this difficult infant temperament, in combination with chronic sleep loss and poor coping strategies, requires intervention and support from family and friends before the infant's safety and well-being are jeopardized.

Clinical Summary

Some women may deliberately plan to bed-share with their infant during the early postpartum period to foster closeness and facilitate breast-feeding. Still others may not plan to do so, but resort to bed-sharing as a trial-and-error strategy to obtain more sleep. Although a pregnant woman may not be planning to bed-share with her infant or may be reluctant to discuss this with her health care provider, all women should be advised of the pros and cons regarding bed-sharing with an infant, and fathers should participate in the discussion as well. New parents have many adjustment to make in their daytime activities and their nightly sleep patterns once the baby in born. Their depressive symptoms may be more a function of chronic

Table 6
Typical Sleep Changes During Pregnancy and Postpartum

	First trimester	Second trimester	Third trimester	Postpartum
Sleep changes	Fragmented sleep due to frequent urination Less deep sleep (stages 3–4 slow-wave sleep) compared with preconception	Sleep less fragmented Less deep sleep	Sleep fragmented by: frequent urination leg cramps heartburn nasal congestion irregular contractions shortness of breath breast tenderness carpal tunnel/ joint pain Less deep sleep	Sleep fragmented by infant feeding More fragmented sleep for first-time mothers than experienced mothers Longer wake episodes for breast-feeding mothers, but they may have more deep sleep than non-lactating mothers More opportunity to nap if not employed outside of the home More deep sleep
Daytime symptoms	Fatigue/sleepiness Morning or evening nausea	More energy Nasal congestion	Increased fatigue/ sleepiness	Fatigue/sleepiness
Clinical evaluation	Check serum iron and folate levels for risk of restless legs syndrome	Assess for sleep disordered-breathing	Assess for: a) restless legs b) sleep-disordered breathing Ask about plans for infant sleeping arrangements	Assess for: a) excessive daytime sleepiness b) cognitive dysfunction c) postpartum depression Ask about infant's sleep and parenting activities during the night

sleep loss than maladjustment to parenthood. Increased sleep, which can be improved with daytime activities such as light exposure and exercise, may be more therapeutic in treating the depressed state than counseling, psychotherapy, or antidepressant medication. Careful clinical evaluation is needed, however, if new mothers or fathers are not coping well with their disrupted sleep patterns, in that there may be increased risk of physical abuse of an infant who is perceived as having a poor temperament.

SUMMARY

Sleep patterns may be disturbed by the 10th week of pregnancy—even earlier than recorded in most research studies—when complaints of urinary frequency and fatigue are first noticed. Compared to prepregnancy and pregnancy or compared to healthy controls, sleep efficiency is lowest during the first postpartum month, particularly for novice mothers compared to experienced mothers, but significant sleep loss is evident for all new parents. The major concern for postpartum women is sleep loss and the resulting physical fatigue, negative mood states, and cognitive impairment (Table 6). How this sleep loss affects women's health, relationships with family, or the health of new fathers has not been a focus of research or clinical practice. Interventions to improve sleep may be minimal and inexpensive, and such treatments should be evaluated from a clinical and cost-effectiveness standpoint.

REFERENCES

1. National Sleep Foundation, Sleep and women poll. 1998; www.sleepfoundation.org; accessed March 2005.
2. Schweiger, M.S., Sleep disturbance in pregnancy. *Am J Obstet Gynecol*, 1972;**114**:879–882.
3. Driver, H.S. and C.M. Shapiro, A longitudinal study of sleep stages in young women during pregnancy and postpartum. *Sleep*, 1992;**15**:449–453.
4. Lee, K.A., M.E. Zaffke, and G. McEnany, Parity and sleep patterns during and after pregnancy. *Obstet Gynecol*, 2000;**95**:14–18.
5. Izci, B., S.E. Martin, K.C. Dundas, W.A. Liston, A.A. Calder, and N.J. Douglas, Sleep complaints: snoring and daytime sleepiness in pregnant and pre-eclamptic women. *Sleep Med*, 2005;**6**:163–169.
6. Lee, K.A., and C.L. Gay, Sleep in late pregnancy predicts length of labor and type of delivery. *Am J Obstet Gynecol*, 2004;**191**:2041–2046.
7. Baratte-Beebe, K.R. and K. Lee, Sources of mid-sleep awakenings in childbearing women. *Clin Nurs Res*, 1999;**8**:386–397.
8. Pien, G.W. and R.J. Schwab, Sleep disorders during pregnancy. *Sleep*, 2004;**27**:1405-1417.
9. Moorcroft, W.H., *Understanding Sleep and Dreaming*. New York: Kluwer Academic/Plenum Publishers, 2003:168–169.
10. Van, P., T. Cage, and M. Shannon, Big dreams, little sleep: dreams during pregnancy after prior pregnancy loss. *Holist Nurs Pract*, 2004;**18**:284–292.
11. Wolfson, A.R., S.J. Crowley, U. Anwer, and J.L. Bassett, Changes in sleep patterns and depressive symptoms in first-time mothers: Last trimester to one-year postpartum. *Behav Sleep Med*, 2003;**1**:54–67.
12. Greenwood, K.M. and K.M. Hazendonk, Self-reported sleep during the third trimester of pregnancy. *Behav Sleep Med*, 2004;**2**:191–204.
13. Hedman, C., T. Pohjasvaara, U. Tolonen, A.S. Suhonen-Malm, and V.V. Myllyla, Effects of pregnancy on mothers' sleep. *Sleep Med*, 2002;**3**:37–42.
14. Gay, C.L., K.A. Lee, and S. Lee, Sleep patterns and fatigue in new mothers and fathers. *Biol Res Nurs*, 2004;**5**:311–318.
15. Lee, K.A., M.E. Zaffke, and K. Barette-Beebe, Restless legs syndrome and sleep disturbance during pregnancy: the role of folate and iron. *J Women's Health Gender-Based Med*, 2001;**10**:335–341.
16. Manconi, M., V. Govoni, A. De Vito, et al. Pregnancy as a risk factor for restless legs syndrome. *Sleep Med*, 2004;**5**:305–308.
17. Nikkola, E., U. Ekblad, E. Ekholm, H. Mikola, and O. Polo, Sleep in multiple pregnancy: breathing patterns, oxygenation, and periodic leg movements. *Am J Obstet Gynecol*, 1996;**174**:1622–1625.
18. Goodman, J.D.S., C. Brodie, and G.A. Ayida, Restless legs syndrome in pregnancy. *Br Med J*, 1988;**297**:1101–1102.
19. Suzuki, K., T. Ohida, T. Sone, et al., The prevalence of restless legs syndrome among pregnant women in Japan and the relationship between restless legs syndrome and sleep problems. *Sleep*, 2003;**26**:673–677.
20. Briggs, G.G., R.K. Freeman, and S.J. Yaffe, *Drugs in Pregnancy and Lactation*. Philadelphia: Lippincott Williams & Wilkins, 2002.
21. Sahota, P.K., S.S. Jain, and R. Dhand, Sleep disorders in pregnancy. *Curr Opin Pulm Med*, 2003;**9**:477–483.
22. Edwards, N., P.G. Middleton, D.M. Blyton, and C.E. Sullivan, Sleep disordered breathing and pregnancy. *Thorax*, 2002;**57**:555–558.

23. Maasilta, P., A. Bachour, K. Teramo, O. Polo, and L.A. Laitinen, Sleep-related disordered breathing during pregnancy in obese women. *Chest*, 2000;**120**:1448–1454.

24. Loube, D.I., J.S. Poceta, M.C. Morales, M.D. Peacock, and M.M. Mitler, Self-reported snoring in pregnancy: association with fetal outcome. *Chest*, 1996;**109**:885–889.

25. Schutte, S., A. Del Conte, K. Doghramji, et al. Snoring during pregnancy and its impact on fetal outcome. *Sleep Res*, 1994;**23**:325.

26. Franklin, K.A., P.A. Holmgren, F. Jönsson, N. Poromaa, H. Stenlund, and E. Svanborg, Snoring, pregnancy-induced hypertension, and growth retardation of the fetus. *Chest*, 2000;**117**:137–141.

27. Taylor, R.N. and J.M. Roberts, Endothelial cell dysfunction. In: *Chesley's Hypertension Disorders in Pregnancy* (M.D. Linhheimer and J.M. Roberts, eds.). Stamford, CT: Appleton & Lange, 1999:395–429.

28. Edwards, N., D.M. Blyton, T. Kirjavainen, G.J. Kesby, and C.E. Sullivan, Nasal continuous positive airway pressure reduces sleep-induced blood pressure increments in preeclampsia. *Am J Respir Crit Care Med*, 2000;**162**:252–257.

29. Ekholm, E.M., O. Polo, E.R. Rauhala, and U.U. Ehblad, Sleep quality in preeclampsia. *Am J Obstet Gynecol*, 1992;**167**:1262–1266.

30. Guilleminault, C., M. Kreutzer, and J.L. Chang, Pregnancy, sleep disordered breathing and treatment with nasal continuous positive airway pressure. *Sleep Med*, 2004;**5**:43–51.

31. Conklin, K.A., Obstetric analgesia and anesthesia. In: *Essentials of Obstetrics and Gynecology* (N.F. Hacker and J.G. Moore, eds.). Philadelphia: WB Saunders, 1998:169–170.

32. Wilkie, G. and C.M. Shapiro, Sleep deprivation and the postnatal blues. *J Psychosom Res*, 1992;**36**:309–316.

33. Heasman, L., J.A.D. Spencer, and M.E. Symonds, Plasma prolactin concentrations after caesarean section or vaginal delivery. *Arch Dis Child Fetal Neonatal Ed*, 1997;**77**:F237–F238.

34. Tribotti, S., N. Lyons, S. Blackburn, M. Stein, and J. Withers, Nursing diagnoses for the postpartum woman. *J Obstet Gynecol Neonatal Nurs*, 1988;**17**:410–417.

35. Zaffke, M.E. and K.A. Lee, Sleep architecture in a postpartum sample: a comparative analysis. *Sleep Res*, 1992;**21**:327.

36. Nishihara, K., S. Horiuchi, H. Eto, and S. Uchida, Comparisons of sleep patterns between mothers in post-partum from 9 to 12 weeks and non-pregnant women. *Psychiatry Clin Neurosci*, 2001;**55**:227–228.

37. Karacan, I., W. Heine, H.W. Agnew, R.L. Williams, W.B. Webb, and J.J. Ross, Characteristics of sleep patterns during late pregnancy and postpartum periods. *Am J Obstet Gynecol*, 1968;**101**:579–586.

38. Coble, P.A., C.F. Reynolds, D.J. Kupfer, P.R. Houck, N.L. Day, and D.E. Giles, Childbearing in women with and without a history of affective disorder. II. Electroencephalographic sleep. *Comp Psychiatry*, 1994;**35**:215–224.

39. Wambach, K.A., Maternal fatigue in breastfeeding primiparae during the first 9 weeks postpartum. *J Hum Lactation*, 1998;**14**:219–229.

40. Quillan, S.I., Infant and mother sleep patterns during 4th postpartum week. *Iss Comprehens Pediatr Nurs*, 1997;**20**:115–123.

41. Noel, G.L., H.K. Suh, and A.G. Frantz, Prolactin release during nursing and breast stimulation in postpartum and nonpostpartum patients. *J Clin Endocrinol Metab*, 1974;**38**:413–423.

42. Nissen, E., K. Uvnas-Moberg, K. Svensson, S. Stock, A.-M. Widstrom, and J. Winberg, Different patterns of oxytocin, prolactin but not cortisol release during breastfeeding in women delivered by Caesarean section or by the vaginal route. *Early Hum Dev*, 1996;**45**:103–118.

43. Blyton, D.M., C.E. Sullivan, and N. Edwards, Lactation is associated with an increase in slow-wave sleep in women. *J Sleep Res*, 2002;**11**:297–303.

44. Petre-Quadens, I. and C. DeLee, Sleep-cycle alterations during pregnancy, postpartum and the menstrual cycle. In: *Biorhythms and Human Reproduction* (M. Ferin, F. Halberg, R.M. Richart, and R.L. Van Wiele, eds.). New York: John Wiley, 1974:335–351.

45. Morelli, G.A., B. Rogoff, D. Oppenhein, and D. Goldsmith, Cultural variation in infants' sleeping arrangements: questions of independence. *Dev Psychol*, 1992;**28**:604–613.

46. Nakamura, S.W., Are cribs the safest place for infants to sleep? Yes: Bed sharing is too hazardous. *West J Med*, 2001;**174**:300.

47. McKenna, J.J., E.B. Thoman, T.F. Anders, A. Sadeh, V.L. Schechtman, and S.F. Glotzbach, Infant-parent co-sleeping in an evolutionary perspective: implications for understanding infant sleep development and the sudden infant death syndrome. *Sleep*, 1993;**16**:263–282.

48. Willinger, M., C.-W. Ko, H.J. Hoffman, R.C. Kessler, and M.J. Corwin, Trends in infant bed sharing in the United States, 1993-2000. *Arch Pediatr Adolesc Med*, 2003;**157**:43–49.

49. McCoy, R.C., C.E. Hunt, S.M. Lesko, et al. Frequency of bed sharing and its relationship to breastfeeding. *J Dev Behav Pediatrics*, 2004;**25**:141–149.

50. Ball, H.L., Breastfeeding, bed-sharing, and infant sleep. *Birth*, 2003;**30**:181–188.

51. Brenner, R.A., B.G. Simons-Morton, B. Bhaskar, M. Revenis, A. Das, and J.D. Clemens, Infant-parent bed sharing in an inner-city population. *Arch Pediatr Adolesc Med*, 2003;**157**:33–39.

52. Gay, C.L., T.M. Ward, and K.A. Lee, Parent-newborn co-sleeping in the San Francisco Bay area. *Sleep*, 2004;**27**(Abstr Suppl):A356.

53. Romito, P., M.J. Saurel-Cubizolles, and M. Cuttini, Mothers' health after the birth of the first child: The case of employed women in an Italian city. *Women Health*, 1994;**21**:1–22.

54. Lee, K.A., G. McEnany, and M.E. Zaffke, REM sleep and mood state in childbearing women: sleepy or weepy? *Sleep*, 2000;**23**:877–885.

55. Kennedy, H.P., C.T. Beck, and J.W. Driscoll, A light in the fog: caring for women with postpartum depression. *J Midwifery Women's Health*, 2002;**47**:318–330.

56. Abou-Saleh, M., R. Ghubash, L. Karim, M. Krymski, and I. Bhai, Hormonal aspects of postpartum depression. *Psychoneuroendocrinology*, 1998;**23**:465–475.

57. Parry, B.L., M.L. Curran, C.A. Stuenkel, et al., Can critically times sleep deprivation be useful in pregnancy and postpartum depressions? *J Affect Disord*, 2000;**60**:201–212.

58. Corral, M., A. Kuan, and D. Kostaras, Bright light therapy's effect on postpartum depression. *Am J Psychiatry*, 2000;**157**:303–304.

59. Sadeh, A., I. Dark, and B.R. Vohr, Newborns' sleep-wake patterns: the role of maternal, delivery and infant factors. *Early Hum Dev*, 1996;**44**:113–126.

16
Pregnancy and Obstructive Sleep Apnea

Helena Schotland

INTRODUCTION

Pregnancy is a period of profound physiological change. During gestation, alterations in sleep and breathing are common. In some cases, these normal physiological alterations may result in sleep-disordered breathing (SDB). The purpose of this chapter is to describe the normal physiological changes seen in sleep and breathing during pregnancy and discuss the pathological implications of these alterations as they relate to snoring and obstructive sleep apnea (OSA).

SLEEP ARCHITECTURE AND QUALITY IN NORMAL PREGNANCY

Estrogen and progesterone levels rise progressively during pregnancy with implications for sleep and wakefulness. Estrogen reduces rapid eye-movement (REM) sleep (1–3), whereas progesterone has a sedating effect (4) and can increase non-REM sleep (5). The alterations in the sleep patterns of a pregnant woman are most notable in the first and third trimesters. During the first trimester there is an increase in total sleep time and daytime somnolence, whereas the third trimester is characterized by a decrease in total sleep time and an increase in nocturnal awakenings (6). The etiology of these awakenings is multifactorial and may be caused by fetal movements, urinary frequency, leg cramps, back pain, heartburn, or generalized discomfort (6,7).

RESPIRATORY CHANGES DURING PREGNANCY

During pregnancy a variety of physical and hormonal factors influence breathing. Some of these factors are detrimental and may predispose pregnant women to SDB, whereas others may be protective. The most obvious mechanical factor appreciated during pregnancy is the enlarging uterus, which alters intra-abdominal pressure and leads to deformation of the diaphragm and intrathoracic structures. Spirometric studies reveal a progressive decrease in functional residual capacity (FRC) and expiratory reserve volume as term approaches (8–11). These alterations can cause closing volume to be greater than FRC, resulting in shunting and hypoxemia (12). The reduced FRC is also associated with reduced lung oxygen stores, which may have obvious implications in the setting of a nocturnal respiratory dis-

From: *Current Clinical Neurology: Sleep Disorders in Women: A Guide to Practical Management*
Edited by: H. P. Attarian © Humana Press Inc., Totowa, NJ

turbance *(13)*, such as OSA. A number of studies have demonstrated that oxygen saturation is reduced in normal late pregnancy *(14–16)*. This effect is magnified when a pregnant woman is in the supine position *(14,17)*. Fortunately, pregnant women have a preference for sleeping in the lateral position *(15,18)*, which may improve oxygenation and protect them from SDB. Pregnancy is also a physiological state in which body weight increases dramatically over a short time period. In nonpregnant individuals, weight gain is directly correlated with severity of SDB over time *(19)*. It is not known whether gestational weight gain is an independent risk factor for SDB during pregnancy, but some authors suggest that it may exacerbate SDB, especially among obese women *(20)*.

In addition to physical alterations of pregnancy affecting respiratory mechanics, hormonal changes may also lead to detrimental mechanical alterations in the respiratory system. For example, the rising estrogen concentration during pregnancy leads to changes in airway mucosa such as hyperemia and mucosal edema *(21)*. This effect is most prominent during the third trimester, when significant nasal obstruction occurs and snoring is observed. Forty-two percent of pregnant women at 36 weeks gestation complain of rhinitis and nasal congestion *(22)*. In addition to the changes seen in the nasopharynx, the oropharynx is also altered during pregnancy. A study of 242 pregnant women revealed an increase in Mallampati scores between 12 and 38 weeks gestation *(23)*.

The hormonal alterations of pregnancy may be associated with mechanisms that protect the pregnant woman from SDB. The rising progesterone concentration of pregnancy is associated with hyperventilation as a result of enhanced respiratory center sensitivity to carbon dioxide *(24,25)*. This augmented respiratory drive also increases the responsiveness of upper airway dilator muscles to chemical stimuli *(26,27)*, theoretically protecting against airway obstruction.

The myriad alterations of pregnancy are associated with profound changes in the respiratory system—some changes protect pregnant women from developing SDB, whereas others predispose pregnant subjects to SDB. The remainder of this chapter is devoted to the discussion of abnormal breathing during sleep—from snoring to OSA.

SNORING AND PREGNANCY

In nonpregnant women, the prevalence of habitual snoring is only 4% *(28,29)*. This is in stark contrast to the prevalence of self-reported snoring in pregnant women, which ranges from 11–23% for self-reported habitual snoring *(28–30)* to 41% for self-reported intermittent snoring during pregnancy *(29)*. Because snoring is a marker for OSA, this increase in snoring during pregnancy has prompted further investigation.

Two questionnaire studies have demonstrated conflicting results regarding fetal outcomes in pregnant snorers. Loube et al. *(28)* found no significant difference in mean birthweight, Apgar scores, or complications in newborns of snorers compared with the newborns of nonsnorers. In contrast, Franklin et al. *(30)* demonstrated that habitual snorers were more likely to have infants with lower Apgar scores and growth retardation than nonhabitual snorers. In this study, witnessed apneas were observed in 11% of the habitual snorers compared with only 2% of the nonhabitual snoring group, but confirmatory polysomnograms were not performed. Thus, it is not possible to definitively link adverse fetal outcomes to OSA directly on the basis of this study. Habitual snoring during pregnancy may also have adverse effects on the health of the mother *(29,30)* as well as the fetus. In addition to their findings of adverse fetal outcomes in habitual snorers, Franklin et al. *(30)* also reported a link between habitual snoring and pregnancy-induced hypertension. There was also an association between habitual snoring and pre-eclampsia in this study, although it did not reach statistical significance.

OBSTRUCTIVE SLEEP APNEA AND PREGNANCY

Although OSA is a common disorder affecting an estimated 2% of women *(31)* and pregnancy is a common occurrence, the prevalence of OSA in pregnancy has not been studied extensively. Several investigators have performed polysomnographic studies in small groups of pregnant women *(32,33)*. The largest reported study was conducted in 267 pregnant women *(29)*. In this study, 267 women underwent nocturnal polygraphic monitoring, including an Edentrace® system. None of these subjects had an apnea–hypopnea index (AHI) score of more than 5 events per hour at 6 months gestation. During the second portion of this study, 26 women were selected for polysomnography. Thirteen of these women were in the "abnormal-breathing" group, which consisted of chronic, loud snorers or women with significant (≥5%) oxygen desaturation on initial ambulatory recording. At full polysomnography, none of these 26 subjects had an AHI of more than 5 events per hour, but the women in the "abnormal-breathing" group had signs of increased upper airway resistance, manifested by either crescendo respiratory effort or abnormal sustained effort *(29)*.

The medical literature regarding OSA in pregnancy has largely been limited to single case reports *(34–42)* and several small series of patients (Table 1) *(43–45)*. In the 33 pregnancies described in Table 1, associated medical complications included gestational hypertension in 3, pre-eclampsia in 4, diabetes mellitus in 1, gestational diabetes mellitus in 2, and pulmonary hypertension in 1.

When the 33 pregnancies in Table 1 are further evaluated, one factor that stands out is the lower mean infant birthweight for mothers with untreated OSA (2440 ± 431 g) compared with mothers who received some form of therapy for their OSA (2956 ± 216 g). This may be confounded by varying amounts of gestational diabetes mellitus and pre-eclampsia (conditions that can affect birthweight) in the treatment and nontreatment groups. The obvious concern in the nontreatment group is that the hypoxemia associated with OSA leads to placental ischemia, resulting in infants who are small for their gestational age. Pregnant animals exposed to chronic or intermittent prolonged hypoxemia have demonstrated fetal growth restriction *(46–48)*. In humans there is an association between maternal hypoxemia and fetal growth restriction in women with parenchymal lung disease and women living at high altitude *(49)*.

The other notable finding in the 33 pregnancies described in Table 1 is the increase in pregnancy-induced hypertension. Pregnancy-induced hypertension is associated

Table 1
Medical Complications in 33 Pregnancies

Authors	Year	N	Polysomnography or other study/observation	Associated conditions	Treatment	Fetal outcomes
Joel-Cohen and Schoenfeld (43)	1978	3	Clinical observations: Patient 1: 20-60-second apneas Patient 2: 70-80-second apneas Patient 3: 40-second apneas	None	None	Patient 1 (2810-g infant): Apgar 5/7 Patient 2 (2740-g infant): Apgar 5/8 Patient 3 (2680-g infant): Apgar 6/8
Conti et al. (34)	1988	1	History of central and obstructive apneas on prior PSG	Gestational hypertension	None	2730-g infant: "good" Apgar
Hastie et al. (35)	1989	1	AHI 19.7/hour Oxygen saturation nadir 84%	Gestational diabetes mellitus	Tracheostomy at 22 weeks gestation	2840-g infant: Apgar 10/10
Kowall et al. (36)	1989	1	AHI 78.6/hour Oxygen saturation nadir 74%	Polyhydramnios Pre-eclampsia	CPAP at 36 weeks gestation	Infant large for gestational age
Schoenfeld et al. (44)	1989	8	Clinical observations: snoring and nocturnal arousals in all 8 subjects	None	None in all 8 subjects	Mean newborn weight 1780 g
Sherrer et al. (37)	1991	1	PSG after delivery Apnea index 144/hour Oxygen saturation nadir 63%	Diabetes mellitus Pre-eclampsia Balanced chromosomal translocation	None during pregnancy	2780-g infant: Apgar 8/9
Charbonneau et al. (38)	1991	1	Apnea hypopnea index 159/h Oxygen saturation nadir 40%	Gestational diabetes mellitus	CPAP and oxygen at 36 weeks	2680-g infant (<10th percentile), polycythemia
Lefcourt et al. (39)	1996	1	PSG after delivery 817 apneas and hypopneas total Oxygen saturation nadir <50%	Pre-eclampsia	None during pregnancy	2300-g infant: Apgar 9/9

Study	Year	No. subjects	Sleep study findings	Complications	Treatment	Infant outcome
Lewis at al. (40)	1998	1	Nocturnal oximetry with desaturation nadir of 70%	Pulmonary hypertension	CPAP and oxygen at 29 weeks gestation	3055-g infant
Brain et al. (41)	2001	1 subject with 2 pregnancies	AHI 30/hour; Oxygen saturation nadir 20%	Pregnancy 1: gestational hypertension; Pregnancy 2: treated hypertension 1 + proteinuria	Pregnancy 1: no treatment; Pregnancy 2: CPAP throughout pregnancy	Pregnancy 1: intrauterine fetal demise at 23 weeks; fetal weight <10th percentile for gestational age; Pregnancy 2: 3250-g infant: Apgar 6/8
Roush and Bell (42)	2004	1	PSG after delivery; AHI 160/hour	Pre-eclampsia; Fetal heart rate decelerations	None during pregnancy	1700-kg infant: Apgar 8/9
Guilleminault et al. (45)	2004	12	AHI 9–31/hour; Oxygen saturation nadir 81–86%	Gestational hypertension in 1 subject	CPAP throughout pregnancy in 7 subjects; CPAP initiated between 8 and 13 weeks gestation in 5 subjects	All infants healthy; All Apgar >8

AHI, apnea–hypopnea index; PSG, polysomnography; CPAP, continuous positive airway pressure.

with increased maternal and fetal morbidity and mortality *(50)*. It is characterized by hypertension after 20 weeks gestation with or without proteinuria (≥300 mg in 24 hours) that regresses following delivery *(50)*. Pregnancy-induced hypertension may be classified into three types: gestational hypertension (5–9% of pregnancies), pre-eclampsia (5–7% of pregnancies in nulliparous women), and eclampsia (<1% of pregnancies) *(51–54)*. In the group of patients described in Table 1, the incidence of pregnancy-induced hypertension was 21%, with gestational hypertension in 3 subjects and pre-eclampsia in 4 subjects.

Several large studies in the general population have demonstrated that SDB is an independent predictor for the development of hypertension *(55,56)*. The relationship between OSA and pregnancy-induced hypertension is not as well described. Using an acoustic reflection method, Izci et al. *(57)* demonstrated that the upper airways of 37 women with pre-eclampsia were narrower than those of nonpregnant controls. Not surprisingly, inspiratory flow limitation during overnight polygraphic monitoring was also seen in 15 subjects with pre-eclampsia compared with normal pregnant and nonpregnant women *(58)*. However, none of these subjects with pre-eclampsia had OSA. In a study of 502 pregnant women, pregnancy-induced hypertension was found to be more common in habitual snorers than in nonsnorers *(30)*. It is not clear whether upper airway alterations and SDB contribute to the development of pregnancy-induced hypertension or whether the edema associated with pre-eclampsia is the underlying cause of the narrowed upper airway and/or flow limitation *(20)*.

Two studies examine the response of blood pressure to SDB events or treatment of such events. One study evaluated 10 pregnant women with OSA and pre-eclampsia and 10 pregnant women with OSA and no evidence of hypertensive disease *(59)*. Sleep architecture and severity of OSA were similar in the two groups, but the blood pressure response to obstructive breathing events was augmented in women with pre-eclampsia and OSA compared to the pregnant women with OSA alone. This same group of investigators demonstrated that continuous positive airway pressure (CPAP) therapy was effective in eliminating the nocturnal blood pressure increases in 11 women with severe pre-eclampsia and upper airway flow limitation *(60)*.

MANAGEMENT OF OBSTRUCTIVE SLEEP APNEA DURING PREGNANCY

Thus far, there is no consensus regarding how to screen and whom to screen for OSA during pregnancy. It may be more appropriate to develop screening parameters once the prevalence of OSA in pregnancy and in conditions such as pregnancy-induced hypertension has been established. Once OSA has been diagnosed in pregnancy, treatment is indicated. In the group of patients described in Table 1, the methods of treatment included CPAP therapy with or without oxygen and tracheostomy. The advantage of CPAP therapy is that it is noninvasive and can be instituted rapidly. It was also shown to be a safe and effective treatment for OSA in pregnancy *(36,38,40,41,45)*. There may be a role for an auto-titrating CPAP device as pregnant patients continue to gain weight during the gestational period. In the era of CPAP therapy, the need for tracheostomy is rare. Although the use of an oral appliance may be appropriate for mild to moderate OSA, the time necessary for the manufacture and adjustment of the appliance may be excessive for pregnant individuals. Surgical treatment options (e.g., uvulopalatopharyngoplasty) for OSA are problematic for pregnant patients given the risks of anesthesia and the suboptimal efficacy of various surgical interventions.

After a pregnant individual with OSA has delivered, follow-up is required. Pien and Schwab *(20)* advocate individualized postpartum management, recommending a repeat polysomnogram after weight stabilization (≥2 months postpartum). An alternative option is the utilization of an auto-titrating CPAP unit to assess CPAP requirements after delivery in the setting of ongoing weight loss.

CONCLUSION

The physical changes of pregnancy may contribute to the onset or exacerbation of OSA. The prevalence of OSA in pregnancy has not been fully evaluated and requires further study. Some small series of patients and case reports of OSA in pregnancy suggest adverse maternal and fetal outcomes. Therefore, the identification and treatment of pregnant patients with OSA is imperative. CPAP is a simple, noninvasive therapeutic option that is well tolerated and appears to be safe during pregnancy.

REFERENCES

1. Branchey, M., L. Branchey, and R.D. Nadler, Effects of estrogen and progesterone on sleep patterns of female rats. *Physiol Behav*, 1971;6(6):743–746.
2. Colvin, G.B., D.I. Whitmoyer, R.D. Lisk, D.O. Walter, and C.H. Sawyer, Changes in sleep-wakefulness in female rats during circadian and estrous cycles. *Brain Res*, 1968;7(2):173–181.
3. Fang, J., and W. Fishbein, Sex differences in paradoxical sleep: influences of estrus cycle and ovariectomy. *Brain Res*, 1996;734(1–2):275–285.
4. Merryman, W., R. Boiman, L. Barnes, and I. Rothchild, Progesterone anesthesia in human subjects. *J Clin Endocrinol Metab*, 1954;14(12):1567–1569.
5. Friess, E., H. Tagaya, L. Trachsel, F. Holsboer, and R. Rupprecht, Progesterone-induced changes in sleep in male subjects. *Am J Physiol*, 1997;272:E885–E891.
6. Schweiger, M.S. Sleep disturbance in pregnancy. A subjective survey. *Am J Obstet Gynecol*, 1972;114(7):879–882.
7. Fast, A., L. Weiss, S. Parikh, and G. Hertz, Night backache in pregnancy. Hypothetical pathophysiological mechanisms. *Am J Phys Med Rehabil*, 1989;68(5):227–229.
8. Cugell, D.W., N.R. Frank, E.A. Gaensler, and T.L. Badger, Pulmonary function in pregnancy. I. Serial observations in normal women.*Am Rev Tuberc*, 1953;67(5):568–597.
9. Weinberger, S.E., S.T. Weiss, W.R. Cohen, J.W. Weiss, and T.S. Johnson, Pregnancy and the lung. *Am Rev Respir Dis*, 1980;121(3):559–581.
10. Knuttgen, H.G. and K. Emerson Jr., Physiological response to pregnancy at rest and during exercise. *J Appl Physiol*, 1974;36(5):549–553.
11. Craig, D.B. and M.A. Toole, Airway closure in pregnancy. *Can Anaesth Soc J*, 1975;22(6):665–672.
12. Holdcroft, A., D.R. Bevan, J.C. O'Sullivan, and M.K. Sykes, Airway closure and pregnancy. *Anaesthesia*, 1977;32(6):517–523.
13. Feinsilver, S.H. and G. Hertz, Respiration during sleep in pregnancy. *Clin Chest Med*, 1992;13(4):637–644.
14. Trakada, G., V. Tsapanos, and K. Spiropoulos, Normal pregnancy and oxygenation during sleep. *Eur J Obstet Gynecol Reprod Biol*, 2003;109(2):128–132.

15. Hertz, G., A. Fast, S.H. Feinsilver, C.L. Albertario, H. Schulman, and A.M. Fein, Sleep in normal late pregnancy. *Sleep*, 1992;**15**(3):246–251.
16. Bourne, T., A.J. Ogilvy, R. Vickers, and K.Williamson, Nocturnal hypoxaemia in late pregnancy. *Br J Anaesth*, 1995;**75**(6):678–682.
17. Awe, R.J., M.B. Nicotra, T.D. Newsom, and R. Viles, Arterial oxygenation and alveolar-arterial gradients in term pregnancy. *Obstet Gynecol*, 1979;**53**(2):182–186.
18. Mills, G.H. and A.G. Chaffe, Sleeping positions adopted by pregnant women of more than 30 weeks gestation. *Anaesthesia*, 1994;**49**(3):249–250.
19. Peppard, P.E., T. Young, M. Palta, J. Dempsey, and J. Skatrud, Longitudinal study of moderate weight change and sleep-disordered breathing. *JAMA*, 2000;**284**(23):3015–3021.
20. Pien, G.W. and R.J. Schwab, Sleep disorders during pregnancy. *Sleep*, 2004;**27**(7):1405–1417.
21. Elkus, R. and J. Popovich Jr., Respiratory physiology in pregnancy. *Clin Chest Med*, 1992;**13**(4):555–565.
22. Bende, M. and T. Gredmark, Nasal stuffiness during pregnancy. *Laryngoscope*, 1999;**109**(7 Pt 1):1108–1110.
23. Pilkington, S., F. Carli, M.J. Dakin, et al., Increase in Mallampati score during pregnancy. *Br J Anaesth*, 1995;**74**(6):638–642.
24. Prowse, C.M. and E.A. Gaensler, Respiratory and acid-base changes during pregnancy. *Anesthesiology*, 1965;**26**:381–392.
25. Contreras, G., M. Gutierrez, T. Beroiza, et al., Ventilatory drive and respiratory muscle function in pregnancy. *Am Rev Respir Dis*, 1991;**144**(4):837–841.
26. Parisi, R.A., T.V. Santiago, and N.H. Edelman, Genioglossal and diaphragmatic EMG responses to hypoxia during sleep. *Am Rev Respir Dis*, 1988;**138**(3):610–616.
27. Wheatley, J.R. and D.P. White, The influence of sleep on pharyngeal reflexes. *Sleep*, 1993;**16**(8 Suppl):S87–S89.
28. Loube, D.I., J.S. Poceta, M.C. Morales, M.D. Peacock, and M.M. Mitler, Self-reported snoring in pregnancy. Association with fetal outcome. *Chest*, 1996;**109**(4):885–889.
29. Guilleminault, C., M. Querra-Salva, S. Chowdhuri, and D. Poyares, Normal pregnancy, daytime sleeping, snoring and blood pressure. *Sleep Med*, 2000;**1**(4):289–297.
30. Franklin, K.A., P.A.. Holmgren, F. Jonsson, N. Poromaa, H. Stenlund, and E. Svanborg, Snoring, pregnancy-induced hypertension, and growth retardation of the fetus. *Chest*, 2000;**117**(1):137–141.
31. Young, T., M. Palta, J. Dempsey, J. Skatrud, S. Weber, and S. Badr, The occurrence of sleep-disordered breathing among middle-aged adults. *N Engl J Med*, 1993;**328**(17):1230–1235.
32. Maasilta, P., A. Bachour, K. Teramo, O. Polo, and L.A. Laitinen, Sleep-related disordered breathing during pregnancy in obese women. *Chest*, 2001;**120**(5):1448–1454.
33. Nikkola, E., U. Ekblad, E. Ekholm, H. Mikola, and O. Polo, Sleep in multiple pregnancy: breathing patterns, oxygenation, and periodic leg movements. *Am J Obstet Gynecol*, 1996;**174**(5):1622–1625.
34. Conti, M., V. Izzo, M.L. Muggiasca, and M. Tiengo, Sleep apnoea syndrome in pregnancy: a case report. *Eur J Anaesthesiol*, 1988;**5**(2):151–154.
35. Hastie, S.J., K. Prowse, W.H. Perks, J. Atkins, and V.A. Blunt, Obstructive sleep apnoea during pregnancy requiring tracheostomy. *Aust NZ J Obstet Gynaecol*, 1989;**29**(3 Pt 2):365–367.
36. Kowall, J., G.Clark, G. Nino-Murcia, and N. Powell, Precipitation of obstructive sleep apnea during pregnancy. *Obstet Gynecol*, 1989;**74**(3 Pt 2):453–455.
37. Sherer, D.M., C.B. Caverly, and J.S. Abramowicz, Severe obstructive sleep apnea and associated snoring documented during external tocography. *Am J Obstet Gynecol*, 1991;**165**(5 Pt 1):1300–1301.
38. Charbonneau, M., T. Falcone, M.G. Cosio, and R.D. Levy, Obstructive sleep apnea during pregnancy. Therapy and implications for fetal health. *Am Rev Respir Dis*, 1991;**144**(2):461–463.
39. Lefcourt, L.A. and J.F. Rodis, Obstructive sleep apnea in pregnancy. *Obstet Gynecol Surv*, 1996;**51**(8):503–506.
40. Lewis, D.F., A.L. Chesson, M.S. Edwards, J.W. Weeks, and C.D.Adair, Obstructive sleep apnea during pregnancy resulting in pulmonary hypertension. *South Med J*, 1998;**91**(8):761–762.

41. Brain, K.A., J.G.T hornton, A. Sarkar, and A.O. Johnson, Obstructive sleep apnoea and fetal death: successful treatment with continuous positive airway pressure. *BJOG*, 2001;**108**(5):543–544.

42. Roush, S.F. and L. Bell, Obstructive sleep apnea in pregnancy. *J Am Board Fam Pract*, 2004;**17**(4):292–294.

43. Joel-Cohen, S.J. and A. Schoenfeld, Fetal response to periodic sleep apnea: a new syndrome in obstetrics. *Eur J Obstet Gynecol Reprod Biol*, 1978;**8**(2):77–81.

44. Schoenfeld, A., Y. Ovadia, A. Neri, and S. Freedman, Obstructive sleep apnea (OSA)-implications in maternal-fetal medicine. A hypothesis. *Med Hypotheses*, 1989;**30**(1):51–54.

45. Guilleminault, C., M. Kreutzer, and J.L. Chang, Pregnancy, sleep disordered breathing and treatment with nasal continuous positive airway pressure. *Sleep Med*, 2004;**5**(1):43–51.

46. Gozal, D., S.R. Reeves, B.W. Row, J.J. Neville, S.Z. Guo, and A.J. Lipton, Respiratory effects of gestational intermittent hypoxia in the developing rat. *Am J Respir Crit Care Med*, 2003;**167**(11):1540–1547.

47. Gozal, D., E. Gozal, S.R. Reeves, and A.J. Lipton, Gasping and autoresuscitation in the developing rat: effect of antecedent intermittent hypoxia. *J Appl Physiol*, 2002;**92**(3):1141–1144.

48. Schwartz, J.E., A. Kovach, J. Meyer, C. McConnell, and H.S. Iwamoto, Brief, intermittent hypoxia restricts fetal growth in Sprague-Dawley rats. *Biol Neonate*, 1998;**73**(5):313–319.

49. Bernstein, I. and S.G. Gabbe, Intrauterine growth restriction. In: *Obstetrics: Normal and Problem Pregnancies*, 3rd ed. Gabbe SG, Niebyl JR, Simpson JL, eds. New York: Churchill Livingstone; 1996:863–886.

50. Zhang, J., J. Zeisler, M.C. Hatch, and G. Berkowitz, Epidemiology of pregnancy-induced hypertension. *Epidemiol Rev*, 1997;**19**(2):218–232.

51. Kyle, P.M., D. Buckley, J. Kissane, M. de Swiet, and C.W. Redman, The angiotensin sensitivity test and low-dose aspirin are ineffective methods to predict and prevent hypertensive disorders in nulliparous pregnancy. *Am J Obstet Gynecol*, 1995;**173**(3 Pt 1):865–872.

52. Sibai, B.M., S.N. Caritis, E. Thom, et al., Prevention of preeclampsia with low-dose aspirin in healthy, nulliparous pregnant women. *N Engl J Med*, 1993;**329**(17):1213–1218.

53. Carroli, G., L. Duley, J.M. Belizan, and J.Villar, Calcium supplementation during pregnancy: a systematic review of randomised controlled trials. *Br J Obstet Gynaecol*, 1994;**101**(9):753–758.

54. Hauth, J.C., R.L. Goldenberg, C.R. Parker Jr., et al., Low-dose aspirin therapy to prevent preeclampsia. *Am J Obstet Gynecol*, 1993;**168**(4):1083–1091.

55. Peppard, P.E., T. Young, M.Palta, and J. Skatrud, Prospective study of the association between sleep-disordered breathing and hypertension. *N Engl J Med*, 2000;**342**(19):1378–1384.

56. Nieto, F.J., T.B. Young, B.K. Lind, et al., Association of sleep-disordered breathing, sleep apnea, and hypertension in a large community-based study. Sleep Heart Health Study. *JAMA*, 2000;**283**(14):1829–1836.

57. Izci, B., R.L. Riha, S.E. Martin, et al., The upper airway in pregnancy and pre-eclampsia. *Am J Respir Crit Care Med*, 2003;**167**(2):137–140.

58. Connolly, G., A.R. Razak, A. Hayanga, A. Russell, P. McKenna, and W.T. McNicholas, Inspiratory flow limitation during sleep in pre-eclampsia: comparison with normal pregnant and non-pregnant women. *Eur Respir J*, 2001;**18**(4):672–676.

59. Edwards, N., D.M. Blyton, T.T. Kirjavainen, and C.E. Sullivan, Hemodynamic responses to obstructive respiratory events during sleep are augmented in women with preeclampsia. *Am J Hypertens*, 2001;**14**(11 Pt 1):1090–1095.

60. Edwards, N., D.M. Blyton, T. Kirjavainen, G.J. Kesby, and C.E. Sullivan, Nasal continuous positive airway pressure reduces sleep-induced blood pressure increments in preeclampsia. *Am J Respir Crit Care Med*, 2000;**162**(1):252–257.

V Menopause

17

Restless Legs Syndrome and Menopause

Nancy S. Collins

INTRODUCTION

There is no known pathophysiological link and, indeed, very little in the literature written about menopause and restless legs syndrome (RLS). Because the cellular mechanisms explaining the causality of RLS are unknown, much literature has focused on numerous associations in order to discover the etiology and pathophysiology of the disorder in men and women. Some widely held generalizations occur in the literature, including characterizions of the disorder as commonly occurring in middle to late age and with higher prevalence in women. Following this line of logic, one would naturally posit a relationship between RLS and menopause. However, as is discussed in this chapter, these widely held generalizations need to be reexamined in the context of recent epidemiological population- and patient-based data so that the information gathered from the clinical and basic sciences can best be integrated and possible mechanisms underlying RLS discovered, including what role, if any, changes associated with menopause may play in the disorder.

As is discussed in this chapter, epidemiological, clinical, and basic science studies suggest that RLS is a chronic disorder in men and women, possibly resulting from complex metabolic dysfunction often involving iron acquisition/regulation and dopaminergic and opiatergic pathways and likely influenced by as-yet-unknown mechanisms, including genetic, circadian, psychosocial, and medical disorders and possibly other changes associated with aging. There may be no direct correlation between RLS and menopause, but RLS as a preexisting condition may become more evident to patients whose sleep is disrupted as a result of other sleep-disrupting conditions during middle to late age. If menopause does contribute to RLS, the influence of hormonal changes, perhaps via a loss of some neuroprotective effect of gonadal steroids on iron acquisition/regulation, dopaminergic and opiatergic pathways, it would join numerous other medical and aging-related conditions that contribute to the chronic underlying condition of RLS.

CONDITIONS ASSOCIATED WITH RLS

Symptoms of RLS were described first in 1672 by Sir Thomas Willis (1). In 1945 Karl Ekbom described the symptom complex. Since the syndrome was described, numerous associations have been made.

From: *Current Clinical Neurology: Sleep Disorders in Women: A Guide to Practical Management*
Edited by: H. P. Attarian © Humana Press Inc., Totowa, NJ

Iron Deficiency or Iron Dysfunctional States Associated With RLS

Several investigators have shown low iron and ferritin *(2–4)* and anemia *(3,5)* in their patients with RLS. The associations were further supported by reports of symptomatology of RLS at its worst when either low levels or relatively low levels of iron or ferritin levels were noted and symptomatology improved when iron was exogenously given or reached elevated levels.

Dopaminergic Dysfunctional States Associated With RLS

Investigators have performed imaging studies in symptomatic individuals with RLS showing decreased activity in dopaminergic areas of the brain *(6)*. Investigators also document improvement in symptomatology of RLS with exogenous dopaminergic medications *(6,7)*, and worsening with dopaminergic antagonists *(6,8)*. Up to 80% of patients with RLS have periodic limb movement disorder, which also responds well to exogenous dopaminergic medications *(9)*.

Other Medical Disorders Associated With RLS

Investigators have reported peripheral neuropathies *(10)*, diabetes *(3,5,11,12)*, uremia *(1,3,11)*, myelopathy, rheumatoid arthritis *(5)*, hyperthyroid *(3,11)*, hypoparathyroid *(9,11)*, and myocardial infarction not explained by age, gender, or diabetes *(3)*.

Circadian Rhythm of Symptoms of RLS and Other Hormonal Secretory Cycles Associated With RLS

RLS has a circadian onset of symptoms, which are worse in the evening and at bedtime. RLS symptoms tend to occur during the falling or acrophase of circadian melatonin secretion. The circadian rhythm of melatonin consists of a decreased rate of production and release during the day and an increased rate of production and release during the night. (*See* section "Roles of Hormonal and Circadian Influences That May Aggravate RLS in Menopause.")

Conditions Specific to Women Associated With RLS

Pregnancy is associated with RLS *(3)*, particularly during the 4 weeks before and 4 weeks after delivery, after which it usually disappears. RLS is more often reported in women with a positive family history of RLS *(13)*. Reports of RLS in pregnancy range from 11 to 19% *(9)*. One investigator found increased reports of RLS in women with increased parity *(3)*.

Psychosocial Disturbances Associated With RLS

RLS is reported in higher numbers in populations with lower incomes *(12)*, poor mental health *(12,14)*, psychiatric disease, such as depression *(11)*, decreased general health *(12,15)*, low exercise levels *(12)*, and less education *(3)*.

Genetics/Family History Associated With RLS

Rates of familial RLS/ family history of RLS range between 40 and 90% of patients with idiopathic RLS *(11,13,16,17)*. Estimates of inherited RLS range from 33 to 65% *(11)*. Some investigators have reported autosomal dominance *(3,17,18)* with variable penetrance. There is a high concordance rate (83%) for primary/idiopathic RLS in identical twins *(4,19)*. No gender linkage *(12)* has been demonstrated; possibilities *(11,12)* have been postulated, but ascertainment bias cannot be excluded *(9,18)*. Reported chromosomal locations include 12q, in a French family *(11)*, 14q in an Italian family *(11)*, and 9p *(9,20)*. Some investigators suggest genetic predisposition or polymorphism *(21)* and genetic susceptibility to RLS in women. One investigator reported genetic studies that suggested increased concentration of monoamine oxidase alleles in women, which may contribute to sensitivity to RLS, but this association is not particularly strong *(9)*. Investigators have reported that women with a family history of RLS suffer more from RLS during pregnancy than women without a family history of RLS *(13)*, and patients with RLS early in life have an increased incidence of relatives affected with RLS *(5)*.

Two Forms of RLS

There appear to be two forms of RLS: primary/idiopathic (without certain co-morbid medical conditions) and secondary (with certain co-morbid medical conditions). There is no significant difference between the primary or secondary forms of the disorder in terms of clinical symptomatology/phenotype. This suggests a similar underlying pathophysiology *(17)*.

EPIDEMIOLOGY

Overall, in studies of patients and populations that include both primary and secondary forms (*see* above section), RLS is widely reported to affect 5–15% of the population *(3,9,22)*. In studies that evaluated the age and gender of patients with RLS, RLS affected more women than men and prevalence increased with age. Seven population-based studies in the United States, Europe, and Asia have reported higher prevalences in women than in men *(3,13,14,18,21,23,24)*. The perimenopausal and menopausal periods generally coincide with the progressive increases in reported RLS prevalence. Reports that women report earlier onset of RLS than men have also been noted *(21)*.

Nevertheless, recent epidemiological studies (population- and patient-based) are not supportive of menopausal condition as contributing to the prevalence of RLS in women. RLS prevalence in men has also been reported to increase over decades in most studies, to which ovarian failure obviously cannot be a contributing factor *(3,13,14,18,21,23,24)*. Investigators are also now challenging the older prevalence data by asking subjects about the first onset of symptoms. Studies show that when people recognize the onset of the disorder by the time they have reached 20 *(10)* or 30 years of age *(12)*, the small differences in prevalence for the 10-year age groups up to 70 years are not statistically significant. Also, most of these studies (population- and patient-based), which showed increased numbers of people with symptoms in middle and later years, included subjects who, in addition to primary RLS, likely had secondary RLS *(10)*. Even so, in many of these studies, when asked, patients admit that symptoms began decades earlier but that they did not seek medical treatment until in their 40s or 50s *(10)*. In an effort to understand more about the onset and etiology of the condition, a few studies looked at prevalence data of RLS in subjects without co-morbid contributing medical conditions. In the one patient-based study in Canada that looked at prevalence in men and women (using the

International Restless Legs Study Group criteria) excluding subjects with targeted co-morbid conditions, no gender differences were reported *(16)*.

One well-designed population-based study in Kentucky, co-written with an epidemiologist, used a single question that included key RLS symptomatic criteria; it found no gender differences. That study was a statewide telephone survey of 1803 people (with a response rate of 84%) and included co-morbid conditions. It showed an overall prevalence of 9.4% of RLS and no significant gender differences. The same study confirmed a prevalence increase with age in both genders, no more in women than in men, and for the 10-year age groups between 30 and 70, the small differences in prevalence (in both genders) were not statistically significant. In that study, by 30–39 years of age, 11% reported RLS; by 30–50 years of age, 9.5% reported RLS; by 50–70 years of age, 12% had reported RLS.

Therefore, although the disorder is largely described as having onset in middle age (i.e., not seeking medical attention until the fourth decade or later *[10]*), a high proportion of patients admit that the symptoms began decades earlier in both the primary and the secondary forms, with symptoms being milder and intermittent at first and becoming more severe and frequent over decades *(10)*. Some reasons why patients don't report symptoms earlier include the mildness of symptoms at the beginning (69%) or the assumption that the symptoms are not treatable (22%) *(10)*. According to one investigator, if the patient's age of onset was less than 20 years, the mean age to seek medical attention was between 32 and 40 years. If the patient's age of onset was greater than 20 years, the mean age to seek medical attention was between 52 and 54 years *(10)*. In addition, investigators have reported that 62% more women than men report early onset of RLS *(21)*.

Patients with both the primary (>50% *[13]*, 63% *[16]*, and 92% *[17]*) and secondary forms of RLS (13% *[17]*, 18% *[13]*) report a definite or possible positive family history in first-degree relatives. Investigators have found that in patients with a definite positive family history, the age of onset is significantly younger *(16)*. Also, in the primary form, the age of onset tends to be earlier, including childhood (sometimes <10 years) (13.5% *[16]*) and adolescence (38% before age of 20 *[16]*). Mean age of onset for primary RLS is about 27 years *(4,16)*, with 45% of patients experiencing their first symptom before the age of 20 *(4,10)*. Genetics are thought to be autosomal dominant with variable expressivity *(25)*. It has been speculated that the primary form may be explained by a genetic predisposition or polymorphism that alters the risk of RLS development in women earlier in life *(21)*.

In the acquired, or secondary form, onset is generally reported later *(19)* and by more men than women *(2,21)*. Late-onset RLS is often associated with medical conditions such as peripheral neuropathies, uremia, diabetes (although milder), and intermittent symptoms may have been experienced decades sooner but not reported until middle age. Hornyak and Trenkwalder reported that patients with RLS early in life show a lower rate of occurrence of small fiber neuropathy compared to those with later onset *(5)*. They also reported that patients with RLS without a family history had a later age of symptom onset, an increased incidence of neuropathy, and lower ferritin levels *(5)*.

Functional and pathological studies of RLS have shown no difference between the primary and secondary forms of the disorder. However, some investigators noted that familial RLS cases required higher doses of dopaminergic agents than sporadic cases and hypothesize that the gradual loss of efficacy of dopaminergic agents in the familial cases may represent a progression of the underlying central nervous system (CNS) process *(17)*.

MENOPAUSE

Menopause is strictly defined as the 1-year period following the cessation of menstruation *(26)*. However, hormonal changes beginning 7–10 years before the final menses include decreased estradiol, decreased disinhibin, increased follicle-stimulating hormone (FSH), increased luteinizing hormone (LH), change in circulating estrogens from estradiol to estrone, and a minimal decrease in testosterone *(26)*. Ovarian follicular loss accelerates logarithmically dramatically (three- to sixfold) during the decade prior to menopause (late 30s, early 40s). Follicular loss slows from age 25 to 38 years, and then resumes at a rapid rate until the follicles are completely exhausted, sometime during a woman's 50s. As the number of ovarian follicles decreases, there is a decrease in progesterone, which decreases inhibition to the hypothalamus and pituitary, resulting in an increase in FSH and a smaller increase in LH and gonadotropins. Circulating estrogens shift from estradiol to estrone *(26)*.

Adult women between the ages of 20 and 45 include those with regular menstrual cycles, women taking oral contraceptives, pregnant and lactating women, and women entering menopause. Each of these states is associated with a unique hormonal environment *(26)*.

SUBCORTICAL NERVOUS SYSTEM DYSFUNCTION IN RLS

The cellular mechanisms behind the primary and secondary forms of RLS are not known. Review of the literature demonstrates that most researchers agree that RLS has its origin in the CNS *(3,19,27)*, although there is involvement of the peripheral nervous system has also been hypothesized *(10,19)*.

Role of Dopaminergic Dysfunction

Evidence and Theories Supporting Role of Dopaminergic Dysfunction

Mounting evidence indicates that dopaminergic dysfunction is involved in the pathophysiology of RLS. Dopamine (DA) is produced in a circadian rhythm. RLS symptoms follow a circadian rhythm, with RLS symptoms at their worst at night when the concentrations of plasma DA are at their lowest *(6)*. RLS symptoms are increased when taking DA antagonists, which cross the blood–brain barrier (BBB) *(9,27)*. No RLS symptoms are affected when taking DA antagonists, which do not cross the BBB *(27)*. Futhermore, RLS symptoms improve with dopaminergic meds *(9)*.

Some studies in RLS patients show a modest decrease in dopamine D2 receptors in the striatum *(4,6–8)* and dopamine transporter (DAT) binding *(23)*. Decreased D2 binding in caudate and putamen (below normal) in 6 of 13 patients and mildly

decreased binding in the putamen of 3 of 13 patients measuring nigrostriatal terminal DA storage with ^{18}F-dopa and striatal D2 receptor binding in ^{11}C-raclopremide
positron emission tomography (PET) was found by one investigator *(6)*, who found
the mean caudate and putamen ^{18}F-dopa mildly reduced in RLS patients compared
with controls. Historically, [(123)I]-iodobenzamide (IBZM) single photon emis-
sion-computed tomography (SPECT) studies have also shown decreased D2 binding in patients with RLS *(6)*. The hypothesis is that the decreased D2 binding is
owing to receptor dysfunction or downregulation or increased levels of site occu-
pancy by endogenous DA *(6)*.

Patients with L-dopa-responsive RLS may have increased cerebrospinal fluid
(CSF) DA and homovanillic acid concentrations *(17)*. Prominent involvement of
the lower limbs and absence of facial involvement suggest impairment of the DA
system caudal to the midpons or in the spinal cord *(19)*.

Evidence and Theories Not Supporting Dopaminergic Dysfunction

In contrast to the evidence in the PET and SPECT studies previously noted, other
SPECT studies using IBZM show no difference *(4,7,8)* based on DAT binding between
patients with RLS compared to controls *(4,28)*. Also, SPECT of DAT and striatal
D2 receptor binding using 2 β-carboxymethoxy-3 β-(4-iodophenyl)tropane (β-CIT)
showed no presynaptic striatal DA deficiency *(9,29)*.

Research Directions for Dopamine Role in RLS

One investigator suggests that future research should focus on ventral tegmental
DA neurons because they play a role in the regulation of sleep and are particularly
sensitive to opiate agonists, which may mediate therapeutic effects of opiates in
RLS *(17)*. He also suggests that future research should focus on diencephalic DA
cells. Their location in the caudal thalamus and midbrain and periventricular gray
matter and their projections to the spinal cord, where they modulate nociception
and possibly affect motor control, make them compelling candidates for future research
(17). One theory *(27)* is that RLS may be related to hypersensitive postsynaptic DA
receptors, possibly as a result of decreased DA function during the night.

Connor's neuropathological studies in seven patients with RLS showed no cell
loss or clearcut morphological cell damage. However, the remarkable findings did show
that iron and H-ferritin staining was markedly impaired in the substantia nigra of RLS
brains *(30)*. Also, transferrin receptor staining on neuromelanin-containing cells was
decreased in RLS brains. Connor's working hypothesis is that iron acquisition in neuromelanin cells is compromised in RLS, which leads to a series of events (i.e., impaired
DA activity) that ultimately manifests as RLS symptoms *(30)*. Indeed, RLS may
not be a traditional neurodegenerative process, but may be a functional disorder
resulting from impaired iron acquisition by the neuromelanin cells in RLS. The
underlying mechanism may be a defect in the regulation of transferrin receptors *(30)*.

Role of Central Nervous System Iron/Ferritin/Transferrin Metabolism Dysfunction

As noted earlier in this chapter, there is neuropathological evidence showing
that a dysfunction in iron acquisition/regulation is likely involved in the patho-

physiology of RLS (*30; see* earlier discussion for work by Connor). It is not known whether decreased iron is a cause of RLS or if it acts as a trigger or aggravating factor (*23*). Further support of the role of iron dysfunction in RLS is a circadian rhythm of iron production, with serum iron levels decreasing at night (*4,31*), the time of day when RLS symptoms are at their worst. Also, iron is an important cofactor for tyrosine hydoxylase, the rate-limiting enzyme in DA synthesis, and if a DA deficiency state contributes to RLS, then low levels of iron may contribute to these low DA levels (*4*).

Ferritin carries iron across the BBB. Decreased serum ferritin has been associated in some studies with RLS severity particularly in older patients (*19*). Also, there are many reports of ferritin concentrations that are decreased in CSF (*4,32*), even with normal serum ferritin (*32*), and high concentrations of CSF transferrin (*27*) of RLS patients. A recent National Institutes of Health study showed that early-onset RLS patients had lower CSF ferritin (2.1 µg/L) than late-onset RLS patients (2.8 µg/L) and found no differences in serum ferritin levels between the groups (*32a*). The lower levels of CSF ferritin in patients with RLS supports the hypothesis of abnormal brain regulation of ferritin and iron in RLS pathophysiology (*32*), and these findings also support the hypothesis that low CSF iron stores may be better correlated to early-onset than late-onset RLS, which may mean that low stores of iron in the brain are genetically influenced, as in early-onset RLS. Therefore, the prevailing hypothesis is that RLS results from decreased concentrations of iron in the brain, which then interferes with DA synthesis (*31*). Altered iron status would affect both the opiate and DA systems because both the dopamine D2 receptor and the µ-opiate receptor are iron dependent (*9*).

The role of iron deficiency/dysfunction in RLS is also supported by conditions associated with secondary RLS, such as iron-deficiency anemia (*5,23*), pregnancy, and end-stage renal disease (*23*) as well as the reports of the therapeutic efficacy of intravenous iron, which demonstrate remission of RLS symptoms (*11*). Furthur support includes reports of oral administration of iron improving RLS symptoms, particularly if pretreatment ferritin is less than 45 mg/L (*11*). In addition, pregnant women have an at least two- to threefold higher risk of experiencing RLS than the general population (*33*). In this population, iron and folate requirements are 3–4 and 8–10 times higher than in the nonpregnant state (*33*).

Magnetic resonance imaging studies have shown decreased iron in the substantia nigra and putamen in patients with RLS (*2,4,11*). In 21-day-old iron-deficient rats, Erikson et al. (*29*) showed that, although the mechanism is not clear, lowered DAT functioning and decreased DA receptor density are consistent with a coupling of iron-related events. Iron deficiency causes increased extracellular DA subsequent to altered clearance. The increased extracellular DA is a result of iron-deficiency-influenced DA reuptake into the presynaptic membrane via alteration of DAT functioning (the route of removal of >70% of extracellular DA from the synaptic space). Iron deficiency in the striatum causes downregulation of D2 receptors and may contribute to decreased functioning of the DAT. The dopamine systems of female rats were less affected than those in male rats (*29*).

Role of Peripheral Nerve, Spinal Cord, and Nociceptive Pathways Dysfunction

The role of endogenous opiates in RLS is supported, with patients reporting that symptoms improve with opiates *(10)* and worsen with the opiate antagonist naloxone *(10)*, suggesting that RLS is associated with dysfunction of the endogenous opiate system *(10)*. Clinical improvement with dopaminergic drugs that interact with dopaminergic, adrenergic, and opioid systems suggests that a disturbance of these neurotransmitters may underlie the condition *(6)*.

In a study of clinicoetiological correlates, 8 of 15 patients with RLS and peripheral neuropathy were asymptomatic for the peripheral neuropathy and were only diagnosed with the neuropathy following electrophysiological testing (using electromyography/nerve conduction velocity). This leads to the speculation that RLS and peripheral neuropathy may have been underrepresented in previous RLS studies in which clinical neurophysiological testing was not systematically performed in all patients *(17)*. Given the clinical homogeneity between primary and secondary RLS, the high frequency of neuropathy in sporadic cases, and the high rate of subclinical neuropathy, Ondo and Jankovic suggest that screening for neuropathy be done in patients who lack a family history of RLS *(17)*. They also point out that alteration in CNS neurotransmitter function by peripheral nerve perturbation has been demonstrated in animal models *(17)*.

Possible pathophysiological pathways have been proposed, including central sensitization of spinal neurons as in chronic neuropathic pain resulting from abnormal peripheral input and/or altered descending inhibition, i.e., involving the supraspinal dopaminergic system *(25)*. Such pathways include the following:

- A supersensitive CNS movement generator in patients with RLS with a low threshold for incoming sensory stimuli *(10)*.
- Alterations of the complex integration between peripheral and CNS structures, that is, an abnormal sensorimotor integration and enhanced spinal cord excitability *(3)* or nociceptor pathway dysfunction *(25)*.
- Decreased spinal cord disinhibition *(8)*.
- Dysfunction of DA and DA-linked systems that converge on spinal flexor reflexes causing disinhibition *(23)*.
- Disturbed supraspinal pain modulation *(23)* and decreased supraspinal inhibition *(27)*.
- Disinhibition of spinal descending inhibitory pathways *(34)*.

MENOPAUSE AND RLS

Roles of Hormonal and Circadian Influences That May Aggravate RLS in Menopause

Estrogen Deficiency

In general, estrogens are thought to be neuroprotective *(22,34)* and act through genomic mechanisms modulating the synthesis, release, and metabolism of many neuropeptides and neurotransmitters *(34)*. Estrogen leads to neuronal repair and assists neuronal survival *(35)*. Estrogen has multiple effects on neuronal function and modulates the expression of several neurotransmitters. It increases the synthesis of acetylcholine, delays the turnover of serotonin, and regulates serotonin transport and binding in the brain *(22)* and has both agonistic and antagonistic effects on the dopaminergic system *(22)*. Animal studies show it upregulates noradrenaline (but γ-aminobutyric acid is largely unaffected) *(35)*. It causes increased turnover of brainstem norepinephrine, and possibly interferes with dopaminergic transmission *(26,33,36,37)*. Long exposure to estrogen increases DA uptake site density in the nigrostriatal DA system *(22)*. It decreases DA concentrations in the striatum and prevents overactivity of the DA receptors *(22)*.

One theory that might explain RLS symptoms worsening in the decreased estrogen condition of menopause might be related to this decrease in the number of DA receptors. Estrogen interferes with catechol-*O*-methyltransferase (COMT), an enzyme that degrades DA *(22)*. Another theory that might explain RLS symptoms worsening in the decreased estrogen condition of menopause in women might be related to decreased COMT interference, allowing increased COMT degradation of DA and, consequently, decreased amounts of central DA.

In the Erikson et al. *(29)* study of 21-day-old, iron-deficient rats, the lowered DAT functioning in the striatum and decreased dopamine D2 receptor density was significant only in the male rats. This might suggest that the male rats mimicked the low estrogen state of menopause in women vs the female rats that were not castrated and were perhaps unaffected as a result of this neuroprotective effect of estrogens on DAT function and DA receptors.

Jourdain's study in mice suggests that neuroprotection of the nigrostriatal neurons by estrogen involves estrogen receptors rather than antioxidant activity *(37a)*. One theory that might explain RLS symptoms worsening in the decreased estrogen environment of menopause could be related to this loss of neuroprotective effect on DA neurons. Sex steroids modulate the noradrenaline and DA systems at the hypothalamic level and at the extrahypothalamic regions, controlling movement and behavior in animals and humans *(37b)*. In animal studies, estrogens cause increased noradrenaline and increased DA turnover rates during the proestrous period. In Genazzani et al.'s study, castrated female rats experienced increased norepinephrine release and decreased DA release. Exogenous estrogen suoplementation resulted in decreased norepinephrine release and increased dopaminergic neuronal activity and increased DA release in the medial and basal hypothalamus *(37b)*. The worsening of RLS symptoms in the decreased estrogen environment of menopause might be related to this decreased DA release. However, in humans, RLS peaks in third trimester of pregnancy, co-occurring with the rising levels of progesterone, prolactin, and estrogen *(3,26,33)*.

Prolactin and Growth Hormone

In young women, prolactin levels and secretory pulse frequency are higher than in postmenopausal women. Increased growth hormone levels have been reported among estrogen users *(22)*.

Manconi et al. *(33)* point out that prolactin secretion has the same circadian rhythmicity as does RLS symptomatology. Pregnancy is associated with increased reports of RLS. During pregnancy, prolactin levels increase and could be related to decrease in DA action (DA is a very potent prolactin inhibitor) *(30)*.

Gonadotropin-Releasing Hormone

It is known that dopaminergic, opiatergic, and noradrenergic neurotransmission have a coordinated interaction for gonadotropin-releasing hormone *(37b)*.

Melatonin

Earlier in this chapter, it was noted that there is a circadian rhythm of iron production, with RLS symptoms occurring during the time when iron levels decrease at night (4,31). RLS symptoms tend to occur during the acrophase (decrease) of circadian melatonin secretion. The circadian rhythm of melatonin tends to a decreased rate of production and release during the day and increased rate of production and release during the night (38,39).

Michaud et al.'s study (38) of melatonin and body temperature in seven patients and seven controls checked every 2 hours using 28-hour modified constant routine and protocols (used for 40 minutes 12 times with 2 hours in between) showed worsening of RLS symptoms by immobility closely linked to circadian variation. Indeed, immobility worsened the symptoms only between 9:20 PM and 8 AM, corresponding to the period of day during which RLS symptoms reach their maximum intensity, with the highest discomfort occurring between 3 and 4 AM (38,39). The peak of RLS symptoms occured at the same time as the nadir of the *core body temperature* (CBT) (slightly different than in previous studies, which showed the worst RLS symptoms during the falling limb of the CBT, but this was likely a result of sampling every 3–4 hours *in those previous studies.*)

Symptoms start to worsen at the time of melatonin secretion, but the worst RLS symptoms are seen about 2 hours after peak melatonin secretion. Michaud et al. suggest that this is congruent with the hypothesis that melatonin secretion may be driving the increase of RLS symptoms in the evening and at night (39). Garcia-Borreguero et al. (27) noted that an untreated patient reaches maximal symptomatology between 11 PM and 4 AM and maximum relief between 6 AM and 12 PM.

It is generally accepted that physiological concentrations of melatonin exert an inhibitory effect on DA secretion in several areas of the mammalian CNS (39). Melatonin causes inhibition of DA release via membranal low-affinity melatonin-binding sites via the suppression of calcium influx into the stimulated nerve endings presynaptically. Melatonin postsynaptically suppresses NMDA receptor-mediated excitatory responses of striatal neurons to glutamate. Therefore, Michaud et al. suggest that it is reasonable to think that the increase in melatonin secretion in the evening may facilitate the occurrence of RLS symptoms by decreasing the activity of the central dopaminergic systems (39). They suggest that because melatonin is known to normally inhibit central DA secretion, and because alteration of nigrostriatal DA function is likely involved in RLS, melatonin might be implicated in the worsening of RLS symptoms every night.

Steroid receptors have been discovered on the pineal gland, raising the question of whether melatonin synthesis may be modulated by gonadal steroids. In humans, the effects of gonadal steroids on the pineal secretion of melatonin remain controversial (37b).

Melatonin may also be involved in sleep maintenance by blocking arousal mechanisms. Decreases in total melatonin are not associated, *per se*, with menopause (37). However, postmenopausal women with insomnia have been generally shown to have lowered melatonin levels (37). Additionally, estrogen may have a reciprocal melatonin-supportive function. Tamoxifen, an antiestrogen, and oophorectomy cause a decrease in melatonin (37).

An age-related decrease in melatonin secretion in humans has been widely documented *(34)*, and the coincidence of this phenomenon of aging with RLS as a chronic condition that worsens over decades, particularly as estrogen levels in women are also dropping, could lend some (or many) to conclude these phenomena may be related *(40)*. However, this conclusion of decreased melatonin with aging has recently been challenged by highly respected circadian investigators *(41)*, who controlled for confounding variables and showed no difference in the levels of melatonin over the life span. These investigators showed that most healthy older adults have plasma melatonin levels comparable to those of young adults, in contrast to a spate of press releases asserting as fact that melatonin secretion decreases with age beginning as early as age 40. The investigators point out that studies suggesting an age-related decrease in melatonin levels did not take into account subjects who were healthy and nonusers of common drugs that suppress melatonin secretion (e.g., aspirin, ibuprofen, β-blockers) and older studies conducted using ambient light (bright light suppresses melatonin) and did not control for posture, which affects melatonin concentrations. Zeitzer et al. *(41)* studied 34 healthy men and women 65–81 years of age vs 98 drug-free 18- to 30-year-old men in a controlled environment in a sleep laboratory run by experienced circadian rhythm researchers. No significant differences were noted between healthy and drug-free older men and women compared with the young men in plasma melatonin concentrations or duration or integrated area of nocturnal peak of melatonin or mean plasma melatonin concentrations. If their findings are true, the circadian nature of melatonin secretion and RLS symptoms may be related to each other, but decreasing levels of melatonin associated with decreasing levels of estrogen may not be a true association or provide a menopausal correlation/causality for RLS symptoms. The prevailing theory of decreased melatonin and menopause is challenged in a study by Fernandez et al. *(42)* of 77 healthy women aged 30–75 years measuring urinary and serum melatonin and serum FSH showing that urinary melatonin was negatively associated with serum FSH during perimenopause, with the sharpest decline in nocturnal excretion of melatonin occurring long before menopause. Serum FSH rose sharply to high levels before age 50 and remained high thereafter. The decrease in melatonin precedes an increase in FSH long before menopause *(42)*.

Theory That Preexisting RLS May Become More Evident During Menopause

Eichling and Sahni's review paper on menopause and sleep disorders *(37)* finds no direct correlation between RLS and menopause but, like other authors, suggests that with the onset of menopause-associated sleep disruption, a preexisting sleep disorder such as RLS may become more evident. Eichling and Sahni cite several etiologies for menopause-related sleep disruption, including vasomotor symptoms and an increased number of polysomnogram (PSG)-documented arousals associated with dropping levels of estrogen. This theory of preexisting RLS becoming more evident to patients in whom sleep is disrupted by other menopausal disorders is supported by a report of the increased prevalence of insomnia in postmenopausal women vs premenopausal women *(26)*: the prevalence in premenopausal women is 33–36%; in postmenopausal women 44–61%. Subjectively, postmenopausal women report being less satisfied with their sleep than premenopausal women, but PSGs often show better sleep in postmenopausal women (better total sleep time, more slow-wave sleep, decreased wake after sleep onset) *(26)*. Four primary causes of menopausal insomnia have been described *(26)*: hot flashes, mood disorders (depression and anxiety), psychophysiological insomnia once hot flashes start, and increased incidence of sleep-disordered breathing postmenopausally.

CONCLUSION

The association between menopause and restless legs has not been systematically reported. As reviewed in this chapter, some widely held clinical generalizations should be reexamined in the context of recent epidemiological population- and patient-based data so that information gathered from the clinical and basic sciences can best be integrated for possible mechanisms underlying RLS, including what role, if any, changes associated with menopause may contribute to the disorder.

The first widely held generalization is that RLS is a disorder of middle to old age in men and women. However, literature over the last 15 years contradicts this assumption. While most studies show an increased incidence of RLS with age in the general population, when investigators inquire about symptom onset, the disorder is often tracked back to the first two decades of life in men and women, particularly in the primary and familial forms of the disorder. Indeed, evidence generally suggests that RLS is a lifelong chronic disorder that often begins with less frequent and milder symptoms in early adulthood and progresses in severity and duration of symptoms with advancing age *(5,10,23)*.

The second common assumption is that the prevalence of RLS is higher in women. Although most studies still confirm this finding, it has been challenged with data in a few well-designed studies, which showed no sex differences. Because menopause is a condition occurring in middle-aged women, menopause could be erroneously construed as a precipitant to RLS. However, given the mounting evidence of clinical symptoms predating menopause by decades in a large proportion of women with RLS and the fact that men, like women, complain of worsening severity and frequency of RLS symptoms over time, it is likely that if menopause does contribute to the disorder, it is likely only one of a number of aging-related phenomena functionally aggravating the disorder.

Very little is known about the physiological mechanisms underlying RLS, and there is little in the literature about what role, if any, menopause may play in RLS. Evidence from recent epidemiological, clinical, and basic science studies suggests that RLS is a chronic disorder resulting from complex metabolic dysfunction involving the subcortical central and possible peripheral nervous system, often involving iron acquisition/regulation, dopaminergic and opiatergic pathways, and influenced by as-yet-unknown mechanisms involved in genetic, circadian, psychosocial, and medical disorders and likely other changes associated with aging. If menopause is involved, the influence of the hormonal changes of aging—perhaps the loss of some neuroprotective effect of gonadal steroids on iron-acquisition/regulation, dopaminergic, and opiatergic pathways—would join numerous other medical and aging-related conditions that likely aggravate the chronic underlying condition.

REFERENCES

1. Kavanagh, D., S. Siddiqui, and C.C. Geddes, Restless legs syndrome in patients on dialysis. *Am J Kidney Dis*, 2004;**43**(5):763–771.
2. Allen, R.P., D. Picchiettti, W.A. Hening, C. Trenkwalder, A.S. Walters, and J. Montplaisir, Restless legs syndrome: diagnostic criteria, special considerations, and epidemiology. A report from the restless legs syndrome diagnosis and epidemiology workshop at the National Institutes of Health. *Sleep Med*, 2003;**4**(2):101–119.
3. Berger, K., J. Luedemann, C. Trenkwalder, U. John, and C. Kessler, Sex and the risk of restless legs syndrome in the general population. *Arch Intern Med*, 2004;**164**(2):196–202.
4. Schapira, A.H., Restless legs syndrome: an update on treatment options. *Drugs*, 2004;**64**(2):149–158.
5. Hornyak, M. and C. Trenkwalder, Restless legs syndrome and periodic limb movement disorder in the elderly. *J Psychosom Res*, 2004; **56**(5):543–548.
6. Turjanski, N., A.J. Lees, and D.J. Brooks, Striatal dopaminergic function in restless legs syndrome: 18F-dopa and 11C-raclopride PET studies. *Neurology*, 1999;**52**(5):932–937.
7. Trenkwalder, C. and W. Paulus, Why do restless legs occur at rest?—pathophysiology of neuronal structures in RLS. Neurophysiology of RLS (part 2). *Clin Neurophysiol*, 2004;**115**(9):1975–1988.
8. Garcia-Borreguero, D., O. Larrosa, J.J. Granizo, Y. de la Llave, and W.A. Hening, Circadian effects of dopaminergic treatment in restless legs syndrome. *Sleep Med*, 2004;**5**(4):413–420.
9. Chesson, A.L., Jr., M. Wise, D. Davila, et al., Practice parameters for the treatment of restless legs syndrome and periodic limb movement disorder. An American Academy of Sleep Medicine Report. Standards of Practice Committee of the American Academy of Sleep Medicine. *Sleep*, 1999;**22**(7):961–968.
10. Walters, A.S., K. Hickey, J. Maltzman, et al., A questionnaire study of 138 patients with restless legs syndrome: the 'Night-Walkers' survey. *Neurology*, 1996;**46**(1):92–95.
11. Garcia-Borreguero, D., P. Odin, and C. Schwarz, *Restless legs syndrome: an overview of the current understanding and management. Acta Neurol Scand*, 2004;**109**(5):303–317.
12. Phillips, B., T. Young, L. Finn, K. Asher, W.A. Hening, and C. Purvis, Epidemiology of restless legs symptoms in adults. *Arch Intern Med*, 2000;**160**(14):2137–2141.
13. Winkelmann, J., T.C. Wetter, V. Collado-Seidel, et al., Clinical characteristics and frequency of the hereditary restless legs syndrome in a population of 300 patients. *Sleep*, 2000;**23**(5):597–602.
14. Rothdach, A.J., C. Trenkwalder, J. Haberstock, U. Keil, and K. Berger, Prevalence and risk factors of RLS in an elderly population: the MEMO study. Memory and Morbidity in Augsburg Elderly. *Neurology*, 2000;**54**(5):1064–1068.
15. Allen, R.P., A.S. Walters, J. Montplaisir, et al., Restless legs syndrome prevalence and impact: REST general population study. *Arch Intern Med*, 2005;**165**(11):1286–1292.
16. Montplaisir, J., S. Boucher, G. Poirier, G. Lavigne, O. Lapierre, and P. Lesperance, Clinical, polysomnographic, and genetic characteristics of restless legs syndrome: a study of 133 patients diagnosed with new standard criteria. *Mov Disord*, 1997;**12**(1):61–65.
17. Ondo, W. and J. Jankovic, Restless legs syndrome: clinicoetiologic correlates. *Neurology*, 1996;**47**(6):1435–1441.
18. Trenkwalder, C., Restless-legs syndrome in primary care: counting patients in Idaho. *Lancet Neurol*, 2004;**3**(2):83.
19. Ondo, W.G., K.D. Vuong, and Q. Wang, Restless legs syndrome in monozygotic twins: clinical correlates. *Neurology*, 2000;**55**(9):1404–1406.
20. Tison, F., A. Crochard, D. Leger, S. Bouee, E. Lainey, and A. El Hasnaoui, Epidemiology of restless legs syndrome in French adults: a nationwide survey: the INSTANT Study. *Neurology*, 2005;**65**(2):239–246.
21. Nichols, D.A., R.P. Allen, J.H. Grauke, et al., Restless legs syndrome symptoms in primary care: a prevalence study. *Arch Intern Med*, 2003;**163**(19):2323–2329.
22. Polo-Kantola, P. and R. Erkkola, Sleep and the menopause. *J Br Menopause Soc*, 2004;**10**(4):145–150.
23. Chaudhuri, K.R., A. Forbes, D. Grosset, et al., Diagnosing restless legs syndrome (RLS) in primary care. *Curr Med Res Opin*, 2004;**20**(11):1785–1795.

24. Sukegawa, T., M. Itoga, H. Seno, et al., Sleep disturbances and depression in the elderly in Japan. *Psychiatry Clin Neurosci*, 2003;**57**(3):265–270.

25. Stiasny-Kolster, K., C. Trenkwalder, W. Fogel, et al., Restless legs syndrome—new insights into clinical characteristics, pathophysiology, and treatment options. *J Neurol*, 2004. **251**(Suppl 6):VI/39–VI/43.

26. Moline, M., L. Broch, and R. Zak, Sleep problems across the life cycle in women. *Curr Treat Options Neurol*, 2004;**6**(4):319–330.

27. Garcia-Borreguero, D., C. Serrano, O. Larrosa, and J.J. Granizo, Circadian variation in neuroendocrine response to L-dopa in patients with restless legs syndrome. *Sleep*, 2004;**27**(4):669–673.

28. Michaud, M., J.P. Soucy, A. Chabli, G. Lavigne, and J. Montplaisir, SPECT imaging of striatal pre- and postsynaptic dopaminergic status in restless legs syndrome with periodic leg movements in sleep. *J Neurol*, 2002;**249**(2):164–1670.

29. Erikson, K.M., B.C. Jones, and J.L. Beard, Iron deficiency alters dopamine transporter functioning in rat striatum. *J Nutr*, 2000;**130**(11):2831–2837.

30. Connor, J.R., P.J. Boyer, S.L. Menzies, et al., Neuropathological examination suggests impaired brain iron acquisition in restless legs syndrome. *Neurology*, 2003;**61**(3):304–309.

31. Lee, K.A., M.E. Zaffke, and K. Baratte-Beebe, Restless legs syndrome and sleep disturbance during pregnancy: the role of folate and iron. *J Womens Health Gend Based Med*, 2001;**10**(4):335–341.

32. Earley, C.J., D. Heckler, and R.P. Allen, Repeated IV doses of iron provides effective supplemental treatment of restless legs syndrome. *Sleep Med*, 2005;**6**(4):301–305.

32a. Moyer, P., Compromised brain iron abnormalities linked to early-onset restless legs syndrome. *Neurology Today*, 2005;**489**.

33. Manconi, M., V. Govoni, A. De Vito, et al., Restless legs syndrome and pregnancy. *Neurology*, 2004;**63**(6):1065–1069.

34. Rijsman, R., A.K. Neven, W. Graffelman, B. Kemp, and A. de Weerd, Epidemiology of restless legs in The Netherlands. *Eur J Neurol*, 2004;**11**(9):607–611.

35. Polo-Kantola, P., M. Dumont, J. Paquet, A. Desautels, M.L. Fantini, and J. Montplaisir, Estrogen replacement therapy and nocturnal periodic limb movements: a randomized controlled trial. *Obstet Gynecol*, 2001;**97**(4):548–554.

36. Manconi, M., M. Dumont, B. Selmaoui, J. Paquet, M.L. Fantini, and J. Montplaisir, Pregnancy as a risk factor for restless legs syndrome. *Sleep Med*, 2004;**5**(3):305–308.

37. Eichling, P. and J. Sahni, Menopause related sleep disorders. *J Clin Sleep Med*, 2005;**1**(3):291–300.

37a. Jourdain, S., M. Morissette, N. Morin, and T. Di Paolo, Oestrogens prevent loss of dopamine transporter (DAT) and vesicular monoamine transporter (VMAT2) is substantia nigra of 1-methyl-4-phenyl-1,2,3,6-tetrahydropyridine mice. *J Neuroendocrinol*, 2005;**17**(8):509–517.

37b. Genazzani, A.R., F. Bernardi, N. Pluchino, et al., Endocrinology of menopausal transition and its brain implications. *CNS Spectr*, 2005;**10**(6):449–457.

38. Michaud, M., E. Rauhala, R. Erkkola, K. Irjala, and O. Polo, Circadian variation of the effects of immobility on symptoms of restless legs syndrome. *Sleep*, 2005;**28**(7):843–846.

39. Michaud, M., V. Govoni, A. De Vito, et al., Circadian rhythm of restless legs syndrome: relationship with biological markers. *Ann Neurol*, 2004;**55**(3):372–380.

40. Okatani, Y., N. Morioka, and A. Wakatsuki, Changes in nocturnal melatonin secretion in perimenopausal women: correlation with endogenous estrogen concentrations. *J Pineal Res*, 2000;**28**(2):111–118.

41. Zeitzer, J.M., J.E. Daniels, J.F. Duffy, Do plasma melatonin concentrations decline with age? *Am J Med*, 1999;**107**(5):432–436.

42. Fernandez, B., J.L. Malde, A. Montero, and D. Acuna, Relationship between adenohypophyseal and steroid hormones and variations in serum and urinary melatonin levels during the ovarian cycle, perimenopause and menopause in healthy women. *J Steroid Biochem*, 1990;**35**(2):257–262.

18

Insomnia During Menopause

Sleep Laboratory Studies on Insomnia Associated With Postmenopausal Syndrome and Hormone Replacement Therapy

Gerda Saletu-Zyhlarz, Peter Anderer, Georg Gruber, Markus Metka, Johannes Huber, Elisabeth Grätzhofer, and Bernd Saletu

INTRODUCTION

Sleep disturbance is a prevalent health problem *(1–3)* that occurs more frequently in women than in men *(2,4–6)*. Insomnia increases particularly as women approach and pass through menopause *(7–10)*.

Insomnia in postmenopausal women, part of the climacteric syndrome, can occur, on the one hand, in association with hormonal changes *(11,12)*; on the other hand, women are more likely to suffer from psychiatric disorders, such as major depression and anxiety disorders, which are also correlated with insomnia *(5,13)*. Organic sleep disorders such as sleep-disordered breathing (SDB) resulting from a decrease of sex hormones in menopause may play an important role as well *(14)*.

Subjective sleep disturbance and fatigue are among the most frequent complaints of perimenopausal women *(3,6,15–18)*. Owens and Mathews *(5)* reported that as many as 42% of the 521 postmenopausal women in their study had sleep disturbances, which were significantly increased in the transition from the pre- to the postmenopausal status in women who chose not to use hormone replacement therapy (HRT) *(5)*. However, there is little literature on the objective sleep quality (i.e., polysomnography) of postmenopausal syndrome patients compared with normal controls.

Moe *(19)* reported longer sleep latencies, increased nocturnal awakenings, and sleep fragmentation as well as decreased slow-wave sleep (SWS). In addition, less SWS was found. A 24-hour polysomnographic study showed that 10% of the accumulated sleep time of postmenopausal women was recorded out of bed and their sleep was observed shortly after arousal from bed in the morning, which indicated

From: *Current Clinical Neurology: Sleep Disorders in Women: A Guide to Practical Management*
Edited by: H. P. Attarian © Humana Press Inc., Totowa, NJ

daytime tiredness *(19,20)*. However, not all studies of sleep in middle-aged women found a significant effect of the menopausal status *(21,22)*.

The sleep changes in postmenopausal women have been partially attributed to the change of sex steroid hormone profile, which can affect sleep either directly or through an effect on body temperature (hot flushes), circadian rhythm, or stress reactivity *(9,11)*, Jaszmann et al. *(23)*, and Ballinger *(24)* inferred that insomnia is a result of hormonal changes because their surveys showed that the incidence of the complaint rose as the estrogen level fell during the period *(23,24)*. The polysomnographic effects of HRT have been studied for a long time. Thompson and Oswald *(25)* observed a reduction in wakefulness, a decrease in the number of awakenings, and an increase in rapid eye-movement (REM) sleep during 8 weeks of estrogen treatment when compared with baseline measures, whereas untreated control patients did not show any improvement *(25)*. In a crossover study, Schiff et al. *(26)* found a significantly shorter sleep-onset time and more REM sleep during treatment with estradiol compared with placebo *(26)*. Erlik et al. (27) reported that postmenopausal women treated with estrogen had fewer hot flashes associated with wakefulness per night than untreated women *(27)*. Recently, it was observed that estrogen replacement therapy restored the normal sleep electroencephalogram (EEG) as it enhanced REM sleep and decreased time awake during the first sleep cycles *(28)*. The normal decrease in SWS and delta activity from the first to the second sleep cycle was also restored by estrogen. On the other hand, Purdie et al. *(29)* found an improvement in menopausal symptoms under combined estrogen–progesterone therapy, with an improvement of psychological well-being but not parameters of sleep quality *(29)*. Polo-Kantola et al. *(30)* observed that estrogen effectively alleviated hot flashes, sweating, and sleep complaints and improved subjective sleep quality by reducing the total frequency of movement arousals, but did not induce any changes in sleep architecture *(30)*. Although estrogen was found to enhance REM sleep *(26)*, progesterone and its metabolite pregnanolone showed a marked sedating effect with a significant increase in non-REM sleep *(31)*. More-over, pregnenolone, a precursor of progesterone, enhanced SWS and reduced EEG activity in high-frequency bands *(32)*.

The aims of the present study were to investigate the differences in sleep and awakening between untreated insomniac postmenopausal syndrome patients and normal controls as well as to compare the effects of continuous combined adminis-tration of 2 mg estradiol valerate plus 3 mg dienogest (Climodien® 2/3; regimen A) with those of estradiol valerate alone and placebo in a first double-blind, controlled phase. This was followed by an open-label phase, in which all patients were treated with a combination of 2 mg estradiol valerate plus 2 mg dienogest (Climodien 2/2; regimen A®), to allow a stratified comparison of the 2/2 mg preparation (A) vs placebo or vs the 2/3 mg preparation (A).

The progestogen chosen for the present study, dienogest (17-*d*-cyanomethyl-17-α-hydroxy-estra-4,9(10)-dien-3-one), is a synthetic 19-norprogestin devised for oral HRT of natural or postsurgical menopause, as well as for prophylaxis of osteoporosis and cardiovascular diseases in postmenopausal women. The fixed combination of 2 mg of natural estradiol valerate and 2 or 3 mg dienogest is intended for continuous use over 28 days (i.e., without hormonal pause) to produce amenorrhea (Kliogest® principle). This preparation is especially suited for patients who do not tolerate monthly bleeding caused by progestin withdrawal, especially for woman at a later stage of menopause. Compared with other progestins of its structural class (19-nandrolone derivatives), dienogest has special pharmacodynamic and pharmacokinetic features:

1. Marked endometrium efficacy.
2. Lack of interaction between steroid hormone-binding globulin and corticosteroid-binding globulin.
3. High bioavailability resulting from high intestinal absorption and short plasma half-life (5–10 hours) after oral administration.
4. Marked antiandrogenicity.
5. Antiproliferative effects.
6. Metabolic neutrality.
7. Good tolerance and safety profile, including lack of liver metabolic alterations
8. Low toxicity in acute and chronic toxicity tests.
9. Lack of teratogenic, embryotoxic, or postnatal developmental effects *(33)*.

At a biochemical level, finally, dienogest does not influence the cytochrome P-450 system *(33)*.

Dienogest has usually been analyzed in a dosage of 2 mg, in combination with ethinylestradiol (0.03 mg) (available in Germany as the contraceptive Valette®). The frequency of menstrual bleeding disorders is extremely low (4.5%), placing this estrogen–progestogen combination at the highest levels of tolerability among internationally used combined contraceptives.

METHODS
Study Design and Patients

Sleep and awakening quality of 55 insomniac postmenopausal patients was investigated in a double-blind, placebo-controlled, comparative, randomized, three-arm trial phase (Climodien 2/3 = estradiol valerate 2 mg + the progestogen dienogest 3 mg = regimen A; estradiol valerate 2 mg = regimen EV; and placebo = regimen P) followed by an open-label phase in which all patients received Climodien 2/2 (estradiol valerate 2 mg + dienogest 2 mg, INN: estradiol valerate: CAS 979-32-8; INN: dienogest: CAS 65928-58-7 = regimen A). Forty-nine women (16, 17, and 16 valid patients per arm) between 46 and 67 years of age (mean 58, 58, and 56 years, respectively) with the diagnosis of insomnia (G 47.0) related to postmenopausal syndrome (N 95.1) were included in the analysis of the double-blind phase. Pretreatment data of 49 patients (mean age 58 ± 5 years) were compared with those of 22 normal age-matched controls (mean age 57 ± 7 years). Forty-five patients (13, 17, and 15 valid patients) completed the open-label phase. Both the double-blind and open-label phases lasted 2 months. The women enrolled in the study took one tablet daily at the same time of day (7 PM).

Inclusion criteria for patients were as follows:

- A sleep complaint characterized primarily by difficulty falling asleep, maintaining sleep or a feeling of nonrestorative sleep, which occurred at least three times per week for at least 1 month.
- The prevailing sleep disorder was serious enough to require clinical attention.
- The sleep disorder was not likely to be a direct physiological consequence of a medical condition (i.e., menopausal syndrome).
- The disorder could not be better explained by another psychological disorder (e.g., adaptive disorder with the cause of stress being a severe physical disease).
- The disorder did not satisfy the criteria for sleep apnea or narcolepsy.
- The sleep disorders caused clinically significant suffering or a disorder in social, professional, or other important field.
- The state of menopause was confirmed by at least 24 months of amenorrhea and estradiol levels below the postmenopausal limit of the respective laboratory (<55 pg/mL; follicle-stimulating hormone [FSH] >19 mU/mL).
- Kupperman index greater than 15 *(34)*.

Exclusion criteria have been described in detail elsewhere *(35)*.

The study protocol was approved by the Ethics Committee of the Medical Faculty of the University of Vienna and the General Hospital of the City of Vienna. Each patient was informed about the study, and a written consent was obtained. The study was performed in accordance with the ethical principles of the Declaration of Helsinki, as revised by the World Medical Assembly in Tokyo and Venice, as well as with the EC Guideline of Good Clinical Practice.

Evaluations were carried out at baseline as well as at the end of the 2-month double-blind and 2-month open-label phases, respectively (each time after 1 adaptation night). Thus, each patient spent 6 nights in the sleep lab. Normal controls were recorded for 2 nights (adaptation and baseline nights).

Evaluation of Objective Sleep Quality

Polysomnographic all-night recordings were obtained between approx 10:30 PM (lights out) and 6 AM (buzzer or alarm clock). Data were recorded by means of a 16-channel polygraph (Jaeger Sleep Lab 1000P) including three EEG channels (C4-A1, CZ-O2, and C3-A2) according to the 10/20 system, two electrooculogram channels (left/right), submental myogram and tibialis anterior electromyogram from both legs, nasal and oral airflow, movement of the chest and abdomen, snoring, transcutaneous oxygen saturation, and pulse rate (CRITICARE Pulse Oxymeter 504).

Evaluation of Subjective Sleep and Awakening Quality

After the morning toilet, the patients completed the Self-Assessment of Sleep and Awakening Quality Scale (SSA) *(36)*. Thymopsychic variables included subjective well-being in the evening and morning, based on the Von Zerssen BF-S Scale *(37)*, as well as drive, mood, affectivity, and drowsiness in the morning, measured by means of 100-mm visual-analog scales. The Pittsburgh Sleep Quality Index *(38)* was evaluated as well.

Evaluation of Objective Awakening Quality (Psychometry)

Noopsychic tests included the Grünberger alphabetical cancellation test (Alphabetischer Durchstreichtest = AD) for quantification of attention (AD/total score), concentration (AD/E%, errors in percentage of the total score), and attention variability (AD/SV; difference between extreme scores) *(39)*, the Numerical Memory Test *(39)*, as well as the Grünberger Fine Motor Activity Test (right and lefthand) for evaluation of changes in psychomotor activity and drive *(39)*. Reaction time, reaction time variability (msecond), and errors of omission and commission were determined by the computer-assisted reaction time apparatus.

Statistics and Sample Size Determination

The statistical analysis was carried out at the Department of Psychiatry, University of Vienna, using the SPSS software package (SPSS Inc., Chicago, IL; version 8.0.0) under Windows NT, based on descriptive data analysis *(40)* with one confirmatory statement on wakefulness during the total sleep period. The analysis included all variables studied in the clinical trial and was based on data grouped by treatment and trial times. The predetermined null hypothesis for the confirmatory statement was: There is no difference between Climodien, estradiol valerate, and placebo in regard to wakefulness during the total sleep period (maximum error probability = 0.05). α-Adjustment by Bonferroni-Holm led to individual error probabilities of $p(1) < 0.0166, p(2) < 0.025$, and $p(3) < 0.05$. All other variables were tested descriptively.

Normal distribution was tested by means of the Kolmogorov Smirnov test. If in no cases the null hypothesis of normal distribution was rejected at $\alpha = 0.10$, t-tests were used. In the case of a violation of the assumption of normal distribution, a nonparametric Wilcoxon test was used for intragroup comparison and a Mann-Whitney U-test for intergroup comparison. The present findings are based on a per-protocol analysis.

The sample size of 17 valid cases per arm was calculated on the basis of a placebo-controlled study carried out with piperazine estrone sulfate in perimenopausal women by Thompson and Oswald *(25)*. The size of the random sample was determined for the change in nocturnal waking times.

RESULTS

Baseline Differences in Sleep and Awakening Quality Between Insomniac Postmenopausal Syndrome Patients and Normal Controls

Baseline data of 49 drug-free insomniac postmenopausal syndrome patients (mean age 58 ± 5 years) were compared with those of 22 age- and gender-matched normal controls (mean age 57 ± 7 years). Figure 1 depicts the sleep profiles of an individual patient and an age- and gender-matched healthy control. Table 1 shows the means and standard deviations of the total groups of patients and normal controls together with the statistically significant intergroup differences (Mann-Whitney U-test). The patients exhibited slight but statistically significant deviations from the norm concerning sleep initiation and maintenance as well as sleep archi-

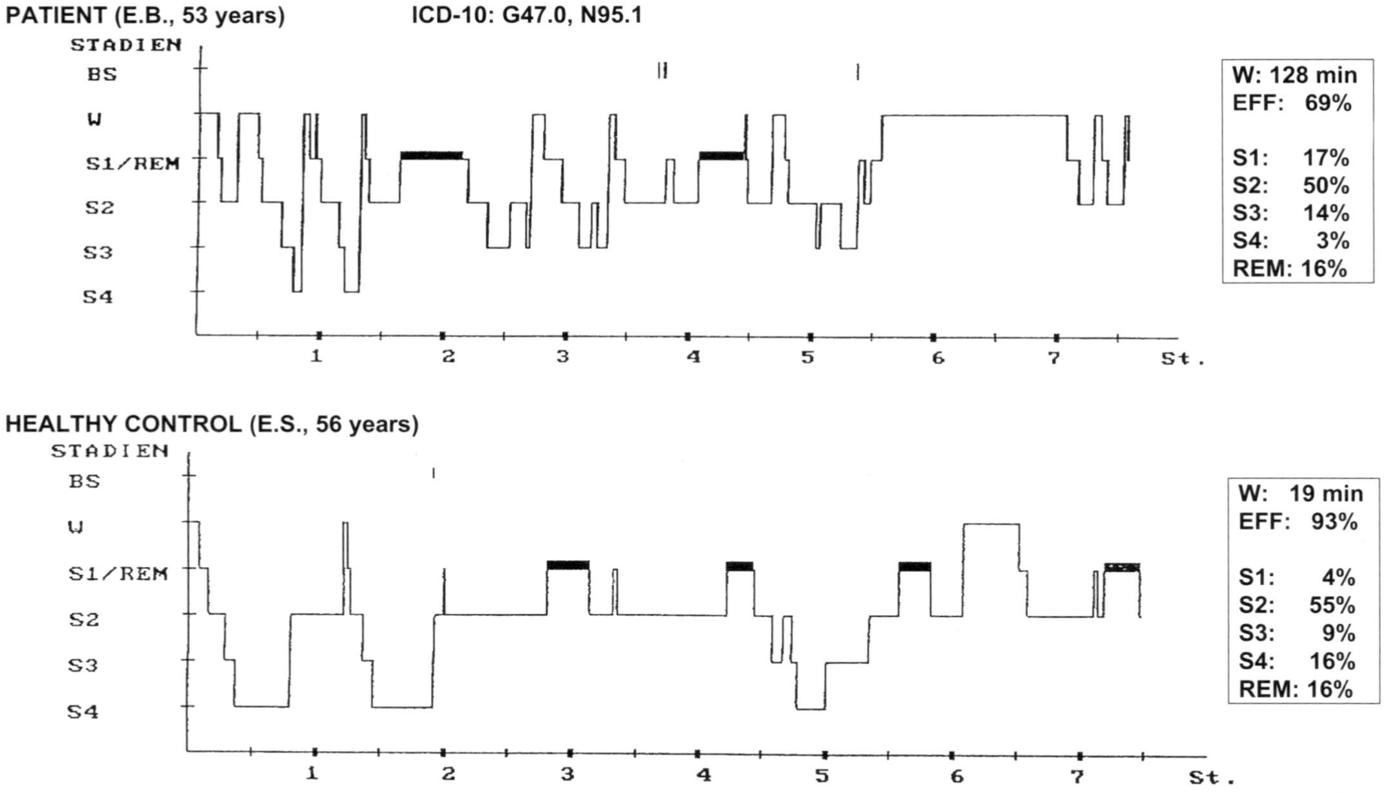
PATIENT (E.B., 53 years)
ICD-10: G47.0, N95.1
STADIEN
BS
W
S1/REM
S2
S3
S4
1
2
3
4
5
6
7
St.
W: 128 min
EFF: 69%
S1: 17%
S2: 50%
S3: 14%
S4: 3%
REM: 16%
HEALTHY CONTROL (E.S., 56 years)
STADIEN
BS
W
S1/REM
S2
S3
S4
1
2
3
4
5
6
7
St.
W: 19 min
EFF: 93%
S1: 4%
S2: 55%
S3: 9%
S4: 16%
REM: 16%

Fig. 1. Sleep profile of an insomniac postmenopausal syndrome patient compared with that of an age- and sex-matched healthy control. Time is shown in the abscissa; sleep stages are depicted in the ordinate. W, nocturnal wake time; EFF, sleep efficiency (sleep time in percentage of time in bed); S1, light sleep; S2, middle deep sleep; S3 + S4, deep sleep; SREM, dream sleep.

Table 1
Insomnia Related to Postmenopausal Syndrome:
Differences From Normal Controls in Objective Sleep Variables

Variables	Patients ($N = 49$; age 58 ± 5)	Controls ($N = 22$; age 57 ± 7)
Sleep initiation + maintenance		
Latency to S1 (min) ↓	16 ± 15	10 ± 9
Latency to S2 (min) ↓	$24 \pm 17^*$	13 ± 9
Wake within TSP (min) ↓	52 ± 32	41 ± 20
Wake before buzzer (min) ↓	$6 \pm 23^{**}$	5 ± 9
Total sleep period (min) ↑	$429 \pm 26^{**}$	464 ± 19
Total sleep time (min) ↑	$375 \pm 40^{**}$	420 ± 24
Sleep efficiency (%) ↑	$83 \pm 9^*$	88 ± 5
Sleep architecture		
Sleep stage 1 (%)	$11 \pm 5^*$	9 ± 3
Sleep stage 2 (%)	$49 \pm 8^*$	54 ± 9
Sleep stage 3 (%)	10 ± 4	8 ± 4
Sleep stage 4 (%)	10 ± 7	8 ± 6
Sleep stage 3 + 4 (%)	21 ± 8	16 ± 8
Sleep stage REM (%)	20 ± 6	22 ± 6
Movement time (min)	2 ± 2	1 ± 1
REM latency (min)	91 ± 55	82 ± 40
Apnea–hypopnea index (*n*/hours sleep)	7 ± 11	3 ± 5

↓↑, Direction of improvement.
The data are presented as means ± SD; $^*p < 0.05$; $^{**}p < 0.01$ vs controls (Mann-Whitney U-test).
S1, light sleep; S2, middle deep sleep; TSP, total sleep period; REM, rapid eye-movement.

tecture (Table 1), with increased latency to S2 (early insomnia) and wakefulness before the buzzer (late insomnia), a shortened sleep period and total sleep time, as well as reduced sleep efficiency. Regarding sleep architecture, S1 was increased, whereas S2 was decreased. No differences between patients and controls were observed in regard to S3 and S4, dream sleep, movement time, REM latency, or the apnea–hypopnea index (AHI).

Subjective sleep quality was reduced (Table 2), as revealed by both the Pittsburgh Sleep Quality Index and the SSA. The latter also showed deteriorated awakening quality and somatic complaints in the morning. In the thymopsyche, well-being in the evening and morning was deteriorated and drive in the morning was reduced, whereas drowsiness was increased. In the noopsyche, numerical memory, reaction time, and reaction time performance were deteriorated.

HRT and Sleep Initiation and Maintenance

The primary efficacy variable wakefulness during the total sleep period showed an improvement of 18 minutes by Climodien, 15 minutes by estradiol, and 4 minutes by placebo . However, neither the changes compared to predrug treatment nor

Table 2
Insomnia Related to Postmenopausal Syndrome:
Differences From Normal Controls in Subjective
Sleep/Awakening Quality, Thymopsychic, and Noopsychic Variables

Variables	Patients ($N = 49$; age 58 ± 5)	Controls ($N = 22$; age 57 ± 7)
Subjective sleep/awakening quality		
Pittsburgh Sleep Quality Index (score) ↓	11 ± 5 **	4 ± 1
SSA 1—sleep quality (score) ↓	16 ± 5 **	10 ± 2
SSA 2—awakening quality (score) ↓	16 ± 5	11 ± 2
SSA 3—somatic complaints (score) ↓	7 ± 2 *	6 ± 1
SSA 4—(total score) ↓	39 ± 9 **	27 ± 4
Thymopsyche		
Well-being evening (score) ↓	18 ± 12 **	9 ± 8
Well-being morning (score) ↓	15 ± 10 **	7 ± 6
Drive (mm) ↓	40 ± 25 *	24 ± 17
Mood (mm) ↑	65 ± 23	76 ± 11
Affectivity (mm) ↑	71 ± 21	81 ± 9
Drowsiness (mm) ↓	41 ± 29 *	22 ± 16
Noopsyche		
Attention (score) ↑	526 ± 117	502 ± 113
Concentration (% errors) ↓	5 ± 4	4 ± 3
Attention variability (score) ↓	15 ± 6	14 ± 5
Numerical memory (N) ↑	5 ± 2 **	6 ± 1
Fine motor activity ri ↑	34 ± 9 **	36 ± 13
Fine motor activity le ↑	27 ± 8	30 ± 10
Fine motor activity ri+le ↑	61 ± 15	66 ± 22
Reaction time (RT) (ms) ↓	616 ± 94 *	536 ± 107
RT variability (ms) ↓	123 ± 37	100 ± 41
RT errors/commission (N) ↓	6 ± 4	4 ± 4
RT errors/omission (N) ↓	2 ± 3*	1 ± 1

↑↓, Direction of improvement.
The data are presented as means ± SD; *$p < 0.05$; **$p < 0.01$ vs controls (Mann-Whitney U-test).

the differences between the changes in the three groups reached the level of statistical significance ($p < 0.05$, Wilcoxon and Mann Whitney U-Test, respectively). In the subsequent open-label phase, in which all patients received Climodien, those treated in the double-blind phase with Climodien 2/3 improved further on Climodien 2/2, whereas the former estradiol and placebo groups showed an increase in wakefulness during the 2 months of treatment with Climodien (Table 3). However, the findings did not reach the level of statistical significance.

Latency to stage 1 showed a nonsignificant shortening following all three compounds (Table 3). In the open-label phase, Climodien induced a significant lengthening of sleep latency in patients before treated with placebo ($p < 0.05$, Wilcoxon

Table 3

Sleep Initiation and Maintenance in Insomniac Postmenopausal Syndrome Patients Before and After 2 Months of Climodien A (2 mg Estradiol Valerate [EV] + 3 mg Dienogest [DNG]) or 2 mg EV Alone or Placebo as Well as After Subsequent 2-Month Therapy With Climodien A (2 mg EV + 2 mg DNG)

Variable	Night	Climodien A (N = 16)	Estradiol B (N = 17)	Placebo C (N = 16)	Intergroup difference $^+p < 0.05$; $^{++}p < 0.01$; U-test
Latency to stage 1 (min)	Pre	21 ± 17	15 ± 14	10 ± 8	
	2MoDRUG	18 ± 18	10 ± 10	9 ± 7	
	+2MoA	17 ± 15	18 ± 23[e]	19 ± 18[c,e]	
Latency to stage 2 (min)	Pre	27 ± 17	25 ± 18	17 ± 11	
	2MoDRUG	28 ± 22	15 ± 10[a]	18 ± 19	
	+2MoA	23 ± 16	22 ± 14[e]	26 ± 18	
Wake/TSP (min)	Pre	59 ± 43	47 ± 28	48 ± 28	
	2MoDRUG	41 ± 24	32 ± 23	44 ± 32	
	+2MoA	34 ± 27	37 ± 23	52 ± 46	
Wake/before buzzer (min)	pre	7 ± 15	13 ± 37	0 ± 1	
	2MoDRUG	8 ± 19	10 ± 17	2 ± 6	
	+2MoA	12 ± 22	3 ± 11	6 ± 13	
Number of awakenings (N/TSP)	Pre	9 ± 5	9 ± 4	10 ± 6	
	2MoDRUG	8 ± 3	9 ± 4	10 ± 6	
	+2MoA	7 ± 3	9 ± 4	8 ± 5	
Total sleep period (min)	Pre	422 ± 20	424 ± 37	442 ± 11	Pre: A:C[++]; B:C[+]
	2MoDRUG	426 ± 24	435 ± 26	441 ± 12	
	+2MoA	421 ± 23[e]	435 ± 20	427 ± 20[c]	
Total sleep time (min)	Pre	362 ± 51	375 ± 35	392 ± 35	
	2MoDRUG	384 ± 31	402 ± 29	395 ± 37	
	+2MoA	386 ± 36	396 ± 29	374 ± 47	
Sleep efficiency (%)	Pre	80 ± 11	83 ± 7	87 ± 7	
	2MoDRUG	85 ± 7	88 ± 6	87 ± 8	
	+2MoA	86 ± 8	88 ± 6	83 ± 10	

[a] $p < 0.05$ change vs pre.
[b] $p < 0.01$ Wilcoxon.
[c] $p < 0.05$ change vs 2MoDRUG.
[d] $p < 0.01$ Wilcoxon.
[e] $p < 0.05$ Difference (2nd–1st period).
[f] $p < 0.01$ Wilcoxon.
TSP, total sleep period.

233

test). The difference between these two treatments was significant ($p < 0.05$, Wilcoxon test). Moreover, the estradiol group showed a latency increase under Climodien that differed significantly from the shortening observed compared with baseline ($p < 0.05$).

Latency to stage 2 showed a significant shortening after 2 months of estradiol ($p < 0.05$), which differed significantly from the lengthening under Climodien in the following open-label phase. There were no significant findings in the Climodien and placebo groups.

Wake before the buzzer (measuring late insomnia) showed neither significant changes nor significant intergroup differences. The same was true for the number of awakenings.

The total sleep period demonstrated a decrease under Climodien in the open-label phase, which differed significantly from the increase under the preceding Climodien treatment ($p < 0.05$). Moreover, compared with placebo, Climodien significantly decreased the total sleep period.

Total sleep time and sleep efficiency increased after Climodien and estradiol, whereas they remained unchanged under placebo. The changes, however, did not reach the level of statistical significance. In the former placebo group, 2 months of treatment with Climodien resulted in a nonsignificant decrease in sleep efficiency.

HRT and Sleep Architecture

Sleep stages 1, 2, 3, and REM did not show any significant changes or any intergroup differences (Table 4).

Sleep stage 4 showed a significant decrease under Climodien compared with the value obtained after 2 months of estradiol ($p < 0.05$).

Movement time, REM latency, and stage shifts did not exhibit any significant changes.

HRT and Respiratory Events and Snoring

The apnea index showed a significant improvement under Climodien ($p < 0.05$), although the index had *a priori* been within normal limits, as specified by the protocol (Table 5). Climodien was in this respect significantly superior to placebo ($p < 0.05$, U-Test).

The AHI also improved significantly under Climodien ($p < 0.05$), whereas with placebo no changes were observed, with intergroup differences reaching the level of statistical significance. In the open-label phase under Climodien, the AHI increased again in the Climodien group, whereas in the group that had been treated with placebo it decreased (although nonsignificantly). It must be emphasised that the AHIs in all three groups were within normal limits, which is in agreement with the selection criteria excluding patients with sleep apnea syndrome.

The desaturation index also showed a nonsignificant improvement under Climodien, as did minimum O_2 levels. The average low O_2 levels decreased minimally under estradiol and increased minimally under placebo, with a significant difference between the different trends.

Table 4
Sleep Architecture in Insomniac Postmenopausal Syndrome Patients Before and After 2 Months of Climodien a (2 mg Estradiol Valerate [EV] + 3 mg Dienogest [DNG]) or 2 mg EV Alone or Placebo as Well as After Subsequent 2-Month Therapy With Climodien A (2 mg EV + 2 mg DNG)

Variable	Night	Climodien A ($N = 16$)	Estradiol B ($N = 17$)	Placebo C ($N = 16$)
Sleep stage 1 (%)	Pre	11 ± 6	11 ± 5	11 ± 6
	2MoDRUG	11 ± 5	10 ± 4	10 ± 4
	+2MoA	11 ± 3	11 ± 6	10 ± 4
Sleep stage 2 (%)	Pre	50 ± 6	48 ± 10	50 ± 8
	2MoDRUG	53 ± 7	50 ± 6	54 ± 5
	+2MoA	53 ± 5	53 ± 8	50 ± 9
Sleep stage 3 (%)	Pre	11 ± 5	10 ± 3	10 ± 4
	2MoDRUG	9 ± 4	11 ± 5	10 ± 4
	+2MoA	9 ± 4	11 ± 5	11 ± 3
Sleep stage 4 (%)	Pre	9 ± 6	11 ± 9	10 ± 7
	2MoDRUG	8 ± 7	10 ± 7	8 ± 5
	+2MoA	6 ± 5	7 ± 7^c	9 ± 6
Sleep stages 3 + 4 (%)	Pre	20 ± 7	21 ± 9	20 ± 6
	2MoDRUG	17 ± 8	21 ± 6	18 ± 6
	+2MoA	14 ± 7	18 ± 8	19 ± 7
Sleep stage REM (%)	Pre	19 ± 6	21 ± 6	19 ± 6
	2MoDRUG	19 ± 6	19 ± 5	19 ± 4
	+2MoA	21 ± 4	18 ± 3	20 ± 5
Movement time (min)	Pre	1 ± 1	2 ± 1	2 ± 2
	2MoDRUG	2 ± 1	1 ± 1	2 ± 2
	+2MoA	2 ± 1	1 ± 1	2 ± 2
REM latency (min)	Pre	97 ± 59	79 ± 50	89 ± 40
	2MoDRUG	72 ± 35	70 ± 34	94 ± 38
	+2MoA	68 ± 31	72 ± 42	89 ± 45
Stage shifts	Pre	61 ± 13	62 ± 10	68 ± 18
	2MoDRUG	61 ± 9	65 ± 15	65 ± 18
	+2MoA	60 ± 11	64 ± 11	59 ± 15

$^a p < 0.05$ change vs pre.
$^b p < 0.01$ Wilcoxon.
$^c p < 0.05$ change vs 2MoDRUG.
REM, rapid eye-movement.
$^d p < 0.01$ Wilcoxon.
$^e p < 0.05$ Difference (2nd–1st period).

The snoring index improved significantly under Climodien compared with the value after 2 months of Climodien (Table 6).

HRT and Periodic Leg Movements

The number of periodic leg movements per hour of total time in bed showed a nonsignificant decrease after Climodien and estradiol, but a nonsignificant increase after placebo (Table 6). However, the difference was nonsignificant, as were the changes after Climodien in the open-label phase.

Table 5
Respiratory Variables in Insomniac Postmenopausal Syndrome Patients Before and After 2 Months of Climodien a (2 mg Estradiol Valerate [EV] + 3 mg Dienogest [DNG]) or 2 mg EV Alone or Placebo as Well as After Subsequent 2-Month Therapy With Climodien A* (2 mg EV + 2 mg DNG)

Variable	Night	Climodien A (N = 16)	Estradiol B (N = 17)	Placebo C (N = 16)	Intergroup difference $^+p < 0.05$; $^{++}p < 0.01$; U-test
Apneas total #	Pre	15 ± 25	20 ± 41	16 ± 36	
	2MoDRUG	8 ± 12	9 ± 13	8 ± 8	
	+2MoA	10 ± 16	9 ± 13	5 ± 6	
Apneas #/hours of sleep	Pre	2 ± 4	3 ± 7	2 ± 6	
	2MoDRUG	1 ± 2[a]	1 ± 2	1 ± 1	2MoDRUG-Pre: A:C+
	+2MoA	2 ± 2	1 ± 2	1 ± 1	
Apneas + hypopneas total #	Pre	51 ± 58	38 ± 71	33 ± 75	
	2MoDRUG	16 ± 21[a]	23 ± 43	32 ± 40	2MoDRUG-Pre: A:C+
	+2MoA	46 ± 87	24 ± 34	16 ± 17	
Apneas + hypopneas #/hours of sleep	Pre	8 ± 9	6 ± 12	5 ± 12	
	2MoDRUG	3 ± 3[a]	4 ± 7	5 ± 6	2MoDRUG: A:C+
	+2moa	7 ± 12	4 ± 6	3 ± 3	
Desaturation total #	Pre	29 ± 34	40 ± 50	64 ± 97	
	2MoDRUG	35 ± 58	25 ± 40	30 ± 56	
	+2MoA	26 ± 47	17 ± 35	23 ± 38	
Desaturation #/hours of sleep	Pre	5 ± 6	7 ± 9	10 ± 15	
	2MoDRUG	6 ± 9	4 ± 6	5 ± 8	
	+2MoA	4 ± 8	3 ± 6	4 ± 6	
Minimum O$_2$	Pre	88 ± 4	73 ± 18	85 ± 8	Pre: A:B++;B:C+
	2MoDRUG	87 ± 7	77 ± 20	86 ± 10	
	+2MoA	88 ± 5	86 ± 8	89 ± 6	
Average low O$_2$	Pre	91 ± 1	90 ± 2	90 ± 3	
	2MoDRUG	91 ± 5	89 ± 5	91 ± 2	2MoDRUG-Pre: B:C+
	+2MoA	91 ± 2	88 ± 8	91 ± 3	

$^ap < 0.05$ change vs pre.
$^bp < 0.01$ Wilcoxon.
$^cp < 0.05$ change vs 2MoDRUG.
$^dp < 0.01$ Wilcoxon.
$^ep < 0.05$ Difference (2nd–1st period).
$^fp < 0.01$ Wilcoxon.

Table 6
Snoring and Periodic Leg Movements in Insomniac Postmenopausal Syndrome Patients Before and After 2 Months of Climodien A (2 mg Estradiol Valerate [EV] + 3 mg Dienogest [DNG]) or 2 mg EV Alone or Placebo as Well as After Subsequent 2-Month Therapy With Climodien A (2 mg EV + 2 mg DNG)

Variable	Night	Climodien A (N = 16)	Estradiol B (N = 17)	Placebo C (N = 16)	Intergroup difference $^+p < 0.05$; $^{++}p < 0.01$; U-test
Snoring events total #	Pre	340 ± 369	113 ± 203	321 ± 312	Pre: A:B$^+$;B:C$^+$
	2MoDRUG	371 ± 360	200 ± 293	296 ± 403	
	+2MoA	226 ± 260^c	225 ± 212	223 ± 217	
Snoring events #/hours of sleep	Pre	59 ± 65	20 ± 40	50 ± 48	Pre: A:B$^+$;B:C$^+$
	2MoDRUG	59 ± 56	31 ± 48	45 ± 60	
	+2MoA	35 ± 40^c	34 ± 33	37 ± 38	
Periodic leg movements #/hours of time in bed	Pre	21 ± 21	18 ± 18	13 ± 15	
	2MoDRUG	14 ± 8	15 ± 11	19 ± 25	
	+2MoA	15 ± 17	14 ± 12	23 ± 36	

$^a p < 0.05$ change vs Pre. $^c p < 0.05$ change vs 2MoDRUG. $^e p < 0.05$ Difference (2nd–1st period).
$^b p < 0.01$ Wilcoxon. $^d p < 0.01$ Wilcoxon. $^f p < 0.01$ Wilcoxon.

HRT and Subjective Sleep and Awakening Quality

Subjective sleep quality, evaluated by means of SSA, improved significantly under Climodien and estradiol, but not under placebo (Table 7). The improvement induced by Climodien and estradiol differed significantly from the nonsignificant deterioration under placebo ($p < 0.01$ and 0.05, respectively). In the open-label phase with Climodien, sleep quality improved further in the Climodien and estradiol groups, with a significant improvement in the Climodien group ($p < 0.05$, Wilcoxon), wheras there was a further nonsignificant deterioration in the placebo group.

Awakening quality improved nonsignificantly under Climodien and Climodien, whereas no changes occurred in the estradiol or placebo groups. Similar results were obtained for somatic complaints.

Thus, the total SSA score improved most pronouncedly with Climodien, followed by estradiol, while there was a slight deterioration with placebo, although the findings did not reach the level of statistical significance. The same results were obtained for the open-label phase.

The Pittsburgh Sleep Quality Index improved significantly with all three compounds compared with baseline. In the open-label phase, Climodien improved the index significantly compared with the preceding placebo treatment.

Well-being in the evening and morning did not yield any significant results. The same was true for morning drive, mood, affectivity, and drowsiness (Table 8).

HRT and Objective Awakening Quality (Psychometry)

Intellectual and Mnestic Performance

Attention did not improve significantly with Climodien, estradiol, or placebo (Table 9).

Table 7
Subjective Sleep and Awakening (SSA) Quality in Insomniac Postmenopausal Syndrome Patients Before and After 2 Months of Climodien A (2 mg Estradiol Valerate [EV] + 3 mg Dienogest [DNG]) or 2 mg EV Alone or Placebo as Well as After Subsequent 2-Month Therapy With Climodien A (2 mg EV + 2 mg DNG)

Variable	Night	Climodien A (N = 16)	Estradiol B (N = 17)	Placebo C (N = 16)	Intergroup difference $^+p < 0.05$; $^{++}p < 0.01$; U-test
Sleep quality (SSA-1) ↓	Pre	17 ± 4	17 ± 5	13 ± 3	Pre: A:C^{++}; B:C$^+$
	2MoDRUG	14 ± 5^a	14 ± 5^a	14 ± 5	2MoDRUG-Pre: A:C^{++}; B:C$^+$
	+2MoA	13 ± 5^c	13 ± 3	15 ± 4	
Awakening quality (SSA-2) ↓	Pre	16 ± 5	15 ± 5	15 ± 4	
	2MoDRUG	15 ± 5	15 ± 6	15 ± 4	
	+2MoA	13 ± 3	15 ± 4	15 ± 3	
Somatic complaints (SSA-3) ↓	Pre	7 ± 2	7 ± 2	6 ± 1	
	2MoDRUG	7 ± 2	7 ± 2	6 ± 2	
	+2MoA	6 ± 1	7 ± 2	6 ± 1	
Total score (SSA) ↓	Pre	40 ± 8	39 ± 11	34 ± 7	Pre: A:C$^+$
	2MoDRUG	35 ± 11	36 ± 11	35 ± 9	
	+2MoA	31 ± 7	34 ± 6	35 ± 6	
Pittsburgh sleep quality index (PSQI)	Pre	11 ± 4	13 ± 3	11 ± 4	
	2MoDRUG	8 ± 4^a	10 ± 4^b	9 ± 3^a	
	+2MoA	8 ± 2	10 ± 4^e	7 ± 3^c	

$^a p < 0.05$ change vs Pre. $^c p < 0.05$ change vs 2MoDRUG. $^e p < 0.05$ Difference (2nd–1st period).

$^b p < 0.01$ Wilcoxon. $^d p < 0.01$ Wilcoxon. $^f p < 0.01$ Wilcoxon.

↓↑, direction of improvement.

Table 8
Morning/Evening Thymopsychic Findings in Insomniac Postmenopausal Syndrome Patients Before and After 2 Months of Climodien A (2 mg Estradiol Valerate [EV] + 3 mg Dienogest [DNG]) or 2 mg EV Alone or Placebo as Well as After Subsequent 2-Month Therapy With Climodien A (2 mg EV + 2 mg DNG)

Variable	Night	Climodien A (N = 16)	Estradiol B (N = 17)	Placebo C (N = 16)	Intergroup difference $^+p < 0.05$; $^{++}p < 0.01$; U-test
Well-being evening ↓	Pre	20 ± 14	14 ± 12	19 ± 11	
	2MoDRUG	15 ± 10	8 ± 7	17 ± 12	
	+2MoA	12 ± 10	8 ± 9	12 ± 10	
Well-being morning ↓	Pre	16 ± 10	12 ± 10	16 ± 12	
	2MoDRUG	17 ± 15	10 ± 10	17 ± 14	
	+2MoA	9 ± 8	9 ± 10	13 ± 9	
Drive (ASES-1) morning ↓	Pre	39 ± 23	30 ± 24	50 ± 25	Pre: B:C+
	2MoDRUG	44 ± 35	32 ± 23	53 ± 31	
	+2MoA	36 ± 21	39 ± 32	41 ± 24	
Mood (ASES-2) morning ↑	Pre	65 ± 19	76 ± 20	57 ± 28	Pre: B:C+
	2MoDRUG	67 ± 24	76 ± 12	56 ± 29	
	+2MoA	71 ± 24	78 ± 17	64 ± 20	
Affectivity (ASES-3) morning ↑	Pre	69 ± 22	79 ± 16	60 ± 28	
	2MoDRUG	64 ± 34	72 ± 20	57 ± 29	
	+2MoA	73 ± 22	79 ± 19	65 ± 16	
Drowsiness (ASES-4) morning ↓	Pre	45 ± 28	38 ± 33	39 ± 27	
	2MoDRUG	43 ± 37	39 ± 30	52 ± 27	
	+2MoA	45 ± 31	45 ± 36	45 ± 26	

$^a p < 0.05$ change vs Pre. $^c p < 0.05$ change vs 2MoDRUG. $^e p < 0.05$ Difference (2nd–1st period).
$^b p < 0.01$ Wilcoxon. $^d p < 0.01$ Wilcoxon. $^f p < 0.01$ Wilcoxon.
↓↑, direction of improvement.

239

Table 9
Morning Intellectual and Mnestic Performance in Insomniac Postmenopausal
Syndrome Patients Before and After 2 Months of Climodien A (2 mg Estradiol
Valerate [EV] + 3 mg Dienogest [DNG]) or 2 mg EV Alone or Placebo as Well
as After Subsequent 2-Month Therapy With Climodien A (2 mg EV + 2 mg DNG)

Variable	Night	Climodien A ($N = 16$)	Estradiol B ($N = 17$)	Placebo C ($N = 16$)
Attention (AD/total score) ↑	Pre	538 ± 124	492 ± 110	537 ± 122
	2MoDRUG	549 ± 110	511 ± 85	566 ± 108
	+2MoA	558 ± 105	535 ± 95	564 ± 132[e]
Concentration (AD/errors [%]) ↓	Pre	4 ± 3	4 ± 3	6 ± 5
	2MoDRUG	4 ± 3	4 ± 5	5 ± 4
	+2MoA	4 ± 3	4 ± 4	5 ± 3
Attention variability (AD/SV) ↓	Pre	13 ± 3	16 ± 7	14 ± 7
	2MoDRUG	14 ± 3	15 ± 6	17 ± 8
	+2MoA	15 ± 3	13 ± 2	13 ± 5
Numerical memory (number) ↑	Pre	5 ± 2	5 ± 2	4 ± 1
	2MoDRUG	6 ± 2[a]	4 ± 1	5 ± 2
	+2MoA	5 ± 2	5 ± 2	5 ± 2

[a]$p < 0.05$ change vs Pre.   [c]$p < 0.05$ change vs 2MoDRUG.
[b]$p < 0.01$ Wilcoxon.   [d]$p < 0.01$ Wilcoxon.
↓↑, direction of improvement.
AD, Alphabetischer Durchstreichtest; SV, attention variability.

In the open-label phase, it increased further in the former Climodien and estradiol groups, but remained unchanged in the placebo group, which was significantly different from the improvement as compared with baseline ($p < 0.05$). Concentration and attention variability showed no significant findings.

Numerical memory improved significantly under Climodien compared with pre-drug treatment ($p < 0.05$), whereas there were no significant changes in the estradiol or placebo groups (Table 9). Under Climodien, mnestic performance did not decline significantly in the former Climodien group, whereas it increased in the estradiol group and remained unchanged in the placebo group.

Psychomotor Performance

Fine motor activity of the right hand improved under Climodien and estradiol, with the changes after the latter reaching the level of statistical significance ($p < 0.01$, Wilcoxon test); under placebo there were no changes (Table 10). Under open-label treatment with Climodien, there was a further improvement in the former Climodien and placebo groups, whereas a nonsignificant decrease occurred in the estradiol group.

Fine motor activity of the left hand showed similar findings, which did not reach the level of statistical significance. Reaction time and reaction time variability did not show any significant changes. However, in regard to the quality of reaction

Table 10
Morning Psychomotor Performance in Insomniac Postmenopausal Syndrome Patients Before and After 2 Months of Climodien A (2 mg Estradiol Valerate [EV] + 3 mg Dienogest [DNG]) or 2 mg EV Alone or Placebo as Well as After Subsequent 2-Month Therapy With Climodien A (2 mg EV + 2 mg DNG)

Variable	Night	Climodien A ($N = 16$)	Estradiol B ($N = 16$)	Placebo C ($N = 16$)
Fine motor activity (right) ↑	Pre	36 ± 10	32 ± 8	34 ± 8
	2MoDRUG	37 ± 9	35 ± 8[b]	34 ± 10
	+2MoA	42 ± 10	34 ± 10	36 ± 9
Fine motor activity (left) ↑	Pre	27 ± 8	26 ± 7	26 ± 7
	2MoDRUG	30 ± 11	25 ± 7	27 ± 9
	+2MoA	33 ± 11	27 ± 8	30 ± 9
Fine motor activity (right + left) ↑	Pre	62 ± 17	58 ± 14	60 ± 14
	2MoDRUG	68 ± 20	61 ± 14	61 ± 18
	+2MoA	75 ± 20	61 ± 17	67 ± 18
Reaction time (RT) (msec) ↓	Pre	617 ± 104	608 ± 96	624 ± 87
	2MoDRUG	623 ± 82	620 ± 100	654 ± 86
	+2MoA	637 ± 77	594 ± 75	614 ± 79
RT variability (msec) ↓	Pre	134 ± 32	142 ± 40	120 ± 37
	2MoDRUG	102 ± 30	120 ± 31	124 ± 29
	+2MoA	98 ± 32	106 ± 36	115 ± 28
RT errors of commission ↓	Pre	6 ± 4	5 ± 5	6 ± 5
	2MoDRUG	3 ± 3[b]	4 ± 2[b]	3 ± 2[b]
	+2MoA	2 ± 2	2 ± 2	4 ± 7
RT errors of omission ↓	Pre	2 ± 3	2 ± 3	1 ± 1
	2MoDRUG	1 ± 1	1 ± 1	1 ± 1
	+2MoA	1 ± 1	0 ± 1	0 ± 1

[a] $p < 0.05$ change vs Pre.　　[c] $p < 0.05$ change vs 2MoDRUG.
[b] $p < 0.01$ Wilcoxon.　　　　[d] $p < 0.01$ Wilcoxon.
↓↑, direction of improvement.

time performance measured by errors of commission, there was a significant improvement after 2 months of Climodien and estradiol, as well as after placebo ($p < 0.01$), with no significant changes after Climodien.

Errors of omission did not yield any significant results.

Psychophysiological Measures

Critical flicker frequency did not change significantly. Muscular strength of the right fingers improved significantly only upon estradiol valerate treatment ($p < 0.01$); muscular strength of the left fingers did not change significantly. Muscular strength of the right hand decreased significantly ($p < 0.01$) after 2 months of Climodien (which was also significantly different from placebo; $p < 0.05$), but increased significantly ($p < 0.05$) after 2 months of Climodien (also in comparison with placebo; $p < 0.05$). The positive effects induced by Climodien differed significantly ($p < 0.05$) from those observed after Climodien. Muscular strength of the left hand decreased slightly under Climodien, whereas it increased after estradiol valerate and placebo. The differences between the drugs reached statistical significance ($p < 0.05$).

Systolic and diastolic blood pressure and pulse rate did not change significantly. The morning pulse rate increased after 2 months of therapy with Climodien in comparison with estradiol valerate ($p < 0.05$).

DISCUSSION

Our polysomnographic investigations as to the differences between patients with insomnia resulting from a postmenopausal syndrome and normal controls demonstrated a significant deterioration of sleep initiation and maintenance as well as increased light sleep stages S1 and decreased sleep stages S2 in patients, whereas deep sleep and REM stages showed no differences compared with controls. These findings are in agreement with the literature on sleep disorders in the menopause *(16,41–43)*. Some authors interpret the changes in terms of an aging effect, because sleep disturbances increase with increasing age in both sexes *(44–46)*. Indeed, sleep architecture changes significantly with the aging process: total sleep time, deep sleep (classified according to Rechtschaffen and Kales *[47]*), and REM stages decrease, whereas nocturnal wakefulness and light sleep stages S1 increase *(48,49)*. Thus, our sleep findings in postmenopausal patients do not merely reflect an enhanced aging process, they also differ from those obtained in other sleep disorders. Insomnia related to depression, for instance, shows shortened REM latency and increased REM density in addition to reduced S4 *(50–53)*; insomnia resulting from generalized anxiety disorder and panic disorder *(54–56)* exhibits predominantly decreased S2, increased S3 and S4, whereas organic insomnia (e.g., consequent to sleep apnea *[57]* and restless legs syndrome *[58,59]* or periodic limb movement disorder *[60]*) shows different sleep architecture patterns.

Our double-blind, placebo-controlled sleep laboratory investigations with Climodien (a new combination of estradiol valerate 2 mg + the progestogen dienogest 3 mg) vs estradiol valerate 2 mg alone in patients with insomnia related to a postmenopausal syndrome showed a moderate improvement in the primary efficacy on variable wakefulness during the total sleep period after 2-month treatment with both Climodien and estradiol compared with baseline, whereas for placebo only minimal changes were observed. Although our findings were in agreement with those obtained by Thompson and Oswald *(25)* concerning the beneficial effect of estrogen therapy (piperazine estrone sulfate 1.5 mgtwice a day given orally over 8 weeks) in perimenopausal women, neither the changes compared with pre-drug treatment nor the differences between the changes in the three groups reached the level of statistical significance. In the subsequent open-label phase, patients on Climodien (estradiol valerate 2 mg + dienogest 2 mg) improved further, whereas the estradiol and placebo groups showed an increase in wakefulness. However, our findings did not reach the level of statistical significance. Similarly, Purdie et al. *(29)* reported a nonsignificant reduction in vasomotor symptoms associated with awakening with the use of 0.625 mg of conjugated equine estrogen with progestogen morgestral 0.15, taken by postmenopausal women for 12 days per 28-day cycle. Recently, estrogen administered by skin patch was found to reduce time awake during the first two sleep cycles to 12 ± 5 in postmenopausal women vs 20 ± 6 minutes in nontreated women *(28)*.

Interesting and partly significant findings were obtained regarding secondary efficacy variables. Concerning sleep initiation, latency to stage 1 showed a nonsignificant shortening after all three compounds. Schiff et al. *(26)* also found a significantly shorter sleep-onset time with estradiol than with placebo. In the open-label phase, Climodien induced a significant lengthening in patients who had before been treated with placebo but also with estradiol. In regard to sleep maintenance, an increase in the total sleep period was induced by Climodien, which differed significantly from the decrease under the subsequent Climodien treatment. Moreover, as compared with placebo treatment, Climodien significantly decreased the total sleep period. Thus, the dienogest dosage seems to play an important role, with 3 mg showing more sleep-promoting properties than 2 mg. Investigating differential effects of two regimens of estrogen–progesterone replacement therapy on the nocturnal sleep of postmenopausal women, Montplaisir et al. *(61)* found increased sleep efficiency after 6-month therapy with oral micronized progesterone, but not with medroxyprogesterone acetate.

Concerning sleep architecture, we observed only a decrease in sleep stage 4 under Climodien compared with the preceding 2 months of estradiol therapy. This was partially in agreement with the results of other studies that reported no change in sleep architecture with HRT *(29,62)*. Investigating HRT with 0.625 mg conjugated equine estrogens in combination with 0.15 mg cyclic norgestrel taken for 12 days per 28-day cycle, Purdie et al. *(29)* did not find improved polysomnographic parameters of sleep quality. On the other hand, Thompson and Oswald *(25)* observed a reduction in wakefulness, a decrease in the number of awakenings, and an increase in REM sleep during 8 weeks of estrogen treatment. However, judging the severity of insomnia by wakefulness in minutes, it seems that our patients were more severely ill, with a wakefulness of almost 1 hour and 9–10 awakenings compared with a wakefulness of 25–40 minutes and 4–5 awakenings in Thompson and Oswald's patients. On the other hand, the latter were more symptomatic than the 33 healthy postmenopausal women of Purdie's group, who showed a wakefulness of only 10–20 minutes. Thus, the data suggest that a moderately ill group may benefit most from HRT, while in more severe cases psychopharmacological agents should be used because, although hormones are subtly sleep-promoting, they are not sleeping pills.

The most interesting findings with Climodien occurred in respiratory variables. The apnea index and the AHI showed a significant improvement under Climodien compared with baseline, although the indices had *a priori* been within normal limits, as required by the protocol. It is noteworthy that in improving respiratory variables during sleep, Climodien was significantly superior to placebo. This confirms the previous findings of Pickett et al. *(63)*, who described a reduced number of apneas and hypopneas in healthy postmenopausal women after 7 days of combined progestogen (medroxyprogesterone acetate 20 mg three times a day) and estrogen (conjugated equine estrogens, Premarin, 1.25 mg twice a day). Because progesterone is decreased in postmenopausal women and is known to be a ventilatory stimulant *(64)*, it has been considered the protective substance in SDB. However, Block et al. *(65)* reported that in contrast to natural progesterone, a synthetic progestogen administered to postmenopausal women reduced the duration of hypopneas, but not the number of episodes of SDB. Several authors reported that progestogen had limited effects in men with SDB *(66–70)*. Thus, progestogen alone obviously cannot develop a protective effect in the absence of estrogen, because estrogen is required to induce progesterone receptors *(71)*. Brodeur et al. *(72)* pointed out that the effects of progesterone might be enhanced by the presence of estrogen.

In a pilot study to test the efficacy of estrogen in sleep apnea syndrome, Keefe et al. *(73)* noticed an improvement within 1 month of initiating therapy with 17β-estradiol alone or in combination with medroxyprogesterone acetate. The respiratory distress index decreased by 25%; the addition of progestogen reduced the sleep apnea syndrome to 50%.

In our study, snoring was reduced by Climodien as compared with Climodien, which reveals that in this regard 2 mg of dienogest are more efficient than 3 mg. Further studies should be conducted to determine whether postmenopausal women with snoring and/or sleep-related breathing disorders such as obstructive snoring and obstructive sleep apnea could benefit from Climodien. Because the results of our study are consistent with the view that female hormones provide protection against SDB, nongenomic female hormones for men suffering from sleep-related breathing disorders may be developed. Recent epidemiological studies in Austria showed that 37% of men and 19% of women snored, whereas 10% of men and 7% of women reported apneas *(74)*. In both males and females there was a substantial age-related increase in snoring and apneas: 54% of men and 34% of women over the age of 50 years snored, whereas 15% of men and 12% of women showed apneas. Snoring and sleep-related breathing disorders lead to abnormalities in sleep architecture and changes in brain function *(57,75,76)*. Moreover, nocturnal respiratory and arousal events are correlated with daytime vigilance decrements *(57)*. Apneas are associated with an increase in morbidity related to cardiovascular and cerebrovascular diseases *(77)*, changes of cerebral hemodynamics *(78)*, and neuropsychological dysfunction *(79,80)*. In a recent study of the prevalence of SDB, Bixler et al. *(81)* pointed out that the menopause is a significant risk factor for sleep apnea in women and that hormone replacement appears to be associated with a reduced risk. On the other hand, concerning the association of hypertension and sleep-related breathing disorders, neither sex nor the menopause changed this relationship *(82)*. In view of the relative paucity of data concerning periodic leg movements and drugs, it is noteworthy that, in contrast to placebo, both Climodien and estradiol tended to attenuate periodic leg movements.

Subjective sleep quality, evaluated by means of the SSA, demonstrated a significant improvement after Climodien and estradiol compared with baseline, with the drug-induced changes being significantly different from the minimal alterations induced by placebo. Thus, the daily ratings of subjective sleep quality seem to be superior to a global rating over a longer period of time; in contrast to the SSA, the Pittsburgh Sleep Quality Index showed no differences between HRT and placebo. Our SSA ratings, performed daily, confirm previous clinical observations of a beneficial influence of estrogen therapy on sleep in postmenopausal women *(83)*. Erlik et al. *(27)* reported that estrogen induced a significant reduction in both hot flashes and waking episodes, whereas Crown and Crisp *(84)* found that only sleep-onset time was sensitive to HRT. In contrast, Purdie et al. *(29)* found no changes in objective or subjective parameters of sleep quality in healthy postmenopausal women during HRT, whereas psychological well-being showed a significant improvement (HRT: 0.625 mg conjugated equine estrogens with 0.15 mg cyclic norgestrel taken for 12 days per 28-day cycle over a study period of 12 weeks). In a 1-year, seven-center trial, 1-month treatment with HRT was found to have a long-term beneficial effect on sleep as assessed by the Sleep Dysfunction Scale *(85)*.

Concerning awakening quality, somatic complaints, and thymopsychic variables in the morning, no significant findings were obtained. Thompson and Oswald's group *(25)* did not observe any differences compared with placebo in regard to mood, whereas the healthy postmenopausal women in Purdie et al.'s study *(29)* showed a significant improvement in free-floating anxiety, somatic anxiety, and depression compared with placebo-treated controls.

Concerning noopsychic variables, numerical memory improved significantly after Climodien compared with pretreatment, whereas after estradiol fine motor activity increased significantly. Errors of commission in the reaction time task improved with all three compounds, which may have been due to a training effect. The observed improvement in numerical memory under Climodien is obviously a result of the increased availability of cognitive information-processing resources, objectified by the P300 amplitude. To our knowledge, our data on noopsychic performance after HRT are the first obtained in the morning after all-night sleep recordings. They are also in agreement with the improvement in vigilance, measured by EEG mapping *(86)*, cognition, measured by event-related potentials *(87)*, and mental performance, evaluated during mid-morning hours *(88)*.

The lack of significant findings in psychophysiological measures reflects the excellent tolerability of all compounds given.

CONCLUSION

The novel estrogen–progestogen combination containing estradiol valerate and dienogest (Climodien, Lafamme®) significantly improved subjective sleep quality and sleep-related breathing disorders, but it had only a slight effect on objective sleep quality and subjective thymopsychic variables. However, the differences between untreated patients and normal controls at baseline were slight, but statistically significant. It may be speculated that the greater improvement in subjective compared to objective sleep variables may be thre result of a halo effect based on an improvement of the postmenopausal syndrome itself, including vegetative disturbances as well as thymopsychic alterations. Psychometric tests have revealed that both an estrogen–progestogen combination and estrogen alone induced a significant improvement in somatic complaints and trait anxiety, whereas state anxiety was more pronouncedly reduced by the combination drug than by estrogen alone *(88)*. Vigilance *(52)* and cognition *(87)* also produced a more pronounced improvement under the combination drug than under estrogen alone, although both preparations were superior to placebo. Thus, the addition of the novel progestogen dienogest to estrogen did not attenuate the effect of the latter, but augmented it, which was also seen for some variables of the present study.

The daytime effects of both HRT preparations seem to be superior to the nighttime effects, which is not surprising, as we have shown in circadian rhythm studies that estradiol, luteinizing hormone, and FSH blood levels are higher during the day than at night *(89,90)*.

Concerning noopsychic performance, numerical memory was significantly improved, whereas fine motor activity was ameliorated with estradiol valerate. Improvements in noopsychic performance were found to have their neurophysiological correlate in a shortening of latency and an augmentation of amplitudes of the cognitive event-related potentials *(87)*. Finally, the mild improvement in sleep with HRT was complemented by a marked vigilance improvement during the day, objectified by computer-assisted EEG-mapping techniques *(86)*. Vigilance improvement is in turn a *sine qua non* for the aforementioned improvement in cognition and psychometric performance *(88)*.

ACKNOWLEDGMENTS

The authors would like to express their thanks to the entire staff of the Sleep Research and Pharmacopsychiatry section of the Department of Psychiatry as well as the Department of Gynecological Endocrinology, University of Vienna, for their cooperative assistance in this project. The pharmacological part of the study was supported by Jenapharm GmbH & Co., KG/Schering AG, Germany.

REFERENCES

1. Hochstrasser, B., [Epidemiology of sleep disorders]. *Ther Umsch*, 1993;**50**(10):679–683.
2. Ohayon, M.M. and T. Roth, What are the contributing factors for insomnia in the general population? J Psychosom Res, 2001;**51**(6): 45–755.
3. Zeitlhofer, J., A. Rieder, G. Kapfhammer, et al., [Epidemiology of sleep disorders in Austria]. *Wien Klin Wochenschr*, 1994;**106**(3):86–88.
4. Brugge, K., D. Kripke, S. Ancoli-Israel, and L. Garfinkel, The association of menopausal status and age with sleep. *Sleep Res*, 1989;**18**:208.
5. Owens, J.F. and K.A. Matthews, Sleep disturbance in healthy middle-aged women. *Maturitas*, 1998;**30**(1):41–50.
6. Saletu, B., N. Brandstatter, R. Frey, et al., [Clinical aspects of sleep disorders—experiences with 817 patients of an ambulatory sleep clinic; comment]. *Wien Klin Wochenschr*, 1997;**109**(11):390–399.
7. Kravitz, H.M., P.A. Ganz, J. Bromberger, L.H. Powell, K. Sutton-Tyrrell, and P.M. Meyer, Sleep difficulty in women at midlife: a community survey of sleep and the menopausal transition. *Menopause*, 2003;**10**(1):19–28.
8. Kuh, D.L., M. Wadsworth, and R. Hardy, Women's health in midlife: the influence of the menopause, social factors and health in earlier life. *Br J Obstet Gynaecol*, 1997;**104**(8):923–933.

9. Lugaresi, E., F. Cirignotta, and M. Zucconi, Good and poor sleepers: an epidemiological survey of San Marino population. In: *Sleep/Wake Disorders: Natural History, Epidemiology, and Long-Term Evolution* (C. Guilleminault and E. Lugaresi, eds.). Raven Press: New York, 1983.

10. Shaver, J.L. and S.N. Zenk, Sleep disturbance in menopause. *J Womens Health Gend Based Med*, 2000;**9**(2):109–118.

11. Manber, R. and R. Armitage, Sex, steroids, and sleep: a review. *Sleep*, 1999;**22**(5):540–555.

12. Moline, M., L. Broch, and R. Zak, Sleep problems across the life cycle in women. *Curr Treat Options Neurol*, 2004;**6**(4):319–330.

13. Krystal, A.D., Insomnia in women. *Clin Cornerstone*, 2003;**5**(3):41–50.

14. Guilleminault, C., L. Palombini, D. Poyares, and S. Chowdhuri, Chronic insomnia, postmenopausal women, and sleep disordered breathing: part 1. Frequency of sleep disordered breathing in a cohort. *J Psychosom Res*, 2002;**53**(1):611–615.

15. Bixler, E.O., A.N. Vgontzas, H.M. Lin, et al., Prevalence of sleep disorders in the Los Angeles metropolitan area. *Am J Psychiatry*, 1979;**136**(10):1257–1262.

16. Hunter, M., R. Battersby, and M. Whitehead, Relationships between psychological symptoms, somatic complaints and menopausal status. *Maturitas*, 1986;**8**(3):217–228.

17. Karacan, I., J.I. Thornby, M. Anch, et al., Prevalence of sleep disturbance in a primarily urban Florida County. *Soc Sci Med*, 1976;**10**(5):239–244.

18. Welstein, L., W. Dement, D. Redington, C. Guilleminault, and M. Mitler, Insomnia in the San Francisco Bay area: a telephone survey. In: *Sleep/Wake Disorders: Natural History, Epidemiology and Long-Term Evolution*, (C. Guilleminault, ed.), New York: Raven Press, 1983:73–85.

19. Moe, K.E., Reproductive hormones, aging, and sleep. *Semin Reprod Endocrinol*, 1999;**17**(4):339–348.

20. Jean-Louis, G., D.F. Kripke, J.D. Assmus, and R.D. Langer, Sleep-wake patterns among postmenopausal women: a 24-hour unattended polysomnographic study. *J Gerontol A Biol Sci Med Sci*, 2000;**55**(3):M120–M123.

21. Asplund, R. and H.E. Aberg, Body mass index and sleep in women aged 40 to 64 years. *Maturitas*, 1995;**22**(1):1–8.

22. Empson, J.A. and D.W. Purdie, Effects of sex steroids on sleep. *Ann Med*, 1999;**31**(2):141–145.

23. Jaszmann, L., N.D. Van Lith, and J.C. Zaat, The peri-menopausal symptoms: the statistical analysis of a survey. *Med Gynaecol Sociol*, 1969;**10**:268–277.

24. Ballinger, C.B., Psychiatric morbidity and the menopause; screening of general population sample. *Br Med J*, 1975;**3**(5979):344–346.

25. Thompson, J. and I. Oswald, Effect of estrogen on the sleep, mood and anxiety of menopausal women. *Br Med J*, 1977;**2**:1317–1319.

26. Schiff, I., Q. Regestein, D. Tulchinsky, and K.J. Ryan, Effects of estrogens on sleep and psychological state of hypogonadal women. *JAMA*, 1979;**242**(22):2405–2404.

27. Erlik, Y., I.V. Tataryn, D.R. Meldrum, P. Lomax, J.G. Bajorek, and H.L. Judd, Association of waking episodes with menopausal hot flushes. *JAMA*, 1981;**245**(17):1741–1744.

28. Antonijevic, I.A., G.K. Stalla, and A. Steiger, Modulation of the sleep electroencephalogram by estrogen replacement in postmenopausal women. *Am J Obstet Gynecol*, 2000;**182**(2):277–282.

29. Purdie, D.W., J.A. Empson, C. Crichton, and L. Macdonald, Hormone replacement therapy, sleep quality and psychological wellbeing. *Br J Obstet Gynaecol*, 1995;**102**(9):735–739.

30. Polo-Kantola, P., R. Erkkola, H. Helenius, K. Irjala, and O. Polo, When does estrogen replacement therapy improve sleep quality? *Am J Obstet Gynecol*, 1998;**178**(5):1002–1009.

31. Schulz, H., M. Jobert, K.W. Gee, and D.W. Ashbrook, Soporific effect of the neurosteroid pregnanolone in relation to the substance's plasma level: a pilot study. *Neuropsychobiology*, 1996;**34**(2):106–112.

32. Steiger, A., L. Trachsel, J. Guldner, et al., Neurosteroid pregnenolone induces sleep-EEG changes in man compatible with inverse agonistic GABAA-receptor modulation. *Brain Res*, 1993;**615**(2):267–274.

33. Teichmann, A.T., *Dienogest—Präklinik und Klinik eines neuen Gestagens [Dienogest—Preclinical and Clinical Characteristics of a New Progestin]*. Berlin/New York: Walter de Gruyter, 1995.

34. Kupperman, H.S., B.B. Wetchler, and M.H. Blatt, Contemporary therapy of the menopausal syndrome. *JAMA*, 1959;**171**:1627–1637.

35. Saletu-Zyhlarz, G., P. Anderer, G. Gruber, et al., Insomnia related to postmenopausal syndrome and hormone replacement therapy: sleep laboratory studies on baseline differences between patients and controls and double-blind, placebo-controlled investigations on the effects of a novel estrogen-progestogen combination (Climodien, Lafamme) versus estrogen alone. *J Sleep Res*, 2003;**12**(3):239–254.

36. Saletu, B., P. Wessely, J. Grünberger, and M. Schulte, Erste klinische Erfahrungen mit einem neuen schlafanstoßenden Benzodiazepin, Cinolazepam, mittels eines Selbstbeurteilungsbogens für Schlaf- und Aufwachqualität (SSA). *Neuropsychiatrie*, 1987;**1**(4):169–176.

37. Von Zerssen, D., D.M. Koeller, and E.R. Rey, Die Befindlichkeitsskala (B-S) - ein einfaches Instrument zur Objektivierung von Befindlichkeitsstörungen, insbesondere im Rahmen von Längsschnittuntersuchungen. *Arzneim Forsch Drug Res*, 1970;**20**:915–918.

38. Buysse, D.J., C.F. Reynolds, 3rd, T.H. Monk, S.R. Berman, and D.J. Kupfer, The Pittsburgh Sleep Quality Index: a new instrument for psychiatric practice and research. *Psychiatry Res*, 1989;**28**(2):93–213.

39. Grünberger, J., *Psychodiagnostik des Alkoholkranken. Ein methodischer Beitrag zur Bestimmung der Organizität in der Psychiatrie*. Vienna: Maudrich, 1977.

40. Abt, K., Descriptive data analysis (DDA) in quantitative EEG studies. In: *Statistics and Topography in Quantitative EEG* (D. Samson-Dollfus et al., eds.). Amsterdam: Elsevier, 1988:150–160.

41. Hunter, M., The south-east England longitudinal study of the climacteric and postmenopause. *Maturitas*, 1992;**14**(2):117–126.

42. Hunter, M.S., Psychological and somatic experience of the menopause: a prospective study (corrected). *Psychosom Med*, 1990;**52**(3):357–367.

43. Kujak, J. and T. Young, The average month-to-month effect of menopausal symptoms on sleep complaints. *Sleep*, 1997;**20**(Suppl 1):384.

44. Feinberg, I., M. Braun, and R.L. Koresko, Vertical eye-movement during REM sleep: effects of age and electrode placement. *Psychophysiology*, 1969;**5**(5):556–561.

45. Tune, G.S., The influence of age and temperament on the adult human sleep-wakefulness pattern. *Br J Psychol*, 1969;**60**(4):31–441.

46. Webb, W.B., The different functional relationships of REM and stage 4 sleep. In: *The Nature of Sleep* (Jovanovic, ed.). Stuttgart: Fischer, 1973:256–258.

47. Rechtschaffen, A. and A. Kales, *A Manual of Standardized Terminology, Technique and Scoring System for Sleep Stages*. San Francisco: Brain Information Service University of California, 1968.

48. Anderer, P., B. Saletu, and R.D. Pascual-Marqui, Effect of the 5-HT(1A) partial agonist buspirone on regional brain electrical activity in man: a functional neuroimaging study using low-resolution electromagnetic tomography (LORETA). *Psychiatry Res*, 2000;**100**(2):81–96.

49. Saletu, B., P. Anderer, R. Frey, M. Krupka, and G. Klüsch, Zur Neurophysiologie des Schlafes/ Some remarks about the neurophysiology of sleep. *Psychiatria Danubina*, 1991;**3**(1–2):31–58.

50. Dietzel, M., B. Saletu, O.M. Lesch, W. Sieghart, and M. Schjerve, Light treatment in depressive illness. Polysomnographic, psychometric and neuroendocrinological findings. *Eur Neurol*, 1986;**25**(Suppl 2):93–103.

51. Reynolds, C.F., 3rd and D.J. Kupfer, Sleep research in affective illness: state of the art circa 1987. *Sleep*, 1987;**10**(3):199–215.

52. Saletu-Zyhlarz, G.M., M.H. Abu-Baker, P. Anderer, et al., Insomnia in depression: differences in objective and subjective sleep and awakening quality to normal controls and acute effects of trazodone. *Prog Neuropsychopharmacol Biol Psychiatry*, 2002;**26**(2):249–260.

53. Saletu-Zyhlarz, G.M., M.H. Abu-Baker, P. Anderer, et al., Insomnia related to dysthymia: polysomnographic and psychometric comparison with normal controls and acute therapeutic trials with trazodone. *Neuropsychobiology*, 2001;**44**(3):139–149.

54. Saletu, B., P. Anderer, N. Brandstatter, et al., Insomnia in generalized anxiety disorder: polysomnographic, psychometric and clinical investigations before, during and after therapy with a long- versus a short-half-life benzodiazepine (quazepam versus triazolam). *Neuropsychobiology*, 1994;**29**(2):69–90.

55. Saletu-Zyhlarz, G., B. Saletu, P. Anderer, et al., Nonorganic insomnia in generalized anxiety disorder. 1. Controlled studies on sleep, awakening and daytime vigilance utilizing polysomnography and EEG mapping. *Neuropsychobiology*, 1997;**36**(3):117–129.

56. Saletu-Zyhlarz, G.M., P. Anderer, P. Berger, G. Gruber, S. Oberndorfer, and B. Saletu, Nonorganic insomnia in panic disorder: comparative sleep laboratory studies with normal controls and placebo-controlled trials with alprazolam. *Hum Psychopharmacol*, 2000;**15**(4):241–254.

57. Saletu, M., C. Hauer, P. Anderer, et al., [Daytime tiredness correlated with nocturnal respiratory and arousal variables in patients with sleep apnea: polysomnographic and EEG mapping studies]. *Wien Klin Wochenschr*, 2000;**112**(6):281–289.

58. Saletu, B., P. Anderer, M. Saletu, et al., Sleep laboratory studies in restless legs syndrome patients as compared with normals and acute effects of ropinirole. 1. Findings on objective and subjective sleep and awakening quality. *Neuropsychobiology*, 2000;**41**(4):181–189.

59. Saletu, M., P. Anderer, B. Saletu, et al., Sleep laboratory studies in restless legs syndrome patients as compared with normals and acute effects of ropinirole. 2. Findings on periodic leg movements, arousals and respiratory variables. *Neuropsychobiology*, 2000;**41**(4):190–199.

60. Saletu, M., P. Anderer, B. Saletu, et al., Sleep laboratory studies in periodic limb movement disorder (PLMD) patients as compared with normals and acute effects of ropinirole. *Hum Psychopharmacol*, 2001;**16**(2):177–187.

61. Montplaisir, J., J. Lorrain, R. Denesle, and D. Petit, Sleep in menopause: differential effects of two forms of hormone replacement therapy. *Menopause*, 2001;**8**(1):10–16.

62. Polo-Kantola, P., R. Erkkola, K. Irjala, S. Pullinen, I. Virtanen, and O. Polo, Effect of short-term transdermal estrogen replacement therapy on sleep: a randomized, double-blind crossover trial in postmenopausal women. *Fertil Steril*, 1999;**71**(5):873–880.

63. Pickett, C.K., J.G. Regensteiner, W.D. Woodard, D.D. Hagerman, J.V. Weil, and L.G. Moore, Progestin and estrogen reduce sleep-disordered breathing in postmenopausal women. *J Appl Physiol*, 1989;**66**(4):1656–1661.

64. Lyons, H.A. and R. Antonio, The sensitivity of the respiratory center in pregnancy and after the administration of progesterone. *Trans Assoc Am Physicians*, 1959;**72**:173–180.

65. Block, A.J., J.W. Wynne, P.G. Boysen, S. Lindsey, C. Martin, and B. Cantor, Menopause, medroxyprogesterone and breathing during sleep. *Am J Med*, 1981;**70**(3):506–510.

66. Dolly, F.R. and A.J. Block, Medroxyprogesterone acetate and COPD. Effect on breathing and oxygenation in sleeping and awake patients. *Chest*, 1983;**84**(4):394–398.

67. Orr, W.C., N.K. Imes, and R.J. Martin, Progesterone therapy in obese patients with sleep apnea. *Arch Intern Med*, 1979;**139**(1):109–111.

68. Rajagopal, K.R., P.H. Abbrecht, and B. Jabbari, Effects of medroxyprogesterone acetate in obstructive sleep apnea. *Chest*, 1986;**90**(6):815–821.

69. Skatrud, J.B., J.A. Dempsey, C. Iber, and A. Berssenbrugge, Correction of CO_2 retention during sleep in patients with chronic obstructive pulmonary diseases. *Am Rev Respir Dis*, 1981;**124**(3):260–268.

70. Strohl, K.P., M.J. Hensley, N.A. Saunders, S.M. Scharf, R. Braun, and R.H. Ingram, Jr., Progesterone administration and progressive sleep apneas. *JAMA*, 1981;**245**(12):1230–1232.

71. Rao, B.R., W.G. Wiest, and W.M. Allen, Progesterone "receptor" in rabbit uterus. I. Characterization and estradiol-17beta augmentation. *Endocrinology*, 1973;**92**(4):1229–1240.

72. Brodeur, P., M. Mockus, R. McCullough, and L.G. Moore, Progesterone receptors and ventilatory stimulation by progestin. *J Appl Physiol*, 1986;**60**(2):590–595.

73. Keefe, D.L., R. Watson, and F. Naftolin, Hormone replacement therapy may alleviate sleep apnea in menopausal women: a pilot study. *Menopause*, 1999;**6**(3):196–200.

74. Zeitlhofer, J., A. Schmeiser, G. Kapfhammer, J. Bolitschek, B. Saletu, and M. Keinze, Epidemiologie von Schlafstörungen in Österreich. *Neuropsychiatrie*, 1996;**10** (1):43.

75. Rumbach, L., J. Krieger, and D. Kurtz, Auditory event-related potentials in obstructive sleep apnea: effects of treatment with nasal continuous positive airway pressure. *Electroencephalogr Clin Neurophysiol*, 1991; **80**(5):454–457.

76. Walsleben, J.A., E.B. O'Malley, K. Bonnet, R.G. Norman, and D.M. Rapoport, The utility of topographic EEG mapping in obstructive sleep apnea syndrome. *Sleep*, 1993;**16**(8 Suppl):S76–S78.

77. Partinen, M. and C. Guilleminault, Daytime sleepiness and vascular morbidity at seven-year follow-up in obstructive sleep apnea patients. *Chest*, 1990;**97**(1):27–32.
78. Siebler, M. and A. Nachtmann, Cerebral hemodynamics in obstructive sleep apnea. *Chest*, 1993;**103**(4):1118–1119.
79. Kales, A., A.B. Caldwell, R.J. Cadieux, A. Vela-Bueno, L.G. Ruch, and S.D. Mayes, Severe obstructive sleep apnea—II: Associated psychopathology and psychosocial consequences. *J Chronic Dis*, 1985;**38**(5):427–434.
80. Millman, R.P., B.S. Fogel, M.E. McNamara, and C.C. Carlisle, Depression as a manifestation of obstructive sleep apnea: reversal with nasal continuous positive airway pressure. *J Clin Psychiatry*, 1989;**50**(9):348–351.
81. Bixler, E.O., A.N. Vgontzas, H.M. Lin, et al., Prevalence of sleep-disordered breathing in women: effects of gender. *Am J Respir Crit Care Med*, 2001;**163**(3 Pt 1):608–613.
82. Bixler, E.O., A.N. Vgontzas, H.M. Lin, et al., Association of hypertension and sleep-disordered breathing. *Arch Intern Med*, 2000;**160**(15):2289–2295.
83. Campbell, S., Double-blind psychometric studies on the effects of natural oestrogens on postmenopausal women. In: *Management of the Menopause and the Postmenopausal Years* (S. Campbell, ed.). Lancaster: MTP Press, 1977:149–158.
84. Crown, S. and A.H. Crisp, *Manual of the Crown-Crisp Experiential Index*. London: Hodder and Stoughton, 1979.
85. Wiklund, I., G. Berg, M. Hammar, J. Karlberg, R. Lindgren, and K. Sandin, Long-term effect of transdermal hormonal therapy on aspects of quality of life in postmenopausal women. *Maturitas*, 1992;**14**(3):225–236.
86. Saletu, B., P. Anderer, D. Gruber, M. Metka, J. Huber, and G. M. Saletu-Zyhlarz, Hormone replacement therapy and vigilance: double-blind, placebo-controlled EEG-mapping studies with an estrogen-progestogen combination (Climodien, Lafamme) versus estrogen alone in menopausal syndrome patients. *Maturitas*, 2002;**43**(3):165–181.
87. Anderer, P., H.V. Semlitsch, B. Saletu, et al., Effects of hormone replacement therapy on perceptual and cognitive event-related potentials in menopausal insomnia. *Psychoneuroendocrinology*, 2003;**28**(3):419–445.
88. Linzmayer, L., H.V. Semlitsch, B. Saletu, et al., Double-blind, placebo-controlled psychometric studies on the effects of a combined estrogen-progestin regimen versus estrogen alone on performance, mood and personality of menopausal syndrome patients. *Arzneimittelforschung*, 2001;**51**(3):238–245.
89. Baumgartner, A., M. Dietzel, B. Saletu, et al., Influence of partial sleep deprivation on the secretion of thyrotropin, thyroid hormones, growth hormone, prolactin, luteinizing hormone, follicle stimulating hormone, and estradiol in healthy young women. *Psychiatry Res*, 1993;**48**(2):153–178.
90. Saletu, B. and G.M. Saletu-Zyhlarz, *Was Sie Schon Immer Über Schlaf Wissen Wollten*. 2001, Vienna: Ueberreuter.

19

Obstructive Sleep Apnea and Menopause

Grace Pien and Sigrid Veasey

INTRODUCTION

A growing body of work supports the concept that menopause is a risk factor for obstructive sleep apnea (OSA). These observations come from clinical and population data examining the relationship between menopausal status and sleep-disordered breathing (SDB), studies examining the clinical characteristics of disease in pre- and postmenopausal women, and laboratory studies of the factors that might place postmenopausal women at increased risk for OSA. This chapter reviews what is known about the increased prevalence of OSA among postmenopausal women, how menopausal status affects the presentation of SDB, and the mechanisms that may underlie the development of sleep apnea among postmenopausal women.

MENOPAUSE AS A RISK FACTOR FOR SLEEP APNEA

Initial reports of the OSA syndrome described a striking predominance of disease among men relative to women, with estimated male-to-female ratios of 8 and 10:1 *(1,2)*. These ratios, however, did not represent general populations. The first study sampled 30 asymptomatic men and 19 women, finding sleep apnea in 20 of the 30 males and very rare events in 3 of the 19 females. In the second study, the ratio of sleep apnea syndrome in males vs females was determined using a sleep clinic population. The findings in these preliminary studies of very few premenopausal women with sleep apnea prompted a comparison of pre- and postmenopausal women *(3)*, which found far more frequent OSA with more significant desaturations in postmenopausal compared to premenopausal women *(3)*. Thus, these studies suggested that there might be both a gender and a menopause effect on the prevalence of sleep apnea.

It was not until 1993, however, that data from the Wisconsin Sleep Cohort Study (WSCS) were published, providing more accurate prevalence data for sleep apnea across several age groups and both genders. In this landmark general population study, undiagnosed SDB was prevalent among both men and women (9 and 4%, respectively, when defined by five or more apnea or hypopnea episodes per hour of sleep) *(4)*. When restricted to individuals with both SDB and excessive daytime

From: *Current Clinical Neurology: Sleep Disorders in Women: A Guide to Practical Management*
Edited by: H. P. Attarian © Humana Press Inc., Totowa, NJ

Potential menopausal risks for sleep apnea progression:

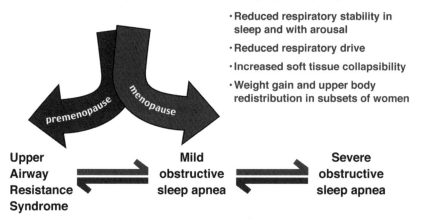

Fig. 1. The causes of obstructive sleep apnea (OSA) are multifactorial, and it is likely that menopausal state by itself does not cause OSA but rather may shift the severity of disease through one or more of the proposed mechanisms shown. Epidemiological studies suggest that the larger menopause shift may occur from upper airways resistance syndrome to mild OSA.

somnolence, 2% of women and 4% of men aged 30–60 years were affected. Thus, the male-to-female ratio of sleep apnea prevalence is high, but not as high as initially believed. Although Young et al. *(4)* did not report information about menopausal status, the prevalence of an apnea–hypopnea index (AHI) of more than five events per hour of sleep among women between ages 30 and 39 years was 6.5%. In women 50–60 years of age, the prevalence was 16%, suggesting that SDB is more common in postmenopausal women. However, the prevalence of SDB increases sharply in men as well for the same age groups—from 17 to 31% *(4)*. Thus, this study was unable to distinguish an age effect on SDB prevalence from a menopausal effect.

Subsequent longitudinal data from women enrolled in the WSCS have more clearly demonstrated that the menopausal transition increases the risk of SDB *(5)*. Compared with premenopausal women, the odds ratios for developing an AHI of five or more events per hour increased to 1.66 for perimenopausal and 2.82 for postmenopausal women. Increased risks for SDB persisted after adjustment for potential confounding factors, including age, body habitus, and smoking, so that at nearly every age between 32 and 53 years, and at every body mass index (BMI) level, SDB prevalence was higher for perimenopausal and postmenopausal women compared with premenopausal women. Furthermore, the odds of having SDB increased with the duration of the postmenopausal state.

The association between menopausal status and SDB was examined by Bixler et al. in a community-based random sample of 1000 women 20–100 years of age from southern Pennsylvania *(6)*. The prevalence of OSA, defined as an AHI of 10 or more events per hour and clinical symptoms of daytime sleepiness, hypertension, or other cardiovascular complications, was 0.6% among premenopausal women compared to 1.9% among postmenopausal women (i.e., a threefold relative risk for postmenopausal women). When defined solely by AHI criteria ($\geq$15 events per hour), the difference in prevalence was even more pronounced, rising from 0.6% of premenopausal women to 3.9% of postmenopausal women. Interestingly, the prevalence of OSA in postmenopausal women was very similar to the prevalence of sleep apnea in age-matched men *(6)*.

Studies in diverse populations from Iceland, Italy, and Hong Kong have offered additional evidence for menopause as a risk factor for OSA *(7–9)*. Together, these studies demonstrate that menopause is a strong risk factor for OSA in women.

HORMONE REPLACEMENT THERAPY AND SLEEP-DISORDERED BREATHING

The increased risk of sleep apnea among menopausal women raises the possibility that hormone replacement therapy (HRT) may reduce this risk. A number of mechanistic studies, discussed later in this chapter, have addressed this issue. Several epidemiological studies have also examined whether the likelihood of having OSA is reduced among users of replacement hormones. It is important to understand that in the studies described here women were not randomized to HRT.

In the southern Pennsylvania cohort previously described, postmenopausal women were categorized by HRT use and compared with premenopausal women *(6)*. Among postmenopausal women currently using HRT, the prevalence of sleep apnea (AHI $\geq$ 10 and clinical symptoms) was similar to that of premenopausal women (0.5% in postmenopausal women on HRT vs 0.6% in premenopausal women). In contrast, the prevalence of sleep apnea among postmenopausal women not using HRT was significantly higher (2.7%). This difference could not be explained by obesity. In fact, women on HRT were twice as likely to be obese. Using an AHI criteria of more than 15, postmenopausal women not using replacement hormones were more than four times as likely to have sleep apnea than premenopausal women; postmenopausal women using HRT did not differ significantly from premenopausal women. The majority of subjects using HRT reported that they were taking estrogen-alone therapy, rather than combination estrogen–progesterone therapy.

Among perimenopausal and postmenopausal subjects in the WSCS, 17–20% reported current HRT use *(5)*. Users of HRT were slightly less likely to have SDB compared with peri- and postmenopausal non-HRT users, but this finding was not statistically significant. The investigators also looked for but did not find a long-term modifying effect that might reduce the likelihood of developing SDB after cessation of HRT.

Data from the Sleep Heart Health Study, a large epidemiological study of the cardiovascular effects of sleep apnea, have also been used to examine the relationship between the use of HRT and SDB *(10)*. Because menopausal status was not recorded at the time of polysomnography, analyses were restricted to women 50 years of age and older. Hormone users comprised 32% of the sample and had approximately half the prevalence of SDB (defined as AHI ≥ 15 events per hour) compared with nonusers, an association that persisted after adjustment for age and BMI (adjusted odds ratio 0.55). The protective effect of HRT was strongest among women 50–60 years of age; it attenuated with age so that women 70 years of age or older had the least protective effect from HRT. However, the effect of HRT appeared to be similar regardless of whether women used estrogen alone or an estrogen–progesterone combination.

Collectively, these data demonstrate that menopause increases the risk of SDB and that HRT may attenuate this risk. The question of whether hormonal therapy may be used to prevent the development of sleep apnea across the menopausal transition has been raised, but it has not been answered with clinical trials *(11)*. Recent results from the Women's Health Initiative (WHI) study, a primary prevention trial of HRT, demonstrated an increased rate of adverse cardiovascular outcomes among women taking estrogen and progestin *(12)*. These findings make a large-scale trial of HRT for the treatment of sleep apnea unlikely. In fact, the WHI study findings appear to have had a substantial impact on women's use of hormonal therapy: 58% of postmenopausal women in a New Zealand population surveyed 6 months after release of the study results reported having stopped their replacement hormones *(13)*. Whether a detectable increase in the overall prevalence of sleep apnea among postmenopausal women will occur owing to widespread cessation of HRT remains to be seen.

IMPACT OF MENOPAUSAL TRANSITION ON CLINICAL CHARACTERISTICS OF SDB

A number of gender differences in the clinical characteristics of OSA have been described. These include differences in disease severity, apnea characteristics, distribution of SDB events during sleep, and clinical presentation. Evidence that some of these characteristics may likewise be affected by menopausal status are reviewed here.

Sleep Apnea Severity

In the Sleep Heart Health Study, mean AHI was observed to be higher among men than women *(14)*. Even when matched by age and BMI, women with sleep apnea have fewer SDB events compared with men *(15)*. In comparing sleep apnea severity on the basis of menopausal status, conflicting reports exist, with data drawn mostly from clinical, rather than population-based, samples. An early report from Guilleminault et al. reported higher mean AHIs among premenopausal than postmenopausal women with OSA *(2)*. However, other authors have observed either no difference in mean AHI between premenopausal and postmenopausal women with OSA *(16)* or more severe disease in postmenopausal women *(17,18)*. These studies have often been limited by selection bias and lack of adjustment for confounding variables such as age and BMI.

Initial data from the WSCS showed that although SDB (AHI five or more events per hour) was more common among women 50–60 years of age than younger women (ages 30–40 and 40–50), the prevalence of more severe disease (AHI ≥ 10, or ≥15 events per hour) was similar in all groups *(4)*. More recent data from this study, using careful classification of menopausal status, demonstrate that whether defined by an AHI of more than 5 or more than 15, the prevalence of SDB approximately triples among peri- and postmenopausal women compared with premenopausal women *(5)*. The latter report may suggest that after taking menopausal status into account, disease severity is similar in premenopausal and postmenopausal women with OSA.

Sleep-Disordered Breathing Characteristics

Compared to men, women with SDB have been observed to have a higher proportion of hypopneas than apneas and to have shorter events associated with less severe oxyhemoglobin desaturation *(15,16,19)*. Differences in the characteristics of SDB events by menopausal status have also been examined in a number of studies. Block et al. examined apnea and hypopnea frequency, duration, and associated desaturation among premenopausal women, postmenopausal women, and men *(3)*. Compared to premenopausal women, postmenopausal women had more frequent events that were longer in duration and more likely to be associated with oxyhemoglobin desaturations of less than 90% *(3)*. When postmenopausal women were compared with men over the age of 50, there were no significant differences in apnea frequency or events associated with oxyhemoglobin desaturation. In contrast, premenopausal women were significantly less likely to have such events than were men younger than 50 years of age. Other studies that have used age as a surrogate marker for menopausal status, which may lead to misclassification bias, have failed to observe differences in the duration of SDB events and oxyhemoglobin desaturation *(16,19)*.

In women, SDB events have been observed to be more frequently concentrated during the rapid eye-movement (REM) sleep period compared with non-REM sleep in women *(15,20)*. Whether this distribution is more likely to occur in pre- or postmenopausal women does not appear to have been examined.

Clinical Presentation of Sleep-Disordered Breathing

Although symptoms of sleep apnea clearly differ between women and men, little is known about whether the menopausal transition also affects the clinical presentation of sleep apnea. Women referred for laboratory evaluation of sleep apnea are as likely as men to report sleepiness and snoring, snorting, gasping, or apneas when asked about these symptoms *(21,22)*. However, compared with men, women with sleep apnea are more likely to complain primarily of insomnia and to have a history of depression or hypothyroidism *(22)*. In one sample, 67% of postmenopausal women with chronic insomnia without excessive daytime sleepiness were found to have sleep apnea (AHI ≥ 5) *(23)*. Studies examining gender differences in reporting of SDB symptoms have not examined potential differences between pre- and postmenopausal women *(21,22,24)*. However, the persistence of gender differences in analyses by age-specific strata *(21)* may suggest that clinical symptoms are likely to be similar regardless of menopausal status.

Given the increased risk of SDB conferred by menopause, the possibility of a relationship between menopausal vasomotor symptoms and SDB has been explored *(25)*. Although nocturnal breathing abnormalities were common among postmenopausal women, vasomotor symptoms (hot flashes) did not predict the occurrence or severity of SDB *(25)*.

In summary, it is clear that differences between women and men exist in the clinical characteristics of SDB. Less is known about how menopausal status affects the clinical presentation of OSA. A small body of work suggests that clinical disease severity is similar in women regardless of menopausal status. However, compared to premenopausal women, apneas and hypopneas in postmenopausal women may more closely resemble the longer, more severe breathing events observed in men. Women with SDB are more likely than men to complain primarily of insomnia or to have complaints aside from somnolence and apneic symptoms that may obscure the diagnosis. Further studies are needed to determine whether the clinical presentation of disease changes after menopause.

MECHANISMS THROUGH WHICH AGING AND MENOPAUSE PREDISPOSE TO THE DEVELOPMENT OR PROGRESSION OF OSA

A substantial body of literature, reviewed in the previous section, supports the idea that menopause may be considered a risk factor for OSA and that the condition itself predisposes to obstructive SDB events. Numerous studies have explored potential mechanisms through which premenopausal women are relatively protected from OSA and why menopause may predispose to increase risk of SDB. This section examines the potential mechanisms underlying menopause as a risk for sleep apnea and reviews this body of literature. Menopausal transition changes in hormonal activities, weight, body mass redistribution, respiratory drive, ventilatory stability, and upper airway mechanics are considered. It is hoped that an improved understanding of what is known and not known of the mechanisms through which menopause contributes to the progression and development of sleep apnea will unveil areas in need of further study and will ultimately lead to novel therapies to prevent and treat OSA in women across all ages.

EFFECTS OF HRT ON OBSTRUCTIVE SDB

Both estrogen and progesterone enhance respiratory chemosensitivity and, thus, have the potential to partly offset the sleep-state-dependent reductions in respiratory drive believed to underlie the pathogenesis of OSA *(26)*. Several studies have examined the effects of progesterone and/or estrogen replacement therapy on OSA in postmenopausal women. One week of medroxyprogesterone and premarin therapy in nine women with mild sleep apnea and previous bilateral ovariectomy and hysterectomy resulted in significant reductions in obstructive events *(27)*. A second smaller study also identified reductions in apnea frequencies with estrogen and progesterone supplementation *(28)*. A third study of six postmenopausal women found a reduction in the respiratory disturbance index from 25 to 12 events ($p < 0.01$) with estrogen-alone therapy *(29)*. In this study, supplementation with progesterone was of no additional benefit and may have worsened the apnea frequency in a sub-set of the subjects *(29)*. A fourth study also supports a positive effect of estrogen and/or progesterone (as estradiol valerate with or without the progestogen dienogest) on the AHI *(30)*. In this randomized placebo-controlled trial, 51 post-menopausal women showed an overall improvement in the AHI on the combined therapy and not on estrogen alone. However, three studies have shown contradic-tory findings. Two of these studies, with sample sizes similar to those listed in the above studies, showed no effects on SDB frequency with either estrogen-alone therapy or estrogen and progesterone therapy subjects with moderate to severe OSA *(31,32)*. In a larger ($N = 62$) randomized, controlled crossover trial, estrogen therapy had minimal effect on sleep apnea or upper airways resistance syndrome in post-menopausal women *(33)*.

Whether these discrepancies in the effect of HRTs represent differences in drugs and doses, severity of apnea, age of women, or physical differences is not known. It is also possible that sample sizes are inadequate to detect consistent small reduc-tions in AHIs. However, in light of an absence of a large positive effect of HRT on sleep apnea in postmenopausal women and the increasingly recognized number of adverse effects of HRT *(34)*, HRT for the treatment of obstructive SDB events in postmenopausal women cannot be justified at present.

The effects of estrogen blockade therapies (e.g., tamoxifen) on obstructive SDB have not been reported. It is conceivable that tamoxifen could worsen sleep apnea. This issue should be advanced. If tamoxifen were found to worsen sleep apnea, this would impact on treatment decisions in select cases of breast cancer and would suggest the need for improved screening for sleep apnea in persons in whom the drug is indicated. At the same time, examining the acute effects of estrogen block-ade would also provide insight into the role intrinsic estrogen plays in upper airway collapsibility and SDB.

Estrogen and progesterone are not the only hormonal changes across menopause. Menopause is associated also with declining levels of circulating testosterone *(35)*. In contrast to the potentially protective effects of estrogen and perhaps progester-one on OSA, testosterone has been implicated in the pathogenesis of OSA in men *(36)*. Testosterone supplementation in women has been shown to raise the hypocapneic ventilatory threshold, an effect that increases respiratory instability and, thus, could increase sleep apnea *(37)*. Therefore, use of androgen supplementa-tion in postmenopausal women may exacerbate sleep apnea. In contrast, age-related declines in androgens would be expected to counter to some degree the climacteric increase in OSA.

Menopause is associated also with increased leptin levels, but only in females who gain weight *(38,39)*. Leptin has significant stimulatory effects on ventilation and ventilatory responses to hypercapnia and hypoxia. Females have higher levels of leptin when matched for BMI, raising the possibility that leptin levels in females protect them in part from sleep apnea *(40)*. What complicates the interpretation of changes in leptin levels and their effects on respiration is that bidirectional alterations in leptin resistance or responsiveness may accompany the change in leptin level. Thus, an increase in leptin levels does not necessarily signify an increase in leptin activity.

Hormonal changes are very likely to contribute to the development and/or progression of OSA in women across the menopausal transition. To really advance this hypothesis, a large-scale prospective study is needed to monitor SDB in women across the menopause transition. To best determine exactly how hormonal changes in menopause contribute to SDB requires following hormonal changes in parallel with SDB changes across menopause, while also addressing the nonhormonal potential menopausal risk factors delineated here.

VENTILATORY RESPONSIVENESS IN MENOPAUSE

Several unique characteristics of respiratory drive and responsiveness to respiratory challenges may protect premenopausal women from sleep-state-dependent respiratory instability. It is not known if gender differences in ventilatory responsiveness are explained completely by hormonal levels, whether there are secondary (long-term) hormonal changes, or whether the gender differences are independent of hormonal differences. Progesterone does have a stimulatory effect on respiration and enhances the respiratory response to acute hypoxia in waking *(41)*, and there is some evidence that physiological changes in hormonal levels alter respiratory responsiveness. Following a voluntary hyperventilation effort, ventilation does not abruptly return to normal but slowly declines. In premenopausal females there is menstrual cycle variation in this ventilatory decline following voluntary hyperventilation, such that ventilation remains elevated longer after a hyperventilation episode during the luteal phase than during the follicular phase *(42)*. This raises the possibility of a novel way through which progesterone might stabilize ventilation during sleep after a sigh or a deep breath. However, the rates of decline in ventilatory responses to acute hypoxia and to hypercarbia (the respiratory changes one expects in sleep apnea) do not vary with gender or with menstrual phase *(43)*. Other groups have looked at the absolute minute ventilation response to hypoxia and hypercarbia *(44,45)*. The small sample sizes in these technically challenging clinical studies cannot exclude small (<30%) differences across gender. Collectively, we may conclude that if there are gender differences in waking responses to hypoxic and hypercapneic challenges, they are small and unlikely to contribute substantially to gender and menopausal differences in sleep apnea severity.

In contrast to the above responses to acute single exposure to hypoxia and hypercarbia, there may be gender differences in responses to episodic hypoxia and hypercapnia, changes that more closely mimic those seen in sleep apnea *(45)*. Specifically, males have a larger ventilatory response to hypercarbia in the presence of episodic hypoxia than do females *(45)*. The significance of the greater ventilatory response upon arousal is that it will drive down carbon dioxide and, thus, at sleep onset would promote a central apnea or respiratory instability. It is not known whether this stabilizing response in premenopausal females diminishes or is attenuated across the development of menopause. It would also be of interest to examine this response before and after estrogen blockade in premenopausal females.

An equally compelling gender difference that may influence respiratory stability in sleep has been reported by Jordan et al. *(46)*, who found that the cardiorespiratory responses to arousal from non-REM sleep were far more pronounced in males than in premenopausal females. Men had higher initial increases in ventilation with arousal, and upon resumption of sleep, men showed more ventilatory suppression, which would clearly promote sleep-state respiratory instability. Cardiovascular responses were measured as well. The amplitude of the finger pulse was greater in males upon arousal (either spontaneous or elicited), raising the possibility that sympathetic drive in response to arousal changes more in males relative to premenopausal females. It will now be important to determine if the amplitude of this ventilatory and/or cardiovascular response predicts SDB in women and if this response changes across menopause with the progression of OSA. We must also determine if this gender difference can be explained by increased sympathetic drive in males relative to females, because this may offer a potential pharmacotherapeutic avenue to reduce the progression of SDB across menopause.

Nasal occlusion in sleep serves as a model of precipitating or increasing the frequency of obstructive sleep-disordered events. Carskadon et al. compared the responses of premenopausal, perimenopausal, and postmenopausal women to nasal occlusion events in sleep *(47)*. There was no major effect of menopausal status on the frequency or severity of apnea and hypopnea events or on the oxygen nadirs for events. This would suggest that changes in hormone levels across menopause are not a major contributor to the increased prevalence of OSA with menopause. In contrast, the key variables for the development of apneas and hypopneas precipitated by nasal occlusion were BMI, neck circumference, and mandibular-hyoid distance *(47)*.

The gender differences identified to date that might protect premenopausal females from OSA are less hyperpnea after episodic hypoxia in females and more stable respiratory effort in non-REM sleep in response to hypercarbia and arousals. It would be of considerable interest to test the effect of acute and longer-term estrogen blockade on these gender differences to determine the role played by hormone activity.

OBESITY AND FAT REDISTRIBUTION WITH MENOPAUSE

Obesity and neck circumference are both well-established independent risk factors for OSA, and obesity increases with aging. A recent follow-up report in the Study of Women's Health Across the Nation of more than 3000 racially and ethnically diverse women followed across the menopausal transition found that menopause overall was not associated with significant weight gain or an increase in abdominal girth *(48)*. Weight over 3 years of observation increased by 3% and waist circumference by just 3% whether women remained premenopausal, shifted into the menopause transition, or completed menopause *(48)*. There was variability in weight gain across women in each group, such that it would be of interest to compare the risk of sleep apnea in women who did gain weight across menopause with that in those who did not gain weight. At the same time, it would be of considerable interest to determine if sleep apnea may occur across menopause without weight gain in some females.

UPPER AIRWAY ANATOMY AND MECHANICS

Gender differences between men and premenopausal women may contribute to the increased prevalence and severity of sleep apnea in men. In males, the upper airway is longer and may be more collapsible *(49)*. A separate study, however, found no difference in collapsibility between normal males and females *(50)*. Moreover, the airway size is smaller in females *(51)*. The increased collapsibility may be a consequence of the increased neck circumference in males *(52)*. Yet neck circumference alone and neck circumference normalized to height explain less than 25% of the gender predisposition to OSA. The length of the upper airway is longer in males, which may predispose to increased collapsibility. There are also soft tissue gender differences that may predispose to OSA. The lateral fad pads are larger in males *(53)*, but the relative role of this particular anatomical feature has not been delineated from neck circumference. Whether any of these anatomical risk factors for OSA are modified across the menopause transition or in parallel to the development of OSA requires studying women across the menopausal transition.

CONCLUSIONS

Although it is clear that the prevalence of OSA increases with menopause, the mechanisms remain unclear. From the above studies, it is likely that changes in both estrogen and progesterone contribute to the risk of obstructive SDB. In addition, there are likely additional important state-dependent ventilatory response patterns and potentially changes in upper airway collapsibility, which may or may not relate directly to hormonal changes. Future studies will be most insightful if cohorts of women are followed completely from well before the menopause transition to well into menopause, examining hormonal, weight, ventilatory, and upper airway dynamics in parallel with sleep studies to best identify important factors contributing to the increased risk of sleep apnea in menopause.

REFERENCES

1. Block, A.J., et al., Sleep apnea, hypopnea and oxygen desaturation in normal subjects. A strong male predominance. *N Engl J Med*, 1979;**300**(10):513–517.
2. Guilleminault, C., et al., Women and the obstructive sleep apnea syndrome. *Chest*, 1988;**93**(1):104–109.
3. Block, A.J., J.W. Wynne, and P.G. Boysen, Sleep-disordered breathing and nocturnal oxygen desaturation in postmenopausal women. *Am J Med*, 1980;**69**(1):75–79.
4. Young, T., et al., The occurrence of sleep-disordered breathing among middle-aged adults. *N Engl J Med*, 1993;**328**(17):230–1235.
5. Young, T., et al., Menopausal status and sleep-disordered breathing in the Wisconsin Sleep Cohort Study. *Am J Respir Crit Care Med*, 2003;**167**(9):1181–1185.
6. Bixler, E.O., et al., Prevalence of sleep-disordered breathing in women: effects of gender. *Am J Respir Crit Care Med*, 2001;**163**(3 Pt 1):608–613.
7. Gislason, T., et al., Snoring, hypertension, and the sleep apnea syndrome. An epidemiologic survey of middle-aged women. *Chest*, 1993;**103**(4):1147–1151.
8. Ferini-Strambi, L., et al., Snoring & sleep apnea: a population study in Italian women. *Sleep*, 1999;**22**(7):859–864.

9. Ip, M.S., et al., A community study of sleep-disordered breathing in middle-aged Chinese women in Hong Kong: prevalence and gender differences. *Chest*, 2004;**125**(1):127–134.

10. Shahar, E., et al., Hormone replacement therapy and sleep-disordered breathing. *Am J Respir Crit Care Med*, 2003;**167**(9):1186–1192.

11. White, D.P., The hormone replacement dilemma for the pulmonologist. *Am J Respir Crit Care Med*, 2003;**167**(9):1165–1166.

12. Rossouw, J.E., et al., Risks and benefits of estrogen plus progestin in healthy postmenopausal women: principal results From the Women's Health Initiative randomized controlled trial. *JAMA*, 2002;**288**(3):321–333.

13. Lawton, B., et al., Changes in use of hormone replacement therapy after the report from the Women's Health Initiative: cross sectional survey of users. *BMJ*, 2003;**327**(7419):845–846.

14. Gottlieb, D.J., et al., Relation of sleepiness to respiratory disturbance index: the Sleep Heart Health Study. *Am J Respir Crit Care Med*, 1999;**159**(2):502–507.

15. Resta, O., et al., Gender difference in sleep profile of severely obese patients with obstructive sleep apnea. *Respir Med*, 2005;**99**:91–96.

16. Leech, J.A., et al., A comparison of men and women with occlusive sleep apnea syndrome. *Chest*, 1988;**94**(5):983–988.

17. Resta, O., et al., Gender, age and menopause effects on the prevalence and the characteristics of obstructive sleep apnea in obesity. *Eur J Clin Invest*, 2003;**33**(12):1084–1089.

18. Dancey, D.R., et al., Impact of menopause on the prevalence and severity of sleep apnea. *Chest*, 2001;**120**(1):151–155.

19. Ware, J.C., R.H. McBrayer, and J.A. Scott, Influence of sex and age on duration and frequency of sleep apnea events. *Sleep*, 2000;**23**(2):165–170.

20. O'Connor, C., K.S. Thornley, and P.J. Hanly, Gender differences in the polysomnographic features of obstructive sleep apnea. *Am J Respir Crit Care Med*, 2000;**161**(5):1465–1472.

21. Redline, S., et al., Gender differences in sleep disordered breathing in a community-based sample. *Am J Respir Crit Care Med*, 1994;**149**(3 Pt 1):722–726.

22. Shepertycky, M.R., K. Banno, and M.H. Kryger, Differences between men and women in the clinical presentation of patients diagnosed with obstructive sleep apnea syndrome. *Sleep*, 2005;**28**(3):309–314.

23. Guilleminault, C., et al., Chronic insomnia, postmenopausal women, and sleep disordered breathing: part 1. Frequency of sleep disordered breathing in a cohort. *J Psychosom Res*, 2002;**53**(1):611–615.

24. Young, T., et al., The gender bias in sleep apnea diagnosis. Are women missed because they have different symptoms? *Arch Intern Med*, 1996;**156**(21):2445–2451.

25. Polo-Kantola, P., et al., Climacteric vasomotor symptoms do not predict nocturnal breathing abnormalities in postmenopausal women. *Maturitas*, 2001;**39**(1):29–37.

26. Hannhart, B., C.K. Pickett, and L.G. Moore, Effects of estrogen and progesterone on carotid body neural output responsiveness to hypoxia. *J Appl Physiol*, 1990;**68**(5):1909–1916.

27. Pickett, C.K., et al., Progestin and estrogen reduce sleep-disordered breathing in postmenopausal women. *J Appl Physiol*, 1989;**66**(4):1656–1661.

28. Keefe, D.L., R. Watson, and F. Naftolin, Hormone replacement therapy may alleviate sleep apnea in menopausal women: a pilot study. *Menopause*, 1999;**6**(3):196–200.

29. Manber, R., et al., The effects of hormone replacement therapy on sleep-disordered breathing in postmenopausal women: a pilot study. *Sleep*, 2003;**26**(2):163–168.

30. Saletu-Zyhlarz, G., et al., Insomnia related to postmenopausal syndrome and hormone replacement therapy: sleep laboratory studies on baseline differences between patients and controls and double-blind, placebo-controlled investigations on the effects of a novel estrogen-progestogen combination (Climodien, Lafamme) versus estrogen alone. *J Sleep Res*, 2003;**12**(3):239–254.

31. Block, A.J., et al., Menopause, medroxyprogesterone and breathing during sleep. *Am J Med*, 1981;**70**(3):506–510.

32. Cistulli, P.A., et al., Effect of short-term hormone replacement in the treatment of obstructive sleep apnoea in postmenopausal women. *Thorax*, 1994;**49**(7):699–702.

33. Polo-Kantola, P., et al., Breathing during sleep in menopause: a randomized, controlled, cross-over trial with estrogen therapy. *Obstet Gynecol*, 2003;**102**(1):68–75.

34. Nelson, H.D., et al., Postmenopausal hormone replacement therapy: scientific review. *JAMA*, 2002;**288**(7):872–881.

35. Meldrum, D.R., et al., Changes in circulating steroids with aging in postmenopausal women. *Obstet Gynecol*, 1981;**57**(5):624–628.

36. Liu, P.Y., et al., The short-term effects of high-dose testosterone on sleep, breathing, and function in older men. *J Clin Endocrinol Metab*, 2003;**88**(8):3605–3613.

37. Zhou, X.S., et al., Effect of testosterone on the apneic threshold in women during NREM sleep. *J Appl Physiol*, 2003;**94**(1):101–107.

38. Di Carlo, C., G.A. Tommaselli, and C. Nappi, Effects of sex steroid hormones and menopause on serum leptin concentrations. *Gynecol Endocrinol*, 2002;**16**(6):479–491.

39. Tufano, A., et al., Anthropometric, hormonal and biochemical differences in lean and obese women before and after menopause. *J Endocrinol Invest*, 2004;**27**(7):648–653.

40. Thomas, T., et al., Relationship of serum leptin levels with body composition and sex steroid and insulin levels in men and women. *Metab Clin Exp*, 2000;**49**(10):1278–1284.

41. Tatsumi, K., et al., Role of endogenous female hormones in hypoxic chemosensitivity. *J Appl Physiol*, 1997;**83**(5):1706–1710.

42. Takano, N., Change in time course of posthyperventilation hyperpnea during menstrual cycle. *J Appl Physiol*, 1988;**64**(6):2631–2635.

43. Jordan, A.S., et al., Ventilatory decline after hypoxia and hypercapnia is not different between healthy young men and women. *J Appl Physiol*, 2000;**88**(1):3–9.

44. Tarbichi, A.G., et al., Lack of gender difference in ventilatory chemoresponsiveness and post-hypoxic ventilatory decline. *Respir Physiol Neurobiol*, 2003;**137**(1):41–50.

45. Morelli, C., M.S. Badr, and J.H. Mateika, Ventilatory responses to carbon dioxide at low and high levels of oxygen are elevated after episodic hypoxia in men compared with women. *J Appl Physiol*, 2004;**97**(5):1673–1680.

46. Jordan, A.S., P.G. D.J. McEvoy, Catcheside, and R. D. McEvoy, Ventilatory response to brief arousal from non-rapid eye movement sleep is greater in men than in women. *Am J Resp Crit Care Med*, 2003;**166**(12):1612–1619.

47. Carskadon, M.A., et al., Effects of menopause and nasal occlusion on breathing during sleep. *Am J Respir Crit Care Med*, 1997;**155**(1):205–210.

48. Sternfeld, B., et al., Physical activity and changes in weight and waist circumference in midlife women: findings from the Study of Women's Health Across the Nation. *Am J Epidemiol*, 2004;**160**(9):912–922.

49. Mohsenin, V., Effects of gender on upper airway collapsibility and severity of obstructive sleep apnea. *Sleep Med*, 2003;**4**(6):523–529.

50. Rowley, J.A., et al., Influence of gender on upper airway mechanics: upper airway resistance and Pcrit. *J Appl Physiol*, 2001;**91**(5):2248–2254.

51. Dancey, D.R., et al., Gender differences in sleep apnea: the role of neck circumference. *Chest*, 2003;**123**(5):1544–1550.

52. Rowley, J.A., et al., Gender differences in upper airway compliance during NREM sleep: role of neck circumference. *J Appl Physiol*, 2002;**92**(6):2535–2541.

53. Schwab, R.J., et al., Upper airway and soft tissue anatomy in normal subjects and patients with sleep-disordered breathing. Significance of the lateral pharyngeal walls. *Am J Respir Crit Care Med*, 1995;**152**(5 Pt 1):1673–1689.

Index